CRAS

Me
and
Nutrition

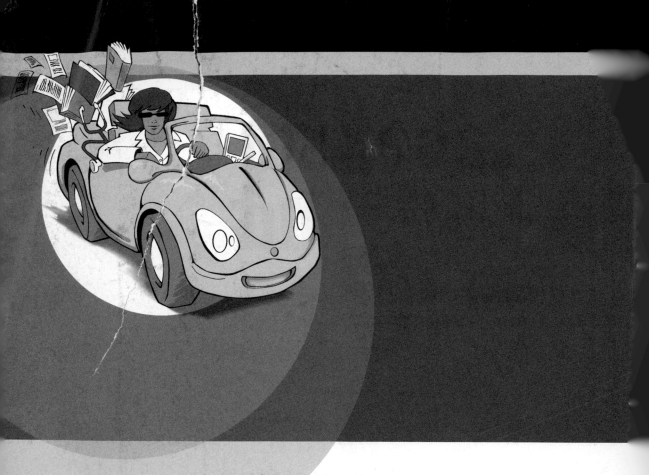

First and second edition authors:

Sarah Benyon
Jason O'Neale Roach

CRASH COURSE

Third edition

Metabolism and Nutrition

Series editor

Daniel Horton-Szar
BSc (Hons), MBBS (Hons), MRCGP
Northgate Medical Practice
Canterbury
Kent, UK

Faculty advisor

Marek Dominiczak
MD, FRCPath, FRCP(Glas)
Consultant Biochemist
Clinical Biochemistry Service
NHS Greater Glasgow and Clyde, UK

Professor in the Medical Faculty,
University of Glasgow, UK
Gartnavel General Hospital
Glasgow, UK

Docent in Laboratory Medicine
University of Turku
Turku, Finland

Ming Yeong Lim

BA (Hons) MB BChir
Addenbrooke's Hospital, Cambridge University, Cambridge, UK

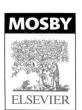

Edinburgh • London • New York • Oxford • Philadelphia • St Louis • Sydney • Toronto 2007

MOSBY
ELSEVIER
An imprint of Elsevier Limited

Commissioning Editor	**Fiona Conn, Alison Taylor**
Development Editor	**Lulu Stader**
Project Manager	**Joannah Duncan**
Cover Design	**Stewart Larking**
Text Design	**Sarah Russell**
Illustrator	**Marion Tasker**

First edition 1998
Second edition 2003
Reprinted 2004
Third edition 2007

ISBN-13: 978 0 7234 3431 3

British Library Cataloguing in Publication Data
A catalogue record for this book is available from the British Library

Library of Congress Cataloging in Publication Data
A catalog record for this book is available from the Library of Congress

Note
Neither the publisher nor the authors assume any responsibility for any loss or injury and/or damage to persons or property arising out of or related to any use of the material contained in this book. It is the responsibility of the treating practitioner, relying on independent expertise and knowledge of the patient, to determine the best treatment and method of application for the patient.

The Publisher

The publisher's policy is to use **paper manufactured from sustainable forests**

Printed in China

Preface

Metabolism and nutrition are words that usually strike fear in first year medical students as metabolic pathways are complicated and require a lot of memory work. Furthermore, it is sometimes difficult to see the importance of studying metabolic pathways, without any clinical emphasis to aid their understanding.

Crash Course : Metabolism and Nutrition aims to bridge together the core facts on metabolic pathways with relevant clinical scenarios, an approach that is in line with current integrated medical courses. Wherever possible, important core information has been presented in a more accessible and student-friendly manner, by using figures and tables to help promote better understanding.

The third edition of this book focuses on improving the clarity of metabolic pathways and updating key concepts to go hand-in-hand with current core medical curricula. My aim was to enhance the book to make it more dynamic to medical students, looking at it from a clinical context. I hope that you will find it useful, not just for passing the exams, but also to understand the importance of metabolic pathways with a clinical emphasis, as they will surely come in handy throughout your medical career.

Ming Yeong Lim

More than a decade has now passed since work began on the first editions of the Crash Course series, and over 4 years since the publication of the second editions. Medicine never stands still, and the work of keeping this series relevant for today's students is an ongoing process. These third editions build upon the success of the preceding books and incorporate a great deal of new and revised material, keeping the series up to date with the latest medical research and developments in pharmacology and current best practice.

As always, we listen to feedback from the thousands of students who use Crash Course and have made further improvements to the layout and structure of the books. Each chapter now starts with a set of learning objectives, and the self-assessment sections have been enhanced and brought up to date with modern exam formats. We have also worked to integrate points of clinical relevance into the basic medical science material, which will not only add to the interest of the text but will reinforce the principles being described.

Despite fully revising the books, we hold fast to the principles on which we first developed the series: Crash Course will always bring you all the information you need to revise in compact, manageable volumes that integrate basic medical science and clinical practice. The books still maintain the balance between clarity and conciseness, and providing sufficient depth for those aiming at distinction. The authors are medical students and junior doctors who have recent experience of the exams you are now facing, and the accuracy of the material is checked by senior faculty members from across the UK.

I wish you all the best for your future careers!

Dr Dan Horton-Szar
Series Editor

Acknowledgement

I would like to thank Dr Dominiczak for his helpful comments whenever I was stuck, as well as my Development Editor, Lulu Stader, for her friendly advice and support throughout this past year.

Thanks also go to my parents and sister, who have always believed in me and encouraged me throughout my medical career.

Figure acknowledgements
Fig 1.2 redrawn with permission from R Bronk. Human Metabolism. Addison Wesley Longman, 1999

Contents

Acyl carrier protein A protein or a domain of a protein that contains thiol groups which provides attachment sites for malonyl CoA and growing fatty acid chains.

Adenosine diphosphate (ADP) A ribonucleotide diphosphate in which two phosphoryl groups are successively linked to the 5′ oxygen atom of adenosine.

Adenosine monophosphate (AMP) A ribonucloetide monophosphate in which a phosphoryl group is linked to the 5′ oxygen atom of adenosine.

Adenosine triphosphate (ATP) A nucleotide containing a purine base (adenine), a five-carbon sugar; ribose, and three phosphate groups.

Adipose tissue Also known as fat tissue. Animal tissue composed of specialized triacylglycerol-storage cells known as adipocytes. There is growing evidence that adipocytes are hormonally active secreting a range of so called adipokines (e.g. leptin is an adipokine).

Aerobic Occuring in the presence of oxygen.

Amino acid An organic acid consisting of an α-carbon atom to which an amino group, a carboxyl group, a hydrogen atom and a specific side chain (R group) are attached.

Anabolism The synthesis of complex molecules from simpler ones. Anabolism is associated with energy entrapment and storage.

Anaemia The blood haemoglobin below the normal range for the patient's age and sex. The normal range in males is 13.5–18.0 g/dL and in females is 11.5–16.0 g/dL.

Anaerobic Occuring in the absence of oxygen.

Atherogenic The ability to start or speed up the process of atherogenesis, which is the inflammation-driven formation of lipid deposits in the arteries leading to thickening and hardening of the arterial wall.

ATPase An enzyme that catalyses hydrolysis of ATP to ADP + Pi.

Autophosphorylation Phosphorylation of a protein kinase catalyzed by the same kinase.

Bioenergetics The study of the energy changes accompanying biochemical reactions.

Beta (β)-oxidation A cyclical sequence of reactions that degrades fatty acids to acetyl CoA. It consists of four steps: oxidation, hydration, further oxidation and thiolysis.

Carbohydrate A complex molecule in which the molar ratio of C:H:O is 1:2:1.

Carnitine shuttle A pathway that shuttles acetyl CoA from the cytosol to the mitochondria through the formation of acyl carnitine.

Catabolism The breakdown of energy-rich complex molecules (e.g. carbohydrate) to simpler ones (e.g. CO_2, H_2O). Catabolism is associated with energy release.

Chaperone A protein that forms complexes with newly synthesized polypeptide chains and assists in their correct folding into biologically functional conformations.

Chylomicron A plasma lipoprotein that transports dietary lipids absorbed from the intestine to the tissues.

Citrate shuttle A pathway that shuttles acetyl CoA from the mitochondria to the cytosol providing a substrate for fatty acid synthesis.

Condensation A reaction involving the joining of two or more molecules accompanied by the elimination of water.

Cori cycle An interorgan metabolic loop that distributes the metabolic burden between the muscle and the liver. Lactate, which builds up in muscle during intense activity, is taken to the liver to be converted back to glucose via gluconeogenesis. This replenishes fuel for the muscle and prevents lactic acidosis. The produced glucose returns to muscle as an energy source, completing the cycle.

C-terminus The amino acid residue bearing a free carboxyl group (–COOH) at one end of a peptide chain.

Cytochrome A haem-containing protein that is an electron carrier in processes such as respiration and photosynthesis.

***De novo* pathway** A metabolic pathway in which a biomolecule is formed 'from scratch', from simple precursor molecules.

Deaminase An enzyme that catalyses the removal of an amino group from a substrate, releasing ammonia.

Dehydrogenase An enzyme catalysing oxidation–reduction reactions involving addition or extraction of hydrogen atoms.

Diabetes mellitus A syndrome caused by the lack, or diminished effectiveness, of insulin, resulting in a raised blood glucose (hyperglycaemia) and the presence of chronic vascular complications.

Dyslipidaemias A group of disorders caused by a defect in lipoprotein formation, transport or degradation.

Electron transport chain A series of enzyme complexes and associated cofactors that are electron carriers, passing electrons from reduced coenzymes or substrates to molecular oxygen (O_2), the terminal electron acceptor of aerobic metabolism.

Endergonic reaction A reaction during which there is a net gain of energy, $\Delta G > 0$. Such reactions do not occur spontaneously.

Endocytosis Process by which matter is engulfed by a plasma membrane and brought into the cell within a lipid vesicle derived from the membrane.

Endothermic reaction A reaction during which there is heat absorption; a positive enthalpy change ($+\Delta H$).

Enthalpy change (ΔH) A measure of the heat released or absorbed during a reaction.

Entropy change (ΔS) A measure of the change in disorder or randomness in a reaction.

Enzyme A biological catalyst, that is almost always a protein.

Essential amino acid An amino acid that cannot be synthesized by the body and must be obtained from the diet.

Essential fatty acid A fatty acid that cannot be synthesized by the body and must be obtained from the diet.

Exergonic reaction A reaction during which there is a net loss of energy, $\Delta G < 0$. Such reactions proceed spontaneously.

Exothermic reaction There is a release of heat during the reaction; a negative enthalpy change ($-\Delta H$).

Fatty acid breakdown The process in which a molecule of fatty acid is degraded by the sequential removal of two carbon units, producing acetyl CoA, which is then oxidized to CO_2 and H_2O by the TCA cycle.

Fatty acid synthesis A cyclical reaction in which a molecule of fatty acid is built up by the sequential addition of two carbons units derived from acetyl CoA.

Feedback inhibition Inhibition of an enzyme that catalyses an early step in a metabolic pathway by an end product of the same pathway.

Free energy change A thermodynamic state that defines the equilibrium in terms of the changes in enthalpy and entropy of a system at constant pressure, $\Delta G = \Delta H - T \times \Delta S$

Free radical A highly reactive atomic or molecular species with unpaired electron.

Gluconeogenesis Production of glucose from non-carbohydrate sources (e.g. amino acids, lactate, glycerol).

Glucose-alanine cycle An interorgan metabolic loop that transports nitrogen (as alanine) to the liver and transports energy (as glucose) from the liver to the peripheral tissues.

Glycation Non-enzymatic reaction resulting in binding of a sugar molecule to a protein.

Glycogen A large, highly branched polymer of glucose molecules joined by α-1,4 linkages with α-1,6 linkages at branch points.

Glycolysis Catabolic pathway consisting of ten enzyme-catalysed reactions by which one molecule of glucose is broken down into two molecules of pyruvate.

Glycoprotein A complex protein molecule containing carbohydrate residues: they are produced through the glycosylation of proteins in the endoplasmic reticulum or in the Golgi apparatus.

Glycosaminoglycan Long unbranched polysaccharides consisting of repeating disaccharide units. The disscharide unit consists of an N-acetyl-hexosamine and a hexose or hexuronic acid, either or both of which may be sulfated.

Glycosides A group of organic compounds, occurring abundantly in plants, that yield a sugar and one or more non-sugar substances on hydrolysis.

Glycosylation The addition of glycosyl groups to a protein to form a glycoprotein.

Haemoglobin A tetrameric, haem-containing globular protein in erythrocytes that carries oxygen to cells and tissues.

High-density lipoprotein (HDL) A type of plasma lipoprotein that is rich in protein and transports cholesterol and cholesteryl esters from tissues to the liver (this is known as the reverse cholesterol transport).

Hydrolase An enzyme that catalyses the hydrolytic cleavage of its substrate.

Hydrophilic 'Water loving'. A molecule that interacts with polar solvents, in particular with water, or with other polar groups.

Hydrophobic 'Water fearing'. Non-polar compounds that do not dissolve in water, such as oil.

Intermediate density lipoprotein (IDL) A type of plasma lipoprotein that is formed during the breakdown of VLDL. IDL are also called remnant lipoproteins and are atherogenic.

Isomerase An enzyme that catalyses a change in geometry or structure within one molecule.

Isozymes Different proteins from a single biological species that catalyse the same reaction.

Ketogenesis A five-step pathway that synthesizes ketone bodies from acetyl CoA in the mitochondrial matrix.

Ketone bodies Small molecules that are synthesized from acetyl CoA in the liver (acetoacetic acid, acetone, 3-hydroxybutyric acid).

Kinase An enzyme that catalyses the transfer of a phosphoryl group to an acceptor molecule.

Lipase An enzyme that catalyses the hydrolysis of triacylglycerols.

Lipid A water-insoluble organic compound found in biological systems.

Lipolysis The hydrolysis of triacylglycerols by lipase. (Note that lipolysis is different from fatty acid breakdown.)

Lipoprotein A macromolecular assembly of lipid and protein molecules with a hydrophobic core and a hydrophilic surface, present in plasma. Lipoproteins transport triglycerides and cholesterol between tissues.

Low density lipoprotein (LDL) A type of plasma lipoprotein that is formed during the breakdown of IDL and is enriched in cholesterol and cholesteryl esters. LDL are atherogenic. The measurement of plasma cholesterol reflects mainly the concentration of LDL.

Lysosome A specialized digestive organelle in eukaryotic cells.

Metabolism An integrated set of chemical reactions occurring in the body. The sum of chemical reactions in the body.

Micelle An aggregation of amphipathic (both water-repellent and water-friendly) molecules in which the hydrophilic portions of the molecules project into the aqueous environment and the hydrophobic portions point into the interior of the structure.

Mitochondrion An organelle that is the main site of oxidative energy metabolism in eurkaryotic cells.

Non-essential amino acid An amino acid that can be produced in sufficient quantity to meet metabolic needs.

N-terminus The amino acid residue bearing a free α-amino group ($-NH_2$) at one end of a peptide chain.

Nucleophilic A chemical compound or group that is attracted to nuclei and tends to donate or share electrons.

Nucleoside A compound containing a purine or pyrimidine and a sugar: purine or pyrimidine N-glycoside of ribose or deoxyribose.

Nucleotide The phosphate ester of a nucleoside, consisting of a nitrogenous base linked to a pentose phosphate.

Oxidase An enzyme that catalyses an oxidation-reduction reaction in which O_2 is the electron acceptor.

Oxidation The loss of electrons by a molecule, atom or ion. Gain of oxygen or loss of hydrogen by a molecule.

Oxidative deamination The removal of an amino group from an amino acid, which leaves behind the carbon skeleton.

Oxidative phosphorylation A process in which ATP is formed as electrons are transferred from NADH and $FADH_2$ to molecular oxygen, via a series of electron carriers that make up the electron transport chain.

Pentose phosphate pathway A pathway by which glucose-6-phosphate is metabolized to generate NADPH and ribose-5-phosphate.

Peptide Two or more amino acids covalently joined in a linear sequence by peptide bonds.

Peptide bond The covalent secondary amide linkage that joins the carbonyl oxygen atom, the amide hydrogen atom, and the two adjacent α-carbon atoms.

Peroxidase An enzyme that catalyses a reaction in which hydrogen peroxide is the oxidizing agent.

Phosphatase An enzyme that catalyses the hydrolytic removal of a phosphoryl group.

Phosphorylase An enzyme that catalyses the cleavage of its substrate via nucleophilic attack by inorganic phosphate.

Phosphorylation A reaction involving the addition of a phosphoryl group to a molecule.

P:O ratio The ratio of molecules of ADP phosphorylated to atoms of oxygen reduced during oxidative phosphorylation.

Polypeptide A polymer of many amino acid residues linked by peptide bonds.

Polysaccharide A polymer of many monosaccharide residues linked by glycosidic bonds.

Protease An enzyme that catalyses hydrolysis of peptide bonds.

Protein A biopolymer consisting of one or more polypeptide chains.

Protein glycosylation The covalent addition of carbohydrate to proteins.

Proteoglycans A special class of glycoproteins that are heavily glycosylated. They consist of a core protein with one or more covalently attached glycosaminoglycan chains.

Purine A nitrogenous base with a two-ring structure in which a pyrimidine is fused to imidazole (e.g. adenine, guanine).

Pyrimidine A nitrogenous base having a heterocyclic ring that consists of four carbon atoms and two nitrogen atoms (e.g. thymine, cytosine).

Reducing agent A substance that provides (as it itself loses) electrons in an oxidation-reduction reaction thereby becoming oxidized.

Reduction The gain of electrons by a molecule, atom or ion. Loss of oxygen or gain of hydrogen by a molecule.

Ribonucleic acid (RNA) A polymer consisting of ribonucleotide residues joined by 3'-5' phosphodiester bonds. The sugar moiety is ribose.

Ribose A five-carbon monosaccharide that is the carbohydrate component of RNA.

Salvage pathway A pathway in which a major metabolite, such as purine or pyrimidine nucleotide, can be synthesized from a preformed molecular entity, such as a purine or pyrimidine, rather than synthesized *de novo*.

Saturated fatty acid A fatty acid that does not contain a carbon-carbon double bond.

Standard redox potential (E_o) A measure of the tendency of a particular redox pair (e.g. NAD^+ and NADH) to lose electrons.

Steroid A lipid characterized by a carbon skeleton with four fused rings. All steroids are derived from the acetyl CoA.

Sterol A steroid containing a hydroxyl group.

Substrate-level phosphorylation Formation of ATP by direct phosphorylation of ADP, without requiring mitochondrial respiratory chain.

Transaminase An enzyme that catalyses the transfer of an α-amino group (NH_3^+) from an amino acid to an α-keto acid.

Triacylglycerol A lipid containing three fatty acyl residues esterified to a glycerol backbone.

Tricarboxylic acid cycle (TCA) A cyclical sequence of eight reactions that completely oxidize one molecule of acetyl CoA to two molecules of CO_2, generating energy either directly as ATP or in the form of reducing equivalents (NADH or $FADH_2$).

Ubiquitin A small basic protein that binds to a protein and targets it for degradation.

Unsaturated fatty acid A fatty acid with at least one carbon-carbon double bond.

Urea cycle A metabolic cycle consisting of five reactions that synthesize the organic compound urea from two inorganic compounds; CO_2 and NH_4^+.

Very low density lipoprotein (VLDL) A type of plasma lipoprotein that transports mostly endogenous triacylglycerols, and also cholesterol and cholesteryl esters from the liver to the tissues.

Vitamin An organic micronutrient that cannot be synthesized by the body and must be obtained from the diet.

Water-soluble vitamin An organic micronutrient that is soluble in water.

BASIC MEDICAL SCIENCE

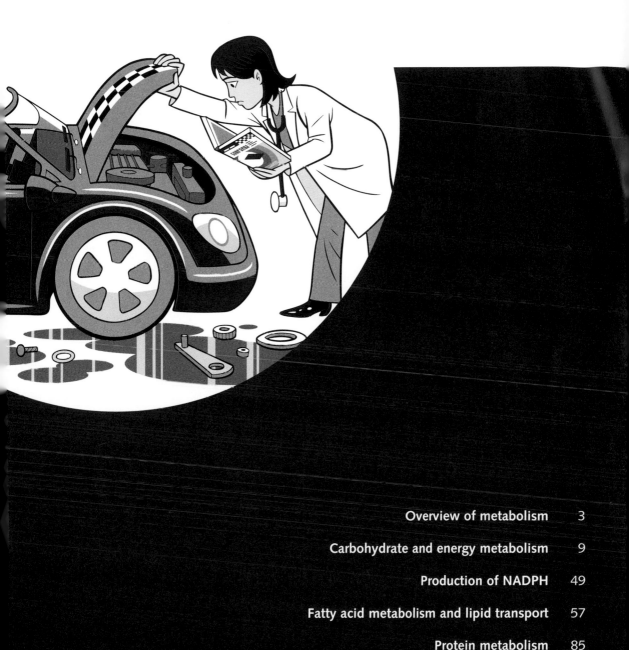

Overview of metabolism

Objectives

You should be able to:

- Define catabolic and anabolic pathways, with examples.
- Understand why metabolic pathways are regulated.
- Discuss the three main mechanisms of control.
- Understand the principles behind predicting the direction of a reaction.
- Define and distinguish between exothermic, endothermic, exergonic and endergonic reactions.
- Define oxidation, reduction and free radicals.

USEFUL DEFINITIONS

Metabolism

Metabolism involves an integrated set of chemical reactions occurring in the body. These reactions enable us to extract energy from the environment and use it to synthesize the building blocks used to make proteins, carbohydrates and fats. Some fundamental points to remember about metabolism are:

- In a metabolic pathway, each reaction provides a substrate (the substance on which an enzyme acts) for the next. It does not occur in isolation.
- Pathways are built up in which the end product forms a substrate for other pathways, producing a continuous process.
- Many people compare metabolism to a 'map', in which the pathways are like roads with 'stop-off points' (intermediates) along the way.
- Roads need traffic lights and speed humps (regulatory mechanisms) to control the amount and speed of traffic.
- Some of the roads are one way, meaning you have to travel a long way round to form some intermediates.
- Remember, when you make any journey, it is important to know where you are going but you do not need to know the names of all the places you travel through.

Metabolic pathways can be classified as either catabolic or anabolic.

Catabolism

Catabolism is the breakdown (degradation) of energy-rich complex molecules such as fat, carbohydrate and protein, to simpler ones, for example CO_2, H_2O and NH_3. The released energy is 'captured' as adenosine triphosphate (ATP) and stored for use in synthetic, anabolic reactions.

Anabolism

Anabolism is the synthesis of complex molecules from simpler ones, for example proteins from amino acids and glycogen from glucose. Synthetic reactions require energy that comes from the hydrolysis of ATP. Some examples of catabolic and anabolic pathways are shown in Fig. 1.1 and a scheme of overall metabolism is given in Fig. 1.2.

Regulation of pathways

Every metabolic pathway usually contains one reaction that is essentially irreversible and is known as the rate-limiting reaction of the pathway. Enzymes catalysing these reactions are subject to strict and sometimes complex regulation to ensure that:

- The speed of the entire pathway is adapted to the cell's needs.

Fig. 1.1 Examples of catabolic and anabolic pathways

Catabolic pathways names end in 'lysis' meaning 'to break down'	Anabolic pathways names end in 'genesis' meaning 'to create'
Glycogenolysis: glycogen breakdown Proteolysis: protein breakdown Lipolysis: triacylglycerol breakdown Glycolysis: glucose breakdown	Glycogenesis: glycogen synthesis Protein synthesis Lipogenesis: triacylglycerol synthesis Gluconeogenesis: glucose synthesis

Metabolic pathways were not just invented to make the first year at medical school very dull! Do not get bogged down remembering every single step and enzyme in a pathway, as you will not be asked to regurgitate this sort of information in an exam. It is much more likely that you will have to discuss the overall functions of a cycle and the tissues in which they are particularly important.

The best way to revise metabolism is to draw simplified cycles of all the pathways, listing the six key criteria in Fig. 1.3 for each: purpose/function, location, site, reaction sequence, key steps and effect of inhibition.

- For any molecule, its synthetic and breakdown pathways are not active at the same time (this would lead to what the biochemists call the 'futile cycle').

Metabolic pathways occur in different cell compartments, different cells and in different tissues of the body at the same time. The pathways are carefully regulated, to ensure that the production of energy and intermediates meets the needs of the individual cell and 'fits in' with the requirements of the rest of the cells in the body. The control of metabolic pathways must also be flexible enough to enable adaptation to different conditions, such as the fed state as opposed to starvation, or periods of exercise. These control mechanisms co-ordinate the pathways in all cells of the body.

Mechanisms of control

There are three main mechanisms of control of metabolic pathways: supply of substrate, allosteric control and hormonal control. Learn these now because they form the basis for control of all metabolic pathways.

Substrate supply

If the concentration of substrate is limiting, then the metabolite flow through the pathway slows down.

Allosteric control

Allosteric effectors bind to key enzymes in pathways. They bind to so called regulatory sites on an enzyme that are distinct from the catalytic (active) site. They may increase or decrease an enzyme's activity. Often, allosteric control is exerted by the end product of a pathway; this may be positive (stimulate pathway) or negative (inhibit pathway).

Hormonal control

There are two mechanisms by which hormones such as insulin or glucagon affect enzyme activity and thus the rate of metabolic pathways:

- Firstly, by reversible phosphorylation of enzymes: this may either increase or decrease their activity. For example, glucagon causes phosphorylation of glycogen synthase and glycogen phosphorylase. Phosphorylation inhibits glycogen synthase but activates glycogen phosphorylase. This ensures that glycogen synthesis and breakdown are not active at the same time; it is discussed fully in Chapter 2.
- Secondly, hormones can affect the rate of a metabolic pathway by enzyme induction. Hormones can increase the amount of enzyme synthesized by stimulating the rate of transcription of its RNA. Similarly, under certain conditions hormones can inhibit transcription and thus the synthesis of certain enzymes—this is called repression.

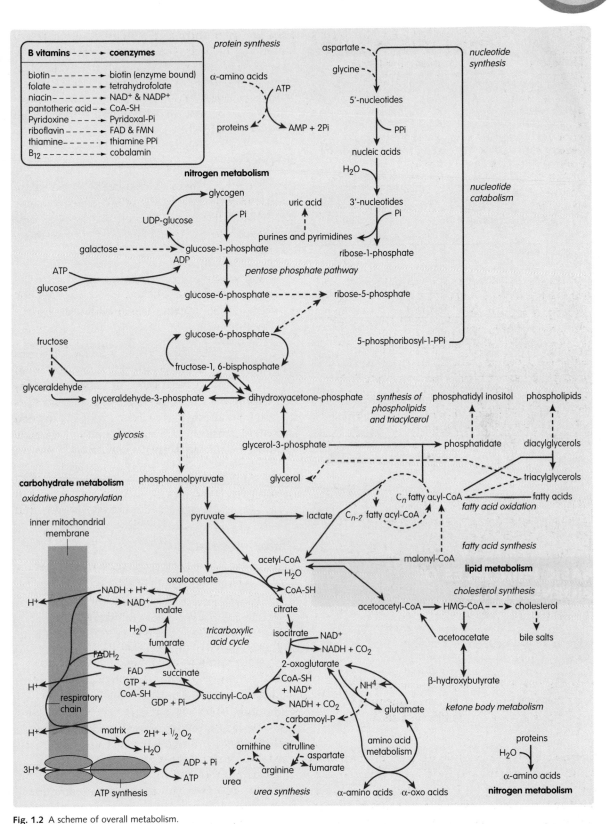

Fig. 1.2 A scheme of overall metabolism.

Fig. 1.3 Key points for remembering a metabolic pathway

Key criteria	Example—glycolysis
What is the purpose of the pathway? Form a working definition of its function knowing: the substrates and products involved and any other key intermediates produced, for example, ATP or NADH	Oxidation of glucose (substrate) to pyruvate (product) with the generation of energy in the form of ATP and NADH
Tissue location: particularly, tissues or cells in the body where the pathway is most important	Glycolysis occurs in all cells of the body but in red blood cells it is the only energy-producing pathway
Cell site: where in the cell it occurs, for example cytosol, mitochondria or both	Glycolysis occurs in the cell cytosol. Pyruvate formed can be transported into mitochondria for addition by the TCA cycle
Sequence of events: know the overall reaction sequence and the number of stages and reactions	Glycolysis has 10 reactions
Key steps: either those which form major control sites or those which are main 'branch points'	Hexokinase reaction Phosphofructokinase reaction Pyruvate kinase
Effect of inhibition of the cycle	Increase in [intermediates] which arise before the site of inhibition Decrease in [intermediates] formed after the block

BASIC PRINCIPLES OF BIOENERGETICS

Bioenergetics is the study of the energy changes accompanying biochemical reactions. It allows us to work out why some reactions occur (they occur because they are energetically favourable) and why some do not. The direction and extent to which a chemical reaction occurs is determined by a combination of two factors:

- Enthalpy change, ΔH, a measure of the heat released or absorbed during a reaction.
- Entropy change, ΔS, a measure of the change in disorder or randomness in a reaction.

Neither enthalpy nor entropy change alone can predict whether a reaction can occur. They are used together, using the formula below, to calculate ΔG, the change in Gibb's free energy of a reaction:

$$\Delta G = \Delta H - T \times \Delta S$$

where T = absolute temperature in degrees Kelvin (K) ($^\circ$C + 273) and ΔG is the energy available to do the work in kJ/mol.

It is ΔG that predicts the favourability and direction of a reaction.

- If $\Delta G < 0$, there is a net loss of energy during the reaction; making this a spontaneous, exergonic reaction.
- If $\Delta G > 0$, there is a net gain of energy during the reaction and the reaction does not occur spontaneously; it is an endergonic reaction, as energy must be added to the system to drive the reaction.
- If $\Delta G = 0$, the reaction is at equilibrium. At equilibrium, the rate of the forward reaction is equal to the rate of the backward reaction and there is no net direction.

Do not confuse exergonic and exothermic, and endergonic and endothermic. Exothermic reactions release heat during a reaction and have a negative enthalpy change ($-\Delta H$). Endothermic reactions absorb heat during a reaction and have a positive enthalpy change ($+\Delta H$). It is not possible to predict favourability or direction of a reaction from enthalpy values. Remember only reactions with a negative ΔG occur spontaneously.

Redox reaction

The word redox comes from the two processes of **red**uction and **ox**idation.

Oxidation means the loss of an electron by a molecule, atom, or ion; loss of hydrogen or gain of oxygen. It also means an increase in oxidation number. An example of an oxidation process:

$$H_2 \rightarrow 2H^+ + 2e^-$$

Reduction means the uptake of an electron by a molecule, atom or ion; loss of oxygen or gain of hydrogen. It also means a decrease in oxidation number. An example of a reduction process:

$$F_2 + 2e^- \rightarrow 2F^-$$

These two processes go together in a chemical reaction, one process cannot occur without the other; electrons lost by one compound must be gained by another. Using the above example,

$$H_2 + F_2 \rightarrow 2H^+ + 2F^-$$

Free radicals are atomic or molecular species with unpaired electrons, and this makes them highly reactive. The two most important oxygen-derived free radicals are superoxide and hydroxyl radical. They are derived from molecular oxygen under reducing conditions and are highly reactive. Because of their reactivity, these free radicals participate in unwanted side reactions, and this results in cell damage.

Carbohydrate and energy metabolism

2

Objectives

You should be able to:

- Understand and describe briefly the function, process and regulation of glycolysis.
- Describe the main pathways of production and utilization of acetyl CoA.
- Understand and describe the process and regulation of the TCA cycle.
- Understand how the electron transport chain produces ATP.
- Describe the synthesis and degradation of glycogen, and how it is regulated.
- Understand the role of the bisphosphoglycerate shunt in erythrocytes.
- Describe briefly the metabolism of fructose, galactose, ethanol and sorbitol.

GLYCOLYSIS AND ITS REGULATION

An overview of glycolysis

Working definition

Glycolysis is a sequence of reactions that breaks down one molecule of glucose (six carbons) to two three-carbon molecules of pyruvate. This sequence involves a net generation of two molecules of ATP and two molecules of NADH (the reduced form of nicotinamide adenine dinucleotide). Glycolysis provides energy and intermediates for other metabolic pathways.

Location

All the cells of the body.

Site

Cell cytosol.

Aerobic and anaerobic glycolysis

Unlike other metabolic pathways, glycolysis can produce ATP under either aerobic or anaerobic conditions.

- Under aerobic conditions, the end-product of glycolysis, pyruvate, enters the mitochondria where it undergoes oxidation by the tricarboxylic acid (TCA) cycle. Reduced nucleotides generated by the TCA cycle take part in oxidative phosphorylation to produce CO_2 and H_2O. This produces large quantities of energy.
- Under anaerobic conditions, pyruvate is reduced in the cytosol by NADH to lactate. This allows the production of ATP in cells that lack mitochondria or are deprived of oxygen, such as erythrocytes. However, this pathway produces a relatively small amount of energy.

Functions and importance of glycolysis

For many tissues glycolysis is an 'emergency' energy-producing pathway when oxygen is sparse. It is most important in:

- Erythrocytes, because they lack mitochondria and therefore glycolysis is their only energy-producing pathway.
- Exercising skeletal muscle, when oxidative metabolism cannot keep up with increased energy demand.
- The brain, because glucose is its main fuel (it needs about 120 g/day).

Glycolysis also contributes to the synthesis of certain specialized intermediates, for example, 2,3-bisphosphoglycerate, an allosteric effector of haemoglobin. It also helps in the metabolism of other sugars, especially fructose and galactose.

9

Glucose entry into cells

Glucose is not small enough to diffuse directly into the cell—it needs help. There are two specific transport mechanisms for glucose.

Facilitated diffusion—glucose transporters

Facilitated diffusion is mediated by a family of glucose transporters. At least five have been identified ; they are named GLUT-1 to GLUT-5 and each has a different tissue distribution (Fig. 2.1). The transporters are integral membrane proteins that bind glucose and transport it through the cell membrane into the cell. Glucose enters the cell down its concentration gradient from an area of high concentration outside the cell to an area of low concentration inside.

Sodium–glucose cotransporter

The second mechanism requires energy to transport glucose against its concentration gradient (i.e. from a low concentration outside the cell to a high concentration inside). This method of glucose transport occurs in the epithelial cells of the intestine (to absorb dietary glucose), renal tubules and the choroid plexus. The movement of glucose is coupled to the concentration gradient of sodium: sodium ions flow down their concentration gradient into the cell, providing the energy to transport glucose into the cell against its gradient.

Trapping glucose in the cell

To be 'trapped' inside the cell, glucose must undergo irreversible phosphorylation. Why? Well, there are two reasons: first, phosphorylated glucose molecules cannot penetrate cell membranes because there are no carriers for them (glucose-6-phosphate is not a substrate for the glucose transporters); secondly, converting glucose to glucose-6-phosphate keeps the concentration of free glucose inside the cell low compared with outside, maintaining the concentration gradient.

Stages of glycolysis

Glycolysis can be divided into two phases: an 'energy investment phase' and an 'energy generating phase'.

Energy investment phase (reactions 1–5 in Fig. 2.2)

Glucose is phosphorylated and cleaved into two molecules of glyceraldehyde-3-phosphate. This process uses two moles of ATP to activate and to increase the energy content of the intermediates (see Figs 2.2 and 2.3).

Energy generating phase (reactions 6–10)

Two molecules of glyceraldehyde-3-phosphate are converted into two molecules of pyruvate with the generation of four moles of ATP (see Figs 2.2 and 2.3).

Fig. 2.1 Examples of glucose transporters		
Transporter	Location	Function
GLUT-1	Erythrocytes and most cell membranes	Insulin-independent: Provides basal glucose transport to cells at a relatively constant rate
GLUT-2	Liver and β cells of pancreas	Insulin-independent: GLUT-2 transporters have a lower affinity for glucose than GLUT-1, therefore, GLUT-2 are only active when there is a high blood glucose, that is, in the fed state
GLUT-3	Brain cells	Insulin-independent
GLUT-4	Muscle and fat cells	Insulin-dependent: muscle and fat cells 'store' GLUT-4 transporters in intracellular vesicles. In the presence of insulin, these vesicles fuse with the cell membrane, resulting in an increase in the number of GLUT-4 transporters in membrane, thus promoting glucose uptake by muscle and fat
GLUT-5	Muscle, liver and fat cells	Insulin-independent: transports fructose

The name of an enzyme can be easily worked out, if you forget it, by knowing the name of the substrate (or the product) and the type of reaction involved (Fig. 2.4). For example, pyruvate is phosphorylated by pyruvate kinase.

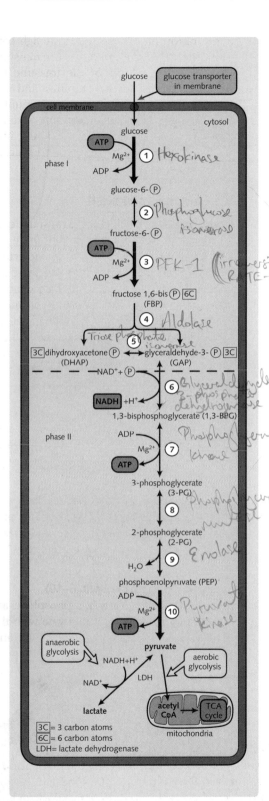

Fig. 2.2 The glycolytic (Embden–Meyerhof) pathway. Glycolysis takes place in the cell cytosol and consists of two distinct phases—energy investment (1–5) and energy generation (6–10). The names of the enzymes catalysing reactions 1 to 10 can be found in Fig. 2.3.

Handwritten annotations on figure:
1 Hexokinase
2 Phosphoglucose isomerase
3 PFK-1 (irreversible RATE-LIMITING)
4 Aldolase
5 Triose phosphate isomerase
6 Glyceraldehyde 3-phosphate dehydrogenase
7 Phosphoglycerate kinase
8 Phosphoglycerate mutase
9 Enolase
10 Pyruvate kinase

Energy yield of glycolysis
Anaerobic glycolysis

The overall reaction can be written as:

$$Glucose + 2Pi + 2ADP \rightarrow 2lactate + 2ATP + 2H_2O$$

The net effect is the generation of two moles of ATP from the anaerobic oxidation of one mole of glucose (Fig. 2.5). There is no net production of NADH because it is used by lactate dehydrogenase to reduce pyruvate to lactate. It is important to remember that, although anaerobic glycolysis only produces a small amount of ATP, it is an extremely valuable energy source for cells when the oxygen supply is limited.

Aerobic glycolysis

The overall reaction can be written as:

$$Glucose + 2Pi + 2NAD^+ + 2ADP \rightarrow$$
$$2pyruvate + 2ATP + 2NADH + 2H^+ + H_2O$$

Two moles of NADH are generated from the oxidation of one mole of glucose; each NADH is oxidized by the electron transport chain to yield about 2.5 ATP. Therefore the net effect of aerobic glycolysis is the generation of 7 ATP per mole of glucose (2 directly by substrate-level phosphorylation and about 5 indirectly by oxidative phosphorylation) (see Fig. 2.5).

Importance of NAD$^+$ regeneration from NADH

NAD$^+$ is the primary oxidizing agent in glycolysis and is an important cofactor for the glyceraldehyde-3-phosphate dehydrogenase reaction (reaction 6 in Fig. 2.2). However, there is only a limited amount of NAD$^+$ available in the cell. Therefore a major problem is its regeneration from NADH, which is essential for glycolysis to continue. There are three possible mechanisms for the regeneration of NAD$^+$:

- Firstly, under anaerobic conditions, pyruvate is reduced to lactate by lactate dehydrogenase, with the simultaneous oxidation of NADH to NAD$^+$ in the cytosol (see Fig. 2.2). This is a reversible reaction in which the direction is determined by the ratio of NADH to NAD$^+$.
- Secondly, under aerobic conditions, NADH is oxidized to NAD$^+$ by the electron transport chain in mitochondria. However, NADH must first enter the mitochondria, either via the

Fig. 2.3 Stages of glycosis. Steps 1 to 10 refer to reactions 1 to 10 in Fig. 2.2

Phase I: Energy investment phase

Step	Enzyme	Type of reaction
1.	Hexokinase: most tissues (glucokinase in liver and β cells of pancreas)	Phosphorylation **irreversible regulatory step**
2.	Phosphoglucose isomerase	Isomerization aldose → ketose
3.	Phosphofructokinase-1 (PFK-1)	Phosphorylation **irreversible rate-limiting step of glycolysis**
4.	Aldolase	Cleavage FBP (6C) → DHAP(3C) → GAP(3C)
5.	Triose phosphate isomerase	Isomerization Note that phase 1 produces two molecules of glyceraldehyde-3-phosphate (GAP)

Phase II: Energy generating phase
each molecule of glyceraldehyde-3-phosphate undergoes the following reactions:

Step	Enzyme	Type of reaction
6.	Glyceraldehyde-3-phosphate dehydrogenase	Oxidative phosphorylation 2 NADH are generated per molecule of glucose oxidized
7.	Phosphoglycerate kinase	Substrate-level phosphorylation
8.	Phosphoglycerate mutase	Transfer of phosphate group from C3 to C2
9.	Enolase	Dehydration
10.	Pyruvate kinase	Substrate-level phosphorylation **irreversible regulatory step**

N.B. All kinases require Mg^{2+} as a cofactor

Fig. 2.4 Enzymes and the types of reactions they catalyse

Enzyme	Type of reaction
Kinase	Phosphorylation
Mutase	Transfer of a functional group from one position to another in the same molecule
Isomerase	Conversion of one isomer into another (isomers are compounds with the same chemical formula, e.g. fructose and glucose are both $C_6H_{12}O_6$)
Synthase	Synthesis of molecule
Carboxylase Decarboxylase	Addition of CO_2 Removal of CO_2
Dehydrogenase	Oxidation-reduction reaction

glycerol-3-phosphate shuttle or the malate–aspartate shuttle (Figs 2.6 and 2.7).

• Thirdly, under anaerobic conditions in yeast (alcoholic fermentation), pyruvate is decarboxylated to CO_2 and acetaldehyde, which is then reduced by NADH to yield NAD^+ and ethanol.

Relevance of a high concentration of lactate in the blood

If anaerobic glycolysis continues, lactate will accumulate. The concentration of lactate in the blood is normally about 1 mmol/L. A blood lactate concentration above this is called hyperlactataemia; increase in the lactate concentration (usually above 5 mmol/L) can cause lactic acidosis. During lactic acidosis the blood pH may decrease (the normal

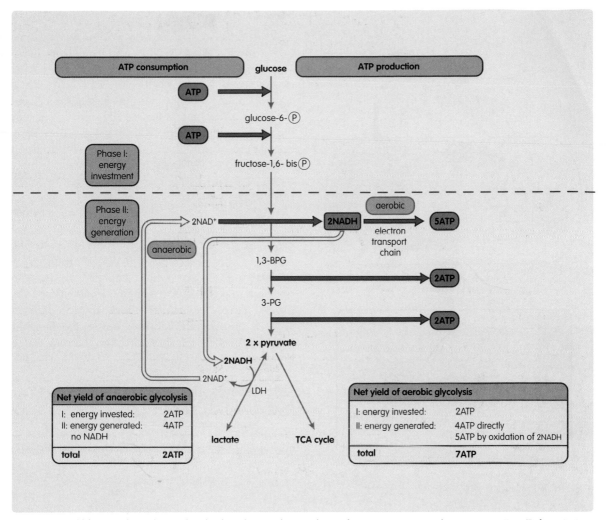

Fig. 2.5 ATP yield from aerobic and anaerobic glycolysis showing the two phases of energy investment and energy generation. (Refer to text for explanation of ATP yields.)

range is 7.35–7.45). Mild lactic acidosis may be caused by intense exercise, such as sprinting; this may lead to muscle cramps (this is covered later in Chapter 7). However, significant tissue hypoxia, occurring for example, because of circulatory collapse or shock (such as may happen after myocardial infarction or massive haemorrhage) may cause severe lactic acidosis.

Functions of the malate–aspartate and glycerol-3-phosphate shuttles

NADH produced by glycolysis must enter the mitochondrial matrix before it can be oxidized by the electron transport chain to yield ATP. The inner mitochondrial membrane is impermeable to NADH and there is no carrier protein in the membrane to transport it across. This is overcome by two mechanisms which enable 'reducing equivalents' to be transferred from the cytosol to the mitochondrial matrix. They are the glycerol-3-phosphate shuttle and the malate–aspartate shuttle. In the glycerol-3-phosphate shuttle (operating mainly in brain and muscle cells), electrons are transferred from NADH to $FADH_2$ (see Fig. 2.6). $FADH_2$, in turn, donates them to ubiquinone (Q) in the electron transport chain to generate 1.5 ATP. In the malate–aspartate shuttle (active mainly in liver and heart cells), electrons from cytosolic NADH are transferred to

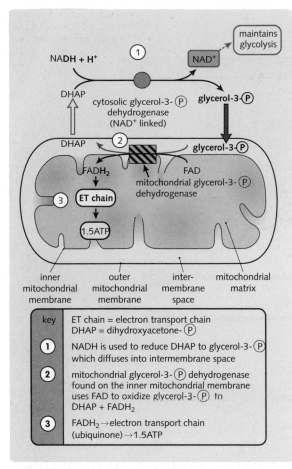

Fig. 2.6 The glycerol-3-phosphate shuttle, located mainly in brain and muscle cells.

mitochondrial NADH (see Fig. 2.7). They are then transferred to the electron transport chain to make about 2.5 moles of ATP.

The functions of the shuttles are therefore to:

- Transport electrons from NADH into mitochondria for ATP generation by the electron transport chain.
- Regenerate NAD$^+$ to allow glycolysis to continue.

Regulation of glycolysis

Regulation sites

Three reactions in glycolysis are essentially irreversible, namely steps 1, 3 and 10 (see Fig. 2.2). These constitute the main regulatory sites of the pathway (ΔG is negative and exergonic for each reaction). The control of these steps and the enzymes catalysing them are now discussed.

Step 1: Hexokinase (ΔG = –17 kJ/mol)

Phosphorylation of glucose to glucose 6-phosphate in the muscle is catalysed by the isoenzyme hexokinase, but in the liver and β cells of the pancreas, by its isoenzyme known as glucokinase. Hexokinase is controlled by product inhibition; high levels of glucose-6-phosphate allosterically inhibit it (see Fig. 2.11). It has a high affinity for glucose (K_m = 0.1 mM) ensuring that even if the intracellular concentration of glucose is low (e.g. during overnight fasting or exercise), the hexokinase reaction can still proceed.

Glucokinase has a lower affinity for glucose (K_m = 10 mM) and is well adapted to cope with the high concentration of glucose in the blood during feeding. Unlike hexokinase, it is not inhibited by glucose 6-phosphate which enables the liver to respond to high blood glucose levels. Therefore, dietary glucose goes to the liver where it is dealt with by glucokinase before it enters the systemic circulation; this prevents hyperglycaemia (high blood glucose concentration).

Step 3: Phosphofructokinase-1 (ΔG = –14 kJ/mol)

Phosphofructokinase-1 (PFK-1) is the most important regulatory enzyme in glycolysis because it catalyses the rate-limiting step. It may be regulated in two ways:

Regulation of PFK-1 by energy levels

High ATP levels allosterically inhibit PFK-1: they indicate an 'energy-rich' cell and therefore there is no need for further energy generation. Increased ATP also lowers the affinity of PFK-1 for its substrate, fructose-6-phosphate.

Citrate, generated by the TCA cycle, enhances the inhibitory effect of ATP. This is because an increased citrate indicates an abundance of metabolic intermediates (e.g. pyruvate, acetyl CoA and oxaloacetate) and no need to break down more glucose.

On the other hand, increased levels of adenosine monophosphate (AMP) that signal that energy stores are depleted, allosterically activate PFK-1 .

Regulation of PFK-1 by fructose 2,6-bisphosphate

Fructose 2,6-bisphosphate (F2,6-BP) is formed by the phosphorylation of fructose-6-phosphate catalysed by phosphofructokinase-2 (PFK-2). It is converted back again by fructose 2,6-bisphosphatase (Fig. 2.8).

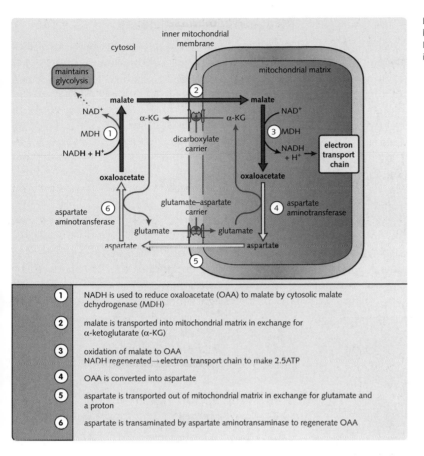

Fig. 2.7 The malate–aspartate shuttle is located mainly in liver and heart cells. N.B. The outer mitochondrial membrane is not shown.

1. NADH is used to reduce oxaloacetate (OAA) to malate by cytosolic malate dehydrogenase (MDH)

2. malate is transported into mitochondrial matrix in exchange for α-ketoglutarate (α-KG)

3. oxidation of malate to OAA
NADH regenerated→electron transport chain to make 2.5ATP

4. OAA is converted into aspartate

5. aspartate is transported out of mitochondrial matrix in exchange for glutamate and a proton

6. aspartate is transaminated by aspartate aminotransaminase to regenerate OAA

F2,6-BP:

- Is the most potent allosteric activator of PFK-1 and glycolysis (Fig. 2.9).

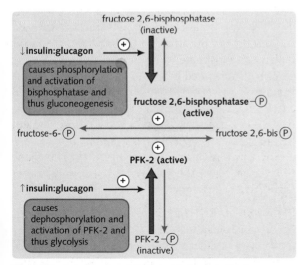

Fig. 2.8 Control of fructose 2,6-bisphosphate production by hormone-dependent reversible phosphorylation of phosphofructokinase-2 (PFK-2) and fructose 2,6-bisphosphatase.

- Increases the affinity of PFK-1 for its substrate, fructose-6-phosphate and it relieves inhibition of PFK-1 by ATP.
- Also inhibits, in the liver, fructose 1,6-bisphosphatase, an enzyme of gluconeogenesis (the pathway responsible for intracellular production of glucose which is unique to the liver; see Fig. 5.19).

The reciprocal action of F2,6-BP ensures that the glycolytic (glucose breakdown) and gluconeogenic

Phosphofructokinase-1 (PFK-1) must be distinguished from phosphofructokinase-2 (PFK-2). PFK-1 is part of the glycolysis pathway and catalyses formation of fructose 1,6-bisphosphate. PFK-2 is not part of the glycolysis pathway but catalyses the formation of fructose 2,6-bisphosphate, which in turn regulates (activates) PFK-1.

(glucose forming) pathways are not active at the same time (see Fig. 2.9).

Regulation of fructose 2,6-bisphosphate

Since F2,6-BP is such an important allosteric activator of glycolysis, its concentration is carefully regulated. Its production is controlled by hormone-dependent reversible phosphorylation of the bifunctional enzyme responsible for its synthesis and breakdown (the enzyme possesses the activity of both PFK-2 and fructose 2,6-bisphosphatase) (Fig. 2.8).

In the liver, an increase in the ratio of insulin to glucagon (e.g. following a meal) leads to enzyme dephosphorylation: this activates PFK-2 and inactivates fructose 2,6-bisphosphatase. This results in an increase in F2,6-BP and thus in the rate of glycolysis. A decrease in the ratio of insulin to glucagon, such as occurs during starvation, leads to phosphorylation of the enzyme, which inactivates PFK-2 and activates fructose 2,6-bisphosphatase: this decreases F2,6-BP and the rate of glycolysis.

Step 10: Pyruvate kinase ($\Delta G = -31$ kJ/mol)

Pyruvate kinase catalyses the final step of glycolysis and is subject to both allosteric regulation and hormone-dependent reversible phosphorylation. Fig. 2.10 illustrates the regulation of pyruvate kinase.

Pyruvate kinase deficiency

This is a rare, autosomal recessive disorder. In homozygotes, pyruvate kinase activity in the erythrocytes is about 5–20% of normal. Because erythrocytes lack mitochondria, they rely on glycolysis for ATP production. ATP is necessary for the maintenance of erythrocytes membrane flexibility and shape, enabling their passage through small vessels. Erythrocytes

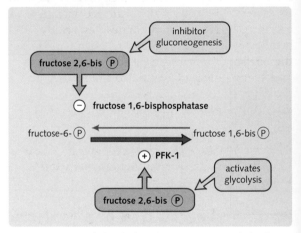

Fig. 2.9 Activation of phosphofructokinase-1 (PFK-1) and glycolysis by fructose 2,6-bisphosphate.

Fig. 2.10 Pyruvate kinase is regulated by allosteric activation and inhibition and also by hormone-dependent reversible phosphorylation of the enzyme.

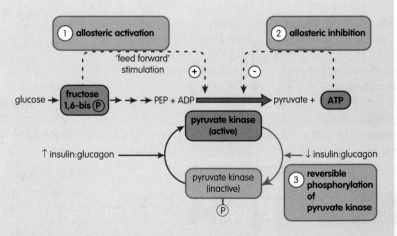

also maintain their osmotic equilibrium via ATP-dependent pumps in its membrane. Pyruvate kinase deficiency is the most common glycolytic enzyme defect and causes a chronic haemolytic anaemia.

Pathogenesis

In pyruvate kinase deficiency the production of ATP is inadequate to meet the energy requirements of the cell and thus to maintain the membrane structure. Alteration in cell shape creates distorted 'prickle-shaped' cells, which are rigid and more sensitive to phagocytosis by cells of the reticuloendothelial system. Therefore, erythrocytes have a shorter life span, leading to increased haemolysis. Inhibition of pyruvate kinase leads to an accumulation of earlier glycolytic intermediates, especially 2,3-bisphosphoglycerate (2,3-BPG). 2,3-BPG decreases the affinity of haemoglobin for oxygen, allowing greater unloading of oxygen to the tissues, which therefore decreases the severity of the hypoxia. The diagnosis of pyruvate kinase deficiency is based on:

- Presence of anaemia.
- Blood film showing prickle cells and an increased number of reticulocytes (red cell precursors).
- Pyruvate kinase activity.

Hormonal regulation of glycolysis

Insulin, released after the consumption of a carbohydrate-rich meal, increases the synthesis of the enzymes glucokinase, PFK-1 and pyruvate kinase; this is known as induction. The increased synthesis of all three enzymes leads to an increase in the rate of glycolysis. On the other hand, when glucagon levels are relatively high (e.g. in starvation or diabetes), there is a decrease in the synthesis of these enzymes (repression) and therefore a decrease in the rate of glycolysis. The overall regulation of glycolysis is mapped out in Fig. 2.11. The branch points of glycolysis, that is, its links to other pathways, are shown in Fig. 2.12. This figure also illustrates how a number of glycolytic intermediates serve as 'entry points' for other sugars into glycolysis.

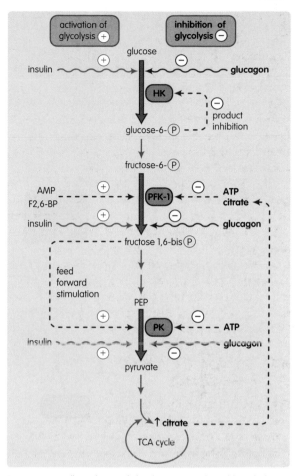

Fig. 2.11 Overall regulation of glycolysis. Remember, although this looks very complicated, the regulation of glycolysis can be divided into the allosteric control and the hormonal control. Refer back to Chapter 1 for a summary of the mechanisms of control if necessary. (F2,6-BP, fructose 2,6-bisphosphate; HK, hexokinase; PFK-1, phosphofructokinase-1; PK, pyruvate kinase.)

ACETYL COA

Structure of acetyl CoA

Acetyl CoA (Fig. 2.13) is formed from coenzyme A (abbreviated to CoA or CoASH). CoA is a complex molecule containing:

- An adenine group.
- A ribose sugar.
- Pantothenic acid (a B vitamin).
- A sulphydryl or thiol group (–SH), the active group.

The thiol group of CoA reacts with carboxyl groups (–COOH) of organic acids to form acyl CoA. If the carboxyl group is part of an acetyl group (CH_3COO^-), acetyl CoA will be formed.

Acetyl CoA is a high-energy compound, which enables it to then serve as a donor of its acetyl group, for example, in fatty acid synthesis and the TCA cycle. Thus, it is a carrier of acetyl groups just like ATP is a carrier of phosphate groups.

Fig. 2.12 The branch points of glycolysis lead off to many other pathways. All these pathways are covered later in the book. (LDH, lactate dehydrogenase; PDH, pyruvate dehydrogenase; GAP, glyceraldehyde phosphate; PEP, phosphoenol pyruvate; 1,3-BPG, 1,3- bisphosphoglycerate; 3-PG, 3-phosphoglycerate.)

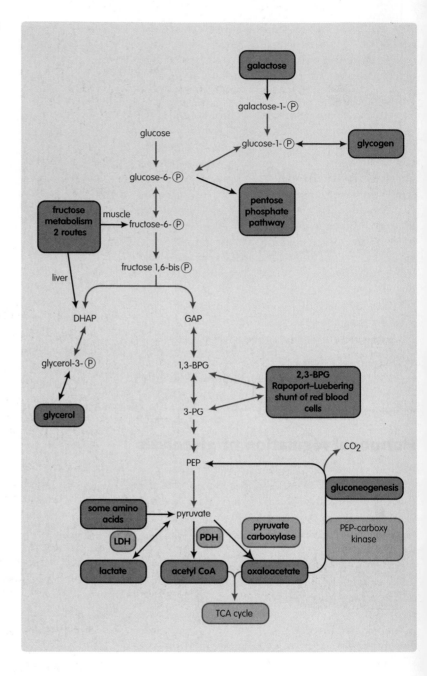

Central role of acetyl CoA

Most energy-generating metabolic pathways of the cell eventually lead to acetyl CoA. It can be formed from carbohydrate, fat and protein. It is also the starting point for the synthesis of fats, steroids and ketone bodies. Its oxidation provides energy for many tissues (Fig. 2.14).

Formation of acetyl CoA from pyruvate

The reaction
Irreversible, oxidative decarboxylation of pyruvate to acetyl CoA by pyruvate dehydrogenase (PDH).

Location
Mitochondrial matrix.

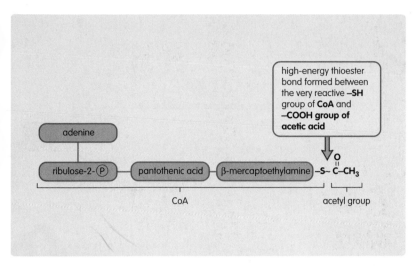

Fig. 2.13 The structure of acetyl CoA. Acetyl CoA is made by the formation of a high-energy thioester bond between the thiol group of CoA and the –COOH group of acetic acid.

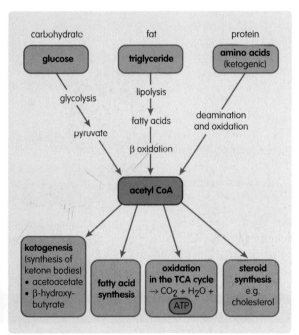

Fig. 2.14 The central role that acetyl CoA plays in metabolism. The main pathways that produce and utilize acetyl CoA.

Significance

The formation of acetyl CoA is irreversible; ΔG = –33.4 kJ/mol. Therefore, pyruvate cannot be formed from acetyl CoA, that is, carbohydrates can be converted to fats but not vice versa. There is no net synthesis of glucose from fatty acids (Fig. 2.15).

Pyruvate dehydrogenase

PDH is a multi-enzyme complex consisting of three enzymes E1, E2 and E3 (a multi-enzyme complex is a group of enzymes that catalyses two or more sequential steps in a metabolic pathway). As the enzymes are physically associated, the reactions occur in sequence without the release of intermediates. PDH also requires five coenzymes (Fig. 2.16).

PDH catalyses a complex, five-step pathway and it is not necessary to know it in detail. Basically, pyruvate is first decarboxylated and the acetyl (two-carbon) group is transferred first to lipoate and then to CoA to form acetyl CoA. Thiamine pyrophosphate (TPP) and CoA are involved in the transfer of the acetyl group. NAD[1], FAD and lipoic acid participate in the oxidation–reduction reactions. The formed NADH enters the electron transport chain to generate 2.5 moles of ATP.

Regulation of pyruvate dehydrogenase

PDH is controlled by two mechanisms; allosteric control and reversible phosphorylation (see Fig. 2.17).

1. Allosteric control—product inhibition
NADH and acetyl CoA compete with NAD^+ and CoA for binding sites on the enzymes within the PDH complex. NADH specifically inhibits E3 and acetyl CoA specifically inhibits E2.

2. Regulation by reversible phosphorylation
The PDH complex can exist in two forms: an active non-phosphorylated form and an inactive

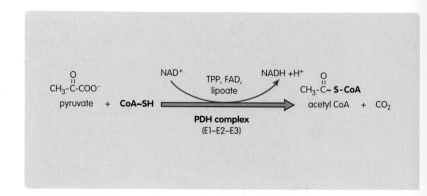

Fig. 2.15 The formation of acetyl CoA. The reaction is irreversible.

Fig. 2.16 Components of the pyruvate dehydrogenase (PDH) complex

Enzyme	Name of enzyme	Coenzymes
E1	Pyruvate decarboxylase	TPP
E2	Dihydrolipoyl transacetylase	Lipoic acid CoA
E3	Dihydrolipoyl dehydrogenase	FAD NAD$^+$

The role of acetyl CoA in metabolism is a common examination question. Be able to discuss briefly the pathways that produce and utilize acetyl CoA (Fig. 2.14) and the conditions under which they are particularly active. For example, ketogenesis becomes very important during prolonged starvation!

phosphorylated form (see Fig. 2.17). Associated with the complex are two additional enzymes, PDH kinase and PDH phosphatase.

PDH kinase catalyses the phosphorylation and thus inactivation of PDH. It is activated by the products NADH and acetyl CoA; this is in addition to their direct, allosteric effect on the PDH complex. PDH kinase is also activated by an increase in the ATP to ADP ratio: this signifies an energy-rich cell and thus a decreased need for energy production by the TCA cycle.

PDH phosphatase dephosphorylates and thus activates PDH. It is activated by insulin and Ca^{2+}.

Deficiency of thiamin

A dietary deficiency of thiamin (vitamin B$_1$) leads to a deficiency of the coenzyme thiamine pyrophosphate. This in turn results in a decrease in the activity of PDH and an accumulation of pyruvate. Excess pyruvate is converted into lactate, which may build up in the blood, leading to lactic acidosis. Vitamin B$_1$ deficiency can lead to:

- Beriberi, a neurological and cardiovascular disorder.
- Wernicke's syndrome, seen in nutritionally deprived alcoholics and also in people with

poor diet who are thiamin deficient. It may progress to Korsakoff's psychosis, an irreversible syndrome characterized by impairment of short-term memory (this is discussed further in Chapter 8).

Inherited PDH deficiency is very rare and presents with lactic acidosis. The build-up of lactate may lead to severe neurological defects.

THE TRICARBOXYLIC ACID CYCLE

The tricarboxylic acid (TCA) cycle is also known as the citric acid cycle or the Krebs cycle.

Working definition

A cyclical sequence of eight reactions that completely oxidize one molecule of acetyl CoA to two molecules of CO$_2$, generating energy, either directly as ATP or in the form of reducing equivalents (NADH or FADH$_2$). The cycle is aerobic; lack of oxygen leads to total or partial inhibition of the cycle.

Location

All mammalian cells that contain mitochondria (i.e. not erythrocytes).

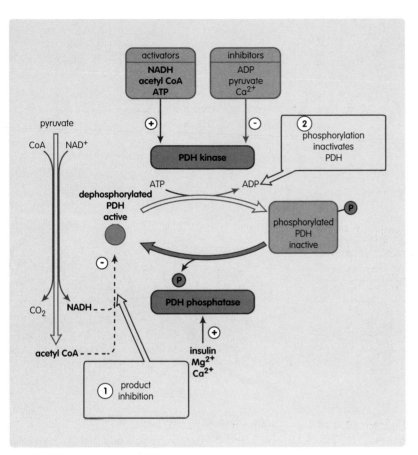

Fig. 2.17 The control of PDH complex by product inhibition and reversible phosphorylation (numbers refer to the text on p. 19).

Site

All the enzymes are found free in the mitochondrial matrix, except succinate dehydrogenase, which is found on the inner face of the inner mitochondrial membrane.

Functions

- The TCA cycle provides a final common pathway for the oxidation of carbohydrate, fat and protein. Glucose, fatty acids and amino acids are all metabolized to acetyl CoA or to other intermediates of the cycle.
- The main function of the cycle is to produce energy, either directly as ATP or as the reducing equivalents NADH or $FADH_2$, which are oxidized by the electron transport chain. Each turn of the cycle produces 10 molecules of ATP; it is the main pathway for energy generation in mammals.
- The cycle provides substrates for the electron transport chain.
- The cycle is also a source of biosynthetic precursors. For example, porphyrins are synthesized from succinyl CoA, and amino acids are synthesized from oxaloacetate and α-ketoglutarate.
- Some of the cycle intermediates also exert regulatory effects on other pathways; for example, citrate inhibits PFK-1 in glycolysis.

Thus, the cycle plays a pivotal role in metabolism. It is considered to be an amphibolic pathway, that is, a pathway that participates both in anabolism (synthetic reactions) and catabolism (oxidation of substrates).

Stages of the TCA cycle

The cycle can be divided into three stages (Figs 2.18 and 2.19).

- Stage I: the attachment of acetyl CoA to the oxaloacetate carrier (reaction 1).
- Stage II: the break-up of the carrier (reactions 2 to 5).
- Stage III: the regeneration of the carrier (reactions 6 to 8).

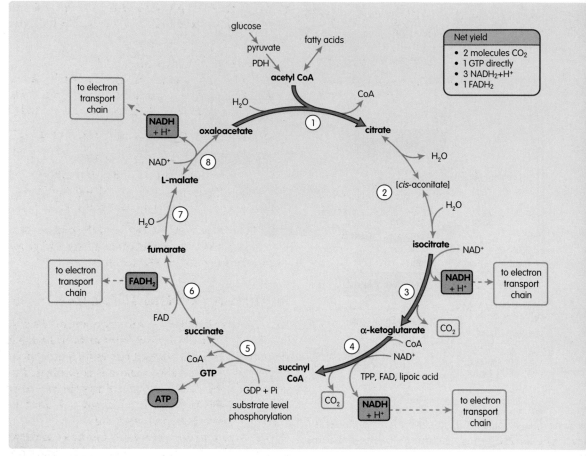

Fig. 2.18 The tricarboxylic acid cycle. Steps 1, 3 and 4 are irreversible, rate-limiting steps. Numbers 1 to 8 correspond to Fig. 2.19. (PDH, pyruvate dehydrogenase.)

It is important to know that:

- Reactions 1, 3 and 4 are irreversible rate-limiting steps.
- The last three reactions of the TCA cycle, which convert succinate to oxaloacetate, involve a characteristic sequence of reactions—oxidation, hydration and oxidation—also found in the β-oxidation of fatty acids. Be aware that the reverse of this is found in fatty acid synthesis.
- In reaction 6, FAD is the electron acceptor because the reducing power of succinate is not sufficient to reduce NAD^+. FAD is covalently bound to succinate dehydrogenase.

Energetics and yield of the TCA cycle

The overall reaction may be written as:

Acetyl CoA + $3NAD^+$ + FAD + GDP + Pi + $2H_2O$
$\rightarrow$ CoA + $2CO_2$ + 3NADH + $FADH_2$ + GTP + $3H^+$

Two carbon atoms enter the cycle as acetyl CoA and two carbon atoms leave it as CO_2 (but they are not the same carbon atoms: this is why it is said that fat cannot be directly converted into carbohydrates). There is no net consumption or production of oxaloacetate or any other intermediates of the cycle.

To learn the intermediates of the TCA cycle it is best to use a mnemonic: e.g. A Certificate In Kama Sutra Should Further My Orgasm

Fig. 2.19 The stages of the tricarboxylic acid (TCA) cycle (numbers 1 to 8 refer to Fig. 2.18)

Types of reaction	Enzyme
stage I:	
1. Condensation: 2C + 4C = 6C	Citrate synthase
stage II:	
2. Isomerization: two steps: dehydration then rehydration	Aconitase
3. Oxidative decarboxylation: 6C → 5C	Isocitrate dehydrogenase
4. Oxidative decarboxylation: 5C → 4C	α-ketoglutarate dehydrogenase complex requires coenzymes TPP, FAD, lipoic acid, NAD^+ and CoA (like PDH)
5. Substrate-level phosphorylation	Succinyl CoA synthetase Nucleoside diphosphate kinase catalyses GTP→ATP
stage III:	
6. Oxidation	Succinate dehydrogenase
7. Hydration	Fumarase
8. Oxidation	Malate dehydrogenase

One molecule of ATP is generated by substrate-level phosphorylation, reaction 5, from guanosine triphosphate (GTP). Three molecules of NADH and one of $FADH_2$ are produced for each molecule of acetyl CoA oxidized by the cycle (reactions 3, 4, 6 and 8). They are then oxidized by the electron transport chain on the inner mitochondrial membrane, generating ATP by oxidative phosphorylation. Remember, the oxidation of NADH by the electron transport chain yields 2.5 ATP and the oxidation of $FADH_2$ yields 1.5 ATP, since it joins the chain further down, bypassing the first oxidative phosphorylation site (see Fig. 2.26).

Therefore the ATP yield for each molecule of acetyl CoA oxidized (i.e. per turn of cycle) is:

- 1 ATP by substrate-level phosphorylation.
- 9 ATP by the oxidative phosphorylation of three NADH (3 × 2.5 ATP) and one $FADH_2$ (1 × 1.5 ATP); this gives a total of 10 ATP.

Fig. 2.20 illustrates the ATP yield from the oxidation of one molecule of glucose under aerobic and anaerobic conditions. Under aerobic conditions, the yield depends upon the shuttle mechanism employed to transport the NADH generated during glycolysis into the mitochondria (see Figs 2.6 and 2.7). Therefore oxidation of 1 molecule of glucose produces:

- Under anaerobic conditions: 2 ATP.
- Under aerobic conditions: approximately 32 ATP if the malate–aspartate shuttle is used or 30 ATP if the glycerol-3-phosphate shuttle is used.

Oxidation of one molecule of glycogen produces:

- Under anaerobic conditions: 3 ATP.
- Under aerobic conditions: 33 ATP if the malate–aspartate shuttle is used and 31 ATP if the glycerol-3-phosphate shuttle is used.

Fig. 2.21 shows the ATP yield from the oxidation of a fatty acid: note that oxidation of a fatty acid yields far more energy than does glucose.

Regulation of the TCA cycle

The TCA cycle is a central pathway of metabolism; it oxidizes acetyl CoA derived from carbohydrate, fat and protein and provides substrates for a number of synthetic reactions. Its regulation is co-ordinated to satisfy the demands of several pathways in a number of tissues. PDH (see Fig. 2.15) 'guards the door' to the cycle, determining pyruvate entry.

The control of the cycle itself can be considered at two levels; allosteric regulation and respiratory control.

Allosteric regulation of enzyme activities

There are three key enzymes:

- Citrate synthase.
- Isocitrate dehydrogenase.
- α-Ketoglutarate dehydrogenase.

All three enzymes are activated by Ca^{2+}. The levels of Ca^{2+} are increased, for example, during muscle contraction, thus increasing ATP generation to cope with the increased energy demand. The enzymes are also regulated by the ATP and NADH content of the cell. An increase in ATP, NADH or the concentration of products signifies a high energy status of the cell. These conditions inhibit the TCA cycle (see Fig. 2.22).

Respiratory control

The overriding control of the TCA cycle is by respiratory control. This is governed by the activity of the

Fig. 2.20 The ATP yield from the oxidation of one molecule of glucose under aerobic and anaerobic conditions. Note that the oxidation of one molecule of glycogen 'saves' an ATP molecule. The extra ATP comes from the fact glycogen is broken down into glucose-1-phosphate, bypassing the need for the first phosphorylation step of glycolysis.

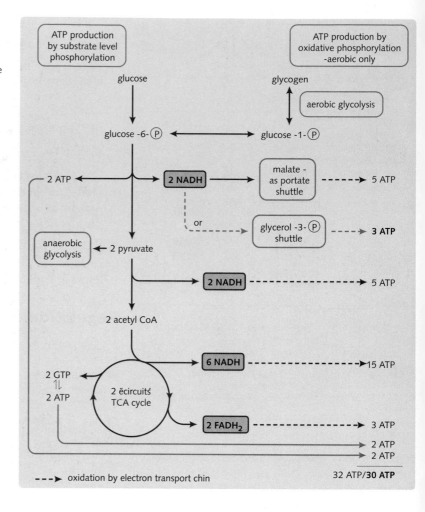

electron transport chain (which oxidizes NADH and FADH$_2$) and the rate of oxidative phosphorylation (ATP synthesis).

How does this occur?

- The activity of the TCA cycle is dependent on a continuous supply of NAD$^+$ and FAD.
- The electron transport oxidizes NADH and FADH$_2$ formed during glycolysis and the TCA cycle to NAD$^+$ and FAD, respectively.
- As the activity of the electron transport chain is tightly coupled to the generation of ATP (see Fig. 2.26), the rate of TCA cycle also depends on the ADP:ATP ratio in the cell.
- Therefore, anything affecting the supply of substrates, namely oxygen, ADP, or reducing equivalents (NAD$^+$ or FAD), would inhibit the cycle.

The TCA cycle is a source of intermediates for biosynthesis

The cycle, as well as being a degradative pathway for the generation of ATP, provides most of its intermediates as substrates for biosynthetic pathways (remember: an amphibolic pathway). The main synthetic pathways that use TCA cycle intermediates are:

- Lipid synthesis: both fatty acids and cholesterol are made from acetyl CoA in the cytosol. Acetyl CoA formed in the mitochondria cannot cross the inner mitochondrial membrane but citrate can. Cytosolic acetyl CoA is recovered from the breakdown of citrate by ATP–citrate lyase (see Fig. 2.23).
- Amino acid synthesis: for example, aspartate being synthesized from oxaloacetate, and glutamate from α-ketoglutarate (see Chapter 5).

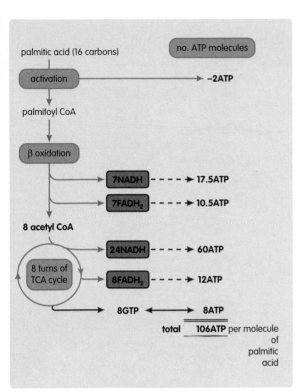

Fig. 2.21 The ATP yield from the oxidation of palmitic acid to acetyl CoA.

Remember the principle of respiratory control: the rate of oxidative phosphorylation is proportional to

$$\frac{[ADP][Pi]}{[ATP]}$$

Thus:

- A low ratio (low concentration of ADP or phosphate and high ATP) decreases the rate of ATP formation. As electron transport and ATP synthesis are coupled, electron transport and thus NADH and FADH$_2$ oxidation will also decrease. Therefore, high ATP:ADP or NADH:NAD$^+$ inhibits the TCA cycle.
- When the concentration of ADP increases, the production of ATP increases until it matches the rate of its consumption by energy-requiring reactions such as muscle contraction or biosynthetic reactions.

The role of the TCA cycle as a source of biosynthetic precursors is a common exam question, so learn it well.

- Porphyrin biosynthesis: from succinyl CoA (see Chapter 6).
- Gluconeogenesis (glucose synthesis): this occurs in the cell cytosol from oxaloacetate. Oxaloacetate cannot cross the inner mitochondrial membrane but malate can. Malate is reconverted to oxaloacetate in the cytosol (see Chapter 5).

The intermediates that are used for synthetic reactions must be replaced for the TCA cycle to be able to continue. For example, if oxaloacetate is used to make amino acids for protein synthesis, it must be reformed. The carboxylation of pyruvate by pyruvate carboxylase supplies the oxaloacetate:

Pyruvate + ATP + CO$_2$ + H$_2$O $\rightleftharpoons$ aloacetate + ADP + Pi

This is an example of an anaplerotic (replenishing) reaction, that fills up the intermediates of the cycle. Others include (see Fig. 2.23):

- The oxidation of odd-chain fatty acids to succinyl CoA.
- The breakdown of various amino acids.

- The transamination and deamination of amino acids to oxaloacetate.

GENERATION OF ATP

ATP is the universal currency of energy in the cell

The body requires a continual supply of energy for its functions such as:

- Muscle contraction.
- Biosynthesis of proteins, carbohydrates and fats.
- Active transport of molecules and ions across cell membranes.

The oxidation of metabolic fuels (protein, carbohydrate and fat) yields energy in the form of ATP. Adenosine triphosphate (Fig. 2.24) is a nucleotide containing:

Fig. 2.22 Regulation of the tricarboxylic acid (TCA) cycle. The three rate-limiting reactions (numbered) of the TCA cycle are all inhibited by ATP and NADH.

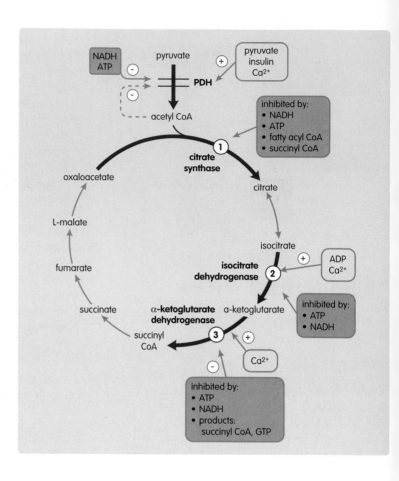

- A purine base, adenine.
- A five-carbon sugar, ribose.
- Three phosphate groups.

ATP is an energy-rich molecule because it contains two phosphoanhydride bonds. When it is hydrolysed to ADP, one of these bonds breaks, releasing a large amount of free energy:

$$ATP + H_2O \rightarrow ADP + Pi$$
$$\Delta G = -30.66\,kJ/mol \text{ (i.e. it is a spontaneous, favourable reaction)}$$

The energy liberated is used to drive chemical reactions. For example, in glycolysis, the hydrolysis of ATP is coupled to the formation of high-energy phosphorylated intermediates such as 1,3-bisphosphoglycerate or phosphoenolpyruvate (see Fig. 2.2). ATP can also be hydrolysed to AMP, releasing pyrophosphate (PPi), which undergoes further spontaneous hydrolysis to two molecules of inorganic phosphate ($2 \times$ Pi), breaking both phosphoanhydride bonds.

Synthesis of ATP

ATP can be synthesized from ADP by two processes: substrate-level phosphorylation and oxidative phosphorylation.

Substrate-level phosphorylation

Substrate-level phosphorylation is defined as the formation of ATP by direct phosphorylation of ADP. It does not require oxygen, making it important for generating ATP when oxygen is in short supply, for example, contracting skeletal muscle. Substrate level phosphorylation occurs in glycolysis and the TCA cycle (Fig. 2.25).

Oxidative phosphorylation

Most ATP is generated by oxidative phosphorylation, and this requires oxygen.

Definition

A process in which ATP is formed as electrons are transferred from NADH and FADH$_2$ to molecular

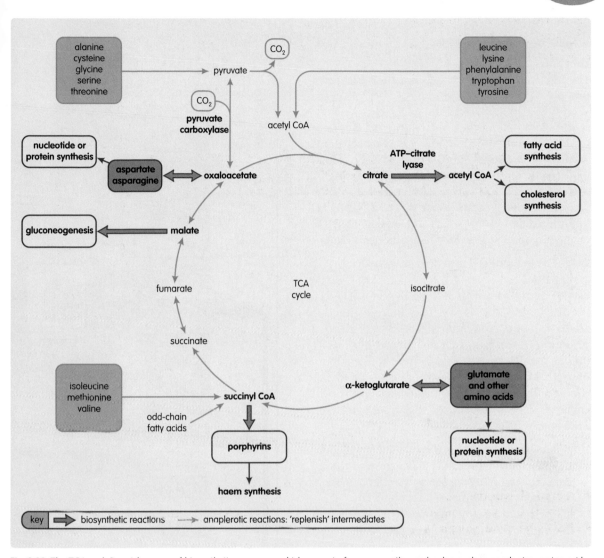

Fig. 2.23 The TCA cycle is a rich source of biosynthetic precursors which go on to form many other molecules, such as porphyrins, amino acids and fatty acids.

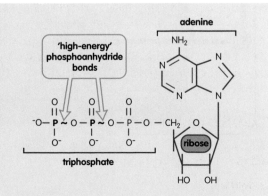

Fig. 2.24 The structure of adenosine triphosphate (ATP). ATP is made up of the purine adenine, the five-carbon sugar ribose, and three phosphate units linked by high-energy phosphoanhydride bonds.

Fig. 2.25 Examples of substrate-level phosphorylation

Example	Reaction	Enzyme
Glycolysis	1,3-BPG + ADP ↔ 3-PG + ATP	Phosphoglycerate kinase
	PEP + ADP → pyruvate + ATP	Pyruvate kinase
TCA cycle	Succinyl-CoA + GDP ↔ succinate + GTP	Succinyl-CoA synthetase

oxygen, via a series of electron carriers that make up the electron transport chain.

Location
The inner surface of the inner mitochondrial membrane.

Pyruvate from glycolysis, fatty acids via β-oxidation, and some amino acids (through trans-amination reactions) provide acetyl CoA, which is oxidized by the TCA cycle to CO_2 and H_2O. During these processes, electrons are donated from metabolic intermediates to the coenzymes NAD^+ and FAD, to form reduced forms NADH and $FADH_2$. Therefore, energy is conserved as these reducing equivalents.

Origin of the reduced intermediates NADH and $FADH_2$
NADH is formed via glycolysis in the cytosol and via the TCA cycle and β-oxidation in mitochondria. $FADH_2$ comes from both the TCA cycle and β-oxidation in the mitochondria. NADH and $FADH_2$ donate their electrons, one at a time, to the electron transport chain. As each electron is passed down the chain, it loses most of its free energy. Part of this energy is captured and used to produce ATP from ADP and inorganic phosphate.

How does this occur?
- The transport of electrons down the electron transport chain is coupled to the transport of protons across the inner mitochondrial membrane, from the mitochondrial matrix into the inner mitochondrial space (Fig. 2.26).
- This occurs at three specific proton-pumping sites and thus creates an electrochemical gradient across the membrane.
- The protons are only allowed back into the mitochondrial matrix via an enzyme, ATP synthase, present in the inner mitochondrial membrane.
- The movement of protons activates ATP synthase to catalyse ATP synthesis.
- Any energy not trapped as ATP is released as heat.

The coupling of the oxidation of NADH and $FADH_2$ by the electron transport chain with the generation of ATP is known as oxidative phosphorylation. (The electron transport chain is sometimes called the respiratory chain because it only works in the presence of oxygen.)

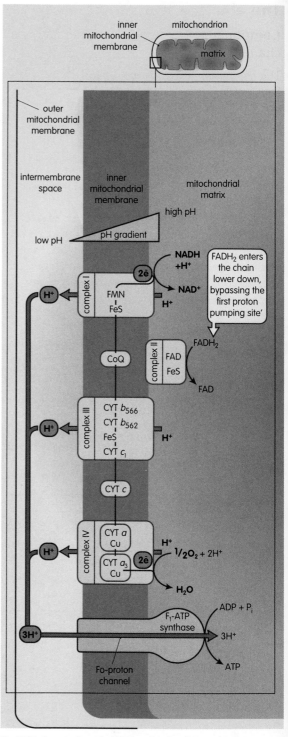

Fig. 2.26 An overview of oxidative phosphorylation, showing components of the electron transport chain (refer also to Fig. 2.27).

The electron transport chain

Components of the electron transport chain

The chain consists of four protein complexes (see Fig. 2.26). These are integral membrane proteins present in the inner mitochondrial membrane, through which electrons pass (Fig. 2.27). The electron-carrying groups within these complexes are either flavins, iron–sulphur proteins, haem groups or copper ions. The complexes are arranged in order of increasing standard redox potential (measured in volts) and increasing electron affinity.

The standard redox potential (E_o) is a measure of the tendency of a particular redox pair (e.g. NAD$^+$ and NADH, or FAD and FADH$_2$) to lose electrons. The more negative the E_o value, the greater the tendency to lose electrons (i.e. lower electron affinity), whereas the more positive the E_o value, the more likely the redox pair is to accept electrons (higher electron affinity). The electrons flow from electron carriers with more negative E_o values to carriers with more positive E_o values, until they are passed to molecular oxygen, which has the highest E_o.

The complexes are linked by two soluble membrane proteins: ubiquinone (coenzyme Q) and cytochrome c, which travel easily along the membrane.

The reactions within the chain

1. The oxidation of NADH or FADH$_2$ initiates electron transport down the chain.
2. Electrons derived from NADH are passed to complex I, whereas electrons of FADH$_2$ go directly to complex II. This is because FADH$_2$ is produced by succinate dehydrogenase, a TCA cycle enzyme, which is actually part of complex II (see Fig. 2.27).
3. Each component of the chain is alternately oxidized and reduced as electrons pass down the chain.

Fig. 2.27 Components of the electron transport chain. Complexes III, IV and cytochrome c are all cytochromes and contain a haem prosthetic group. The iron atom of the haem group is reversibly oxidized and reduced, that is, it alternates between Fe^{2+} and Fe^{3+} as part of its normal function as an electron carrier

Electron carrier	Components	Function
Complex I: NADH ubiquinone reductase	Two types of redox proteins: • flavin mononucleotide (FMN) reduced by NADH → FMNH$_2$ • 1–5 iron–sulphur proteins (FeS) reduced by NADH	Enzyme catalyses the oxidation of NADH **proton pumping site**
Complex II: Succinate ubiquinone reductase	TCA cycle enzyme succinate dehydrogenase FAD 1–3 iron–sulphur proteins	Catalyses the oxidation of FADH$_2$ by CoQ
CoQ (ubiquinone)	Quinone derivative	Shuttles electrons from complexes I and II to III
Complex III: CoQ–cytochrome c reductase	b cytochromes (b_{562} and b_{566}) Ubiquinol–cytochrome c_1 Iron–sulphur proteins	Catalyses the oxidation of CoQ by cytochrome c **proton pumping site**
Cytochrome c	Cytochrome c	Shuttles electrons between complexes III and IV
Complex IV: Cytochrome c oxidase	Cytochromes a and a_3 two copper atoms	Catalyses the four-electron reduction of oxygen to H$_2$O **proton pumping site**

4. Finally, electrons are donated to molecular O_2, reducing it to water.

Why a chain of electron carriers instead of one reaction?

The oxidation of NADH leads to the pumping of protons at three sites across the membrane. When protons re-enter the matrix via ATP synthase, ATP is generated. Oxidation of NADH generates 2.5 molecules of ATP. If only a single reaction were employed, a lot of energy would be wasted, since there would be fewer proton pumping sites and thus less energy generation.

The oxidation of $FADH_2$ leads to the pumping of protons at only two sites across the membrane, bypassing the first site. This leads to only about 1.5 molecules of ATP being produced.

It is useful to note that until fairly recently it was thought that oxidation of NADH by the electron transport chain generated 3 ATP and oxidation of $FADH_2$ produced 2 ATP. However, recent studies on the ATP yield of oxidative phosphorylation have shown that the values are about 2.5 ATP for NADH and 1.5 for $FADH_2$. The reasons for the difference are complex, but basically the lower values compensate for additional protons used for phosphate transport into the mitochondrial matrix and the exchange of mitochondrial ATP for cytosolic ADP by ATP–ADP translocase.

Because of the ongoing debate amongst biochemists about the exact yields, the numbers differ slightly in different textbooks. The values 2.5 ATP for NADH and 1.5 for $FADH_2$ are used throughout this book.

Generation of ATP via a proton gradient

The mechanism of oxidative phosphorylation can be explained by Mitchell's chemiosmotic theory. The flow of electrons down the electron transport chain does not lead directly to ATP synthesis. Instead, electron transport is coupled to pumping of protons across the inner mitochondrial membrane into the intermembrane space at complexes I, III and IV. Proton translocation creates an electrochemical gradient across the membrane (both electrical and pH components), which is about 150–250 mV. It is this potential difference that provides the energy for ATP synthesis when the protons are returned to the matrix through ATP synthase.

Structure of ATP synthase

ATP synthase consists of two subunits (see Fig. 2.26): F_0, a proton channel, and F_1, the enzyme, ATP synthase. Protons re-enter the mitochondrial matrix normally only through the F_0 proton channel. The movement of these protons activates ATP synthesis by the F_1 subunit. A flow of approximately three protons through ATP synthase is required to make each ATP. Therefore, electron transport and phosphorylation are coupled by the proton gradient.

Uncoupling of the electron transport chain from phosphorylation

Any substance that increases the permeability of the inner mitochondrial membrane to protons, so that they can re-enter the mitochondrial matrix at sites other than ATP synthase, causes uncoupling. As a result the re-entry of protons dissipates the proton gradient without ATP production.

Uncouplers

2,4-Dinitrophenol (DNP) is a lipid-soluble proton carrier that can diffuse freely across the inner mitochondrial membrane (see Fig. 2.28). It carries protons across the membrane, dissipating the proton gradient. This results in a decreased flow of protons through ATP synthase and thus decreased ATP production (it short-circuits ATP synthase). Therefore, electron transport occurs normally but with no consequent ATP production. The energy produced by electron transport is released as heat. Another uncoupling agent is trifluoro-carbonylcyanide methoxyphenylhydrazone (FCCP), which acts similarly to DNP.

Uncoupling occurs physiologically in brown adipose tissue. Newborn babies and hibernating mammals contain brown fat, usually in their neck and upper back. The mitochondria of brown fat contain the uncoupling protein thermogenin in their inner mitochondrial membrane. This acts as a proton channel and allows the dissipation of the proton gradient and thus the release of energy as heat, enabling them to keep warm.

Inhibitors of the respiratory chain

Inhibitors bind to a component of the chain and block the transfer of electrons at specific sites

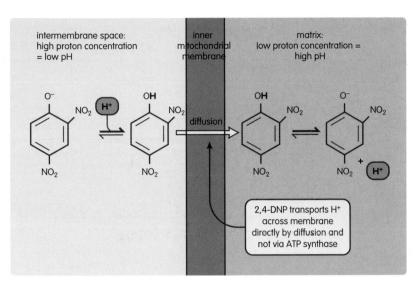

Fig. 2.28 The action of the uncoupler, 2,4-dinitrophenol (2,4-DNP) is to transport protons across the mitochondrial membrane without the production of ATP, dissipating the proton gradient.

intermembrane space: high proton concentration = low pH

inner mitochondrial membrane

matrix: low proton concentration = high pH

diffusion

2,4-DNP transports H⁺ across membrane directly by diffusion and not via ATP synthase

(Fig. 2.29). All the electron carriers of the chain before the block are reduced, whereas those after the block remain oxidized. As the electron transport chain and oxidative phosphorylation are tightly coupled, inhibition leads to a decrease in ATP synthesis.

Tetramethyl-*p*-phenyldiamine (TMPD) is an artificial electron donor: it transfers electrons directly to cytochrome *c*. Vitamin C (ascorbate) is required to reduce TMPD, and they are both often used in combination to study the chain.

Control of ATP generation: respiratory control

The principle of respiratory control is discussed on pp. 23–24 and it would be useful to recap on this now.

A supply of ADP (substrate) is necessary for ATP synthesis; a low concentration of ADP will result in decreased production of ATP. Since electron transport and ATP synthesis are tightly coupled, electron transport and thus oxidation of NADH and $FADH_2$ will also be inhibited.

GLYCOGEN METABOLISM

Role of glycogen

Excess dietary glucose is stored as glycogen. Glucose can be rapidly mobilized from glycogen when the need arises; for example, between meals or during

Fig. 2.29 Inhibitors of the electron transport chain

Inhibitors	Action
Rotenone, amytal and piericidin	Inhibit electron transfer from NADH dehydrogenase (complex I) to ubiquinone
Antimycin A and myxothiazol	Inhibits electron transfer from reduced cytochrome b_{562} to cytochrome c_1 (complex III), therefore preventing proton pumping
Cyanide, carbon monoxide, or azide	Inhibit electron transfer in cytochrome oxidase (complex IV)
Oligomycin and dicyclohexylcarbodiimide (DCCD)	Block the proton channel part (Fo) of ATP synthase, decreasing ATP synthesis

exercise. A constant supply of glucose is essential for life because it is the main fuel of the brain and the only energy source that can be used by cells lacking mitochondria or by contracting skeletal muscle (during anaerobic glycolysis). Glycogen is therefore an excellent short-term storage material that can provide energy immediately.

Glycogen stores

The main stores of glycogen are in muscle and in the liver, where they have different functions (Fig. 2.30).

Fig. 2.30 Comparison of the roles of liver and muscle glycogen

	Liver glycogen	Muscle glycogen
Main function	**Maintenance of blood glucose concentration**, particularly between meals and early stages of fasting	Fuel reserve for muscle contraction
Other roles	**Used as a fuel by any tissue** Liver contains glucose-6-phosphatase, which removes the phosphate group from glucose-6-phosphate, allowing glucose to leave the liver	None: **cannot leave muscle** muscle lacks glucose-6-phosphatase therefore glucose-6-phosphate cannot leave the cell; it enters glycolysis to generate energy instead
Size of stores	Approximately 10% wet weight of liver; **stores last only about 12–24 h**	Approximately 1–2% wet weight of muscle (however, humans have much more muscle than liver glycogen; and therefore about twice as much muscle glycogen as liver glycogen)
Hormonal control	Glucagon and adrenaline promote glycogen breakdown Insulin promotes synthesis	Adrenaline promotes glycogen breakdown Insulin promotes synthesis

Remember that muscle glycogen cannot leave muscle and therefore cannot contribute to the concentration of glucose in the blood. Fig. 2.31 is a graph showing the variation in liver glycogen stores and blood glucose plotted against time of day.

Structure of glycogen

Glycogen is a large, highly branched polymer of glucose. There are two types of linkage found between the glucose molecules (see Fig. 2.32a):

- They are joined by an α-1,4 linkage, to make straight chains.
- An α-1,6 linkage occurs every 8 to 12 glucose residues, to make branch points.

Glycogen is present in the cytosol as granules (the diameter varies between 100 and 400 Å). Besides glycogen, the granules also contain enzymes that catalyse glycogen synthesis and degradation.

Why is it an advantage to have a branched structure?

A branched structure creates a large number of exposed, terminal glucose molecules (i.e. many ends) that are easily accessible to the enzymes catalysing glycogen breakdown. This enables rapid degradation

and glucose release when necessary (e.g. as part of a 'fight-or-flight' response). Branching therefore serves to increase the rate of glycogen synthesis and degradation. It also increases the solubility of glycogen.

Glycogen synthesis (glycogenesis)

Glycogen synthesis takes place in the cytosol. The process requires:

- Three enzymes: uridine diphosphate (UDP)-glucose pyrophosphorylase, glycogen synthase and the branching enzyme, amylo(1,4→1,6)transglycosylase.
- The glucose donor, UDP-glucose.
- A primer to initiate glycogen synthesis if there is no pre-existing glycogen molecule.
- Energy.

There are three stages to glycogenesis (Fig. 2.32b).

Stage I: Initiation—formation of glucose donor

UDP-glucose pyrophosphorylase catalyses the synthesis of UDP-glucose (an activated form of glucose) from glucose-1-phosphate and UTP (see Fig. 2.32b). The reaction is reversible but is driven

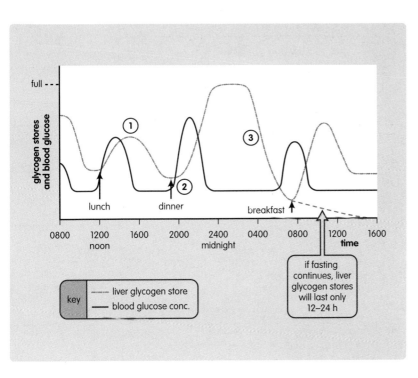

Fig. 2.31 A graph showing the approximate variation of liver glycogen stores and blood glucose against the time of day.
1. After a meal, glycogen stores rise; between meals glycogen stores fall as glucose is released from liver glycogen to help maintain the concentration of glucose in the blood.
2. After a meal there is an increase in blood glucose; between meals it stabilizes.
3. Overnight glycogen stores are mobilized to help maintain blood glucose concentration.

forward by the rapid hydrolysis of pyrophosphate by pyrophosphatase.

Stage II: Elongation of the glycogen chain

Glycogen synthase transfers the glucosyl group from UDP-glucose to the C4 position of an existing glycogen chain to form an α-1,4 glycosidic linkage. The enzyme can only add glucose molecules to a chain already containing at least four glucose residues; that is, it cannot initiate chain synthesis: a primer is required for this. The primer can be either a glycogen fragment or the protein glycogenin.

Stage III: Formation of glycogen branches

Glycogen synthase forms only linear, straight-chain glycogen molecules. A branching enzyme called amylo(1,4→1,6)transglycosylase is required to form branches. When the growing chain contains 11 or more residues, this enzyme transfers a number of them, usually seven, from the non-reducing end of the glycogen chain, to a neighbouring chain, establishing a branch point. Therefore an α-1,4 link is broken but an α-1,6 linkage is formed. The branching enzyme is specific with regard to the length of chain it transfers (usually between five and eight residues). The new branch point must be at least four residues away from an existing branch.

Glycogen degradation (glycogenolysis)

Glycogen degradation takes place in the cytosol. There are two stages (Fig. 2.33).

Stage I: Shortening of the glycogen chain

Glycogen phosphorylase catalyses the sequential removal of glucose residues from the non-reducing end of glycogen. The enzyme requires pyridoxal phosphate (PLP) as a cofactor. Phosphorylase cleaves the terminal α-1,4 glycosidic link, to release glucose-1-phosphate. This process is known as phosphorolysis, which is similar to hydrolysis but uses phosphate instead of water to split the bond. The glucose-1-phosphate produced can be converted to glucose-6-phosphate by phosphoglucomutase, and can either enter glycolysis or, in the liver, be converted to glucose by glucose-6-phosphatase. Phosphorylase continues to degrade glycogen until it reaches a residue four molecules away from a branch point, where it stops.

Fig. 2.32a The branched structure of glycogen, showing the two types of linkages found between glucose molecules. Most glucose molecules are joined by α-1,4 linkages, making straight chains. α-1,6 linkages occur about every 8–12 glucose residues and enable branch points to be formed. Numbers refer to the appropriate carbon atoms in the component glucose molecules.

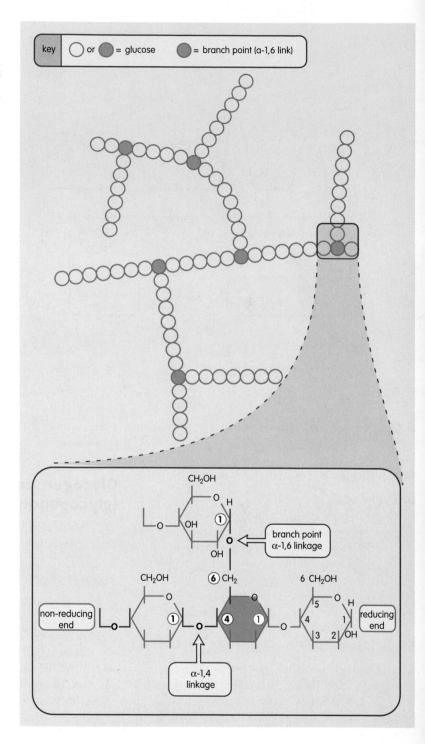

Stage II: Removal of branches

This involves two enzymes: a transferase ([α-1,4→ α-1,4] glucan transferase) that transfers the terminal three glucose residues (a trisaccharide) from one outer branch to another, exposing the α-1,6 branch point; and a debranching enzyme, amylo-α-1,6-glucosidase, which hydrolyses the α-1,6 link to release free glucose. Together, the two enzymes

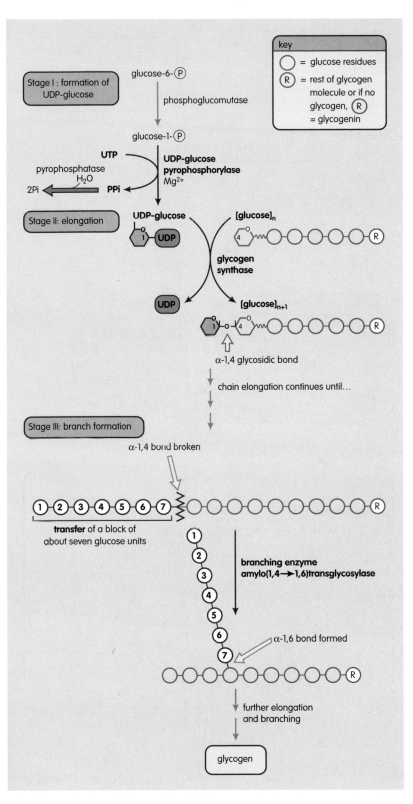

key

○ = glucose residues

Ⓡ = rest of glycogen molecule or if no glycogen, Ⓡ = glycogenin

Stage I : formation of UDP-glucose

glucose-6-Ⓟ

phosphoglucomutase

glucose-1-Ⓟ

UTP

pyrophosphatase
H_2O

UDP-glucose pyrophosphorylase
Mg^{2+}

2Pi ← PPi

Stage II: elongation

UDP-glucose

$[glucose]_n$

glycogen synthase

$[glucose]_{n+1}$

α-1,4 glycosidic bond

chain elongation continues until…

Stage III: branch formation

α-1,4 bond broken

transfer of a block of about seven glucose units

branching enzyme amylo(1,4→1,6)transglycosylase

α-1,6 bond formed

further elongation and branching

glycogen

Fig. 2.32b Glycogen synthesis consists of three stages, starting with the formation of UDP-glucose, which then takes part in the elongation of the glycogen molecule. When the growing glycogen chain is long enough, a polysaccharide of between five and eight units is broken off and transferred to a neighbouring chain to form a branch chain.

Fig. 2.33 Degradation of a glycogen molecule, showing the two stages necessary for its catabolism to monosaccharide units. Shortening of the glycogen chain releases glucose-1-phosphate, while hydrolysis of a branch point releases free glucose.

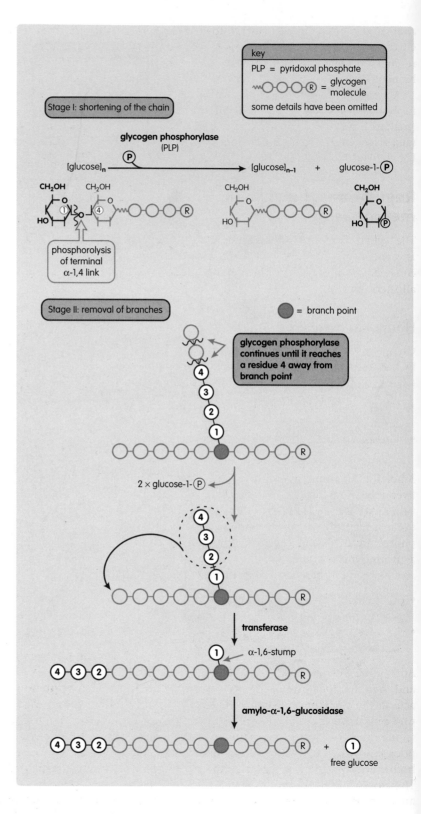

convert the branched structure into a linear one. Glycogen phosphorylase can now proceed until it reaches a residue four molecules away from the next branch point.

A small amount of glycogen breakdown occurs in lysosomes via the enzyme α-1,4 glucosidase (maltase). Deficiency of this enzyme can lead to a fatal glycogen storage disorder, Pompe's disease (see Fig. 2.36).

Regulation of glycogen metabolism

The regulation of glycogen synthesis and degradation is very complex and not fully understood. It can be considered on two levels: hormonal regulation and allosteric control.

Hormonal regulation

Glycogen synthase and phosphorylase are regulated by hormone-dependent reversible phosphorylation. Glycogen phosphorylase exists in two forms:

- Phosphorylase a, the active, phosphorylated form.
- Phosphorylase b, the inactive, dephosphorylated form.

Adrenaline (in muscle and liver) and glucagon (in liver only) stimulate glycogen breakdown. They activate cAMP-dependent protein kinase A which, via the reaction cascade shown in Fig. 2.34, causes the phosphorylation of glycogen phosphorylase, thereby activating this enzyme.

Glycogen synthase also exists in two forms:

- Glycogen synthase a, the active, dephosphorylated form.
- Glycogen synthase b, the inactive phosphorylated form.

Adrenaline and glucagon are catabolic hormones and therefore they inhibit glycogen synthesis. They activate the cAMP-dependent protein kinase A, which phosphorylates glycogen synthase, inactivating it (remember, the opposite happens to glycogen phosphorylase, i.e. it is activated; this ensures that both pathways are not active at the same time). Therefore, glycogen synthase and phosphorylase are reciprocally regulated. The actions of adrenaline and glucagon in glycogen metabolism are shown in Fig. 2.34.

Insulin is an anabolic hormone. It stimulates glycogen synthesis and inhibits glycogen breakdown. It does so by promoting the activation of protein phosphatase-I, which removes the phosphate group by hydrolysis. This leads to dephosphorylation of both glycogen synthase and phosphorylase.

Further details on the mechanism of action of insulin can be found in Chapter 7.

Amplification cascade
The mechanism of action of adrenaline and glucagon in glycogen metabolism shown in Fig. 2.34 is an example of an amplification pathway, in which the large number of steps involved amplifies the hormonal signal, allowing the rapid release of glucose. Only one or two molecules of hormone bind to their receptors, but they each cause the activation of a number of protein kinase molecules (100), which in turn activate many phosphorylase b kinase molecules (1000). This produces large numbers of active glycogen phosphorylase molecules (10 000) to degrade glycogen. If the binding of adrenaline directly activated glycogen phosphorylase it would require huge quantities of hormone for the same response.

Allosteric control

Liver glycogen phosphorylase
Glucose allosterically inhibits liver glycogen phosphorylase a. Phosphorylase a (phosphorylated, active form) contains two binding sites for glucose. The binding of glucose causes a conformational change; this exposes the phosphate groups, enabling their removal by protein phosphatase-I, thus converting it to phosphorylase b (the inactive form). Therefore, the product, glucose, inhibits glycogen breakdown. Glucose-6-phosphate also inhibits phosphorylase but activates glycogen synthase (Fig. 2.35).

Muscle glycogen phosphorylase
The main allosteric control is effected by 5' AMP and Ca^{2+}. Calcium ions released during muscle contraction bind to calmodulin, a subunit of phosphorylase b kinase, activating it. For maximal activation, the enzyme also requires phosphorylation (Fig. 2.34).

AMP is also an indicator of the energy status of the cell. High levels of AMP signal a low energy status (i.e. low ATP), for example, during intense exercise. Therefore AMP allosterically activates phosphorylase b; this increases glycogen breakdown to provide energy for muscle contraction.

Fig. 2.34 The action of adrenaline and glucagon on glycogen metabolism. The mechanism of action is as follows:

1. The binding of adrenaline or glucagon activates adenyl cyclase via a G-protein-coupled pathway (not shown).
2. Adenyl cyclase catalyses the formation of cAMP, which activates a cAMP-dependent protein kinase (protein kinase A).
3. This enzyme contains two regulatory (R) and two catalytic (C) subunits. cAMP binds to the regulatory subunits, allowing the active catalytic subunits to dissociate.
4. cAMP-dependent protein kinase catalyses phosphorylation of:
   a. phosphorylase b kinase, activating it;
   b. glycogen synthase, inhibiting it;
   c. protein phosphatase-inhibitor-I, activating it, thus enabling it to inhibit protein phosphatase-I. (Ca^{2+} released by contracting muscle also helps activate phosphorylase b kinase.)
5. Phosphorylation and activation of glycogen phosphorylase by phosphorylase b kinase activates glycogen breakdown.

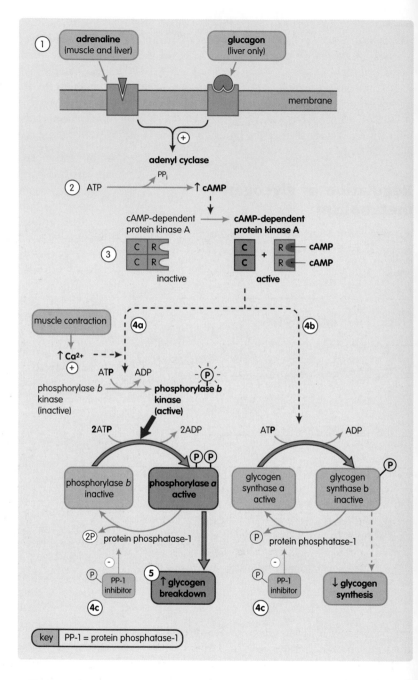

Glycogen storage diseases

This group of inherited diseases is caused by a defect in an enzyme required for either glycogen synthesis or degradation; they are very rare. They are all inherited as autosomal recessive disorders, except for type VIII, which is sex-linked. These diseases either result in the production of an abnormal amount or an abnormal type of glycogen. The main glycogen storage diseases are summarized in Fig. 2.36.

Type I: von Gierke's disease

von Gierke's disease affects mainly the liver and the kidneys. It is caused by a deficiency of glucose-6-phosphatase, the gluconeogenic enzyme that

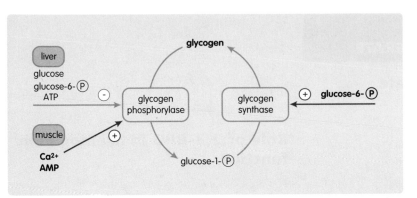

Fig. 2.35 Allosteric control of glycogen metabolosm by glucose, glucose-6-phosphate, calcium ions, AMP and ATP.

Fig. 2.36 The main glycogen storage diseases. They either result in the production of an abnormal amount or an abnormal type of glycogen

Type	Name	Enzyme deficiency	Glycogen structure and amount	Tissues affected
I	von Gierke's disease	Glucose-6-phosphatase	Normal structure, ↑ amount	Liver and kidney are loaded with glycogen; results in hypoglycaemia since glucose cannot leave the liver
II	Pompe's disease	Lysosomal α-1,4-glucosidase	Normal structure, ↑↑↑ amount	Accumulation of glycogen in lysosomes in all organs; prominent cardiomyopathy
III	Cori's disease	Amylo-1,6-glucosidase (debranching enzyme)	Outer chains missing or very short, ↑ amount	Accumulation of branched polysaccharide in liver and muscle; like type I but milder
IV	Andersen's disease	Branching enzyme	Very long unbranched chains, normal amount	Liver failure causes death in the first year of life
V	McArdle's disease	Glycogen phosphorylase	Normal structure, ↑ amount	Muscle has abnormally high glycogen content (2.5–4.1%); diminished exercise tolerance
VI	Hers' disease	Glycogen phosphorylase	Normal structure, ↑ amount	↑ liver glycogen; tendency towards hypoglycaemia
VII	Tarul's disease	Phosphofructokinase	Normal structure, ↑ amount	Muscle as for type V

catalyses the hydrolysis of glucose-6-phosphate in the liver, releasing free glucose into the blood.

The deficiency leads to an increased concentration of glucose-6-phosphate in the liver and kidneys, which in turn results in an increased amount of normal glycogen stored. It also means that the liver is unable to release glucose between meals to regulate and maintain the blood glucose in response to glucagon, leading to a fasting hypoglycaemia.

The main clinical features are: liver enlargement, fasting hypoglycaemia, failure to thrive and raised levels of lactate, ketone bodies, lipid and urate as the body tries to use other fuels.

Type V: McArdle's syndrome

McArdle's syndrome is caused by a deficiency of muscle glycogen phosphorylase; the liver enzyme is normal. The muscle has a high level of glycogen because it cannot break it down. During exercise, the decreased level of muscle phosphorylase means that glycogen stores cannot be used as fuel. The usual increase in blood lactate is not seen after exercise because of insufficient glycolysis. These patients have a decreased exercise tolerance: they tire easily on intense exercise. Otherwise, they have a normal life span and development.

ROLE OF 2,3-BISPHOSPHOGLYCERATE

The bisphosphoglycerate (2,3-BPG) shunt

Location

In erythrocytes.

Pathway

There are two steps in the shunt (Fig. 2.37):

1. Bisphosphoglycerate mutase converts 1,3-BPG into 2,3-BPG.
2. 2,3-bisphosphoglycerate phosphatase hydrolyses 2,3-BPG to 3-phosphoglycerate.

ATP yield

Glycolysis is important to erythrocytes because it is their only energy source (they have no mitochondria and must rely on anaerobic glycolysis). However, the shunt bypasses the energy-generating reaction, meaning there is effectively no net production of ATP.

Regulation of the shunt

Both reactions of the shunt are nearly irreversible. 3-phosphoglycerate stimulates bisphosphoglycerate mutase, thus increasing 2,3-BPG production. 2,3-BPG is a potent inhibitor of its own formation (i.e. negative feedback by the product).

Role of 2,3-BPG in haemoglobin function

Haemoglobin (Hb) is the oxygen-carrying protein found in erythrocytes. It has a high affinity for binding oxygen and transports oxygen from the lungs to the tissues where it is needed. When Hb gets to the tissues, it has to release or 'unload' the oxygen. A low pH (acid; high hydrogen ion concentration) or an increased CO_2 concentration in the tissue favours unloading, as both decrease the affinity of haemoglobin for oxygen; this is known as the Bohr effect.

2,3-BPG present in high concentration in erythrocytes also helps unload oxygen from haemoglobin. Specifically, it is an allosteric effector that

Fig. 2.37 The bisphosphoglycerate shunt in erythrocytes produces 2,3-bisphosphoglycerate (2,3-BPG) with no net energy production.

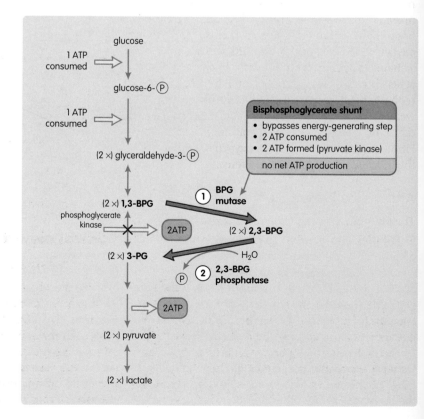

binds to and stabilizes deoxyhaemoglobin, reducing its affinity for oxygen, therefore favouring the release of oxygen (Fig. 2.38). 2,3-BPG fits in a 'pocket' between the two β chains of haemoglobin, but only in the deoxygenated configuration. This pocket contains positively charged amino acids that form salt bridges with the negatively charged phosphate groups of 2,3-BPG, resulting in cross-linking of the β chains. 2,3-BPG cannot bind to oxyhaemoglobin as the gap between the β chains is too small in the presence of oxygen. The reaction may be written as follows:

$$HbO_2 + 2,3\text{-}BPG \rightarrow Hb\text{-}2,3\text{-}BPG + O_2$$
Oxyhaemoglobin   Deoxyhaemoglobin

The oxygen is therefore released for use by the tissues.

Main physiological effects of 2,3-BPG

Fetal haemoglobin

Fetal haemoglobin (HbF) contains two α chains and two γ chains ($\alpha_2\gamma_2$) and is the major type of haemoglobin found in the fetus and in the newborn. HbF has a lower affinity for 2,3-BPG than normal adult haemoglobin (HbA) and therefore it has a higher affinity for oxygen (i.e. holds on to its oxygen). HbF only binds 2,3-BPG weakly as its two γ chains lack some of the positively charged amino acids found in the β chains of HbA. As 2,3-BPG reduces the affinity of haemoglobin for oxygen, the weak interaction between HbF and 2,3-BPG means that HbF has a higher oxygen affinity than normal HbA. This facilitates placental oxygen exchange from the mother's circulation to the fetus.

Altitude acclimatization

The body responds to the chronic hypoxia observed at high altitude by increasing the concentration of

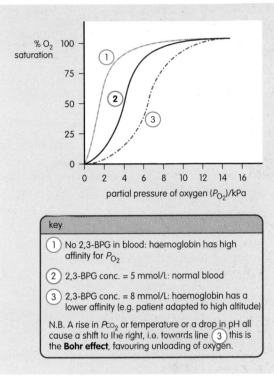

Fig. 2.38 The effect of 2,3-BPG on haemoglobin is to decrease its affinity for oxygen, causing a shift to the right in the oxygen saturation curve.

2,3-BPG in erythrocytes. This adaptation takes a few days. High levels of 2,3-BPG decrease the affinity of haemoglobin for oxygen, allowing greater unloading of oxygen to the tissues so that they receive enough oxygen despite its decreased availability. On return to low altitude, the concentration of 2,3-BPG, which has a half-life of about 6 hours, returns to normal quite quickly. Similarly, high concentrations of 2,3-BPG are observed in patients with chronic obstructive airways disease (COAD).

Clinical significance of 2,3-BPG

Blood transfusions

Storing blood in an acid–citrate–glucose medium leads to a decrease in the concentration of 2,3-BPG to low levels in about 1–2 weeks. The resulting blood has an abnormally high affinity for oxygen and, if given to a patient, it will not be able to unload oxygen to the tissues. The loss of 2,3-BPG can now be prevented by addition of substrates, e.g. inosine, to the storage medium. Inosine enters the erythrocytes

It is useful to be able to draw the oxygen dissociation curve and relate the effect of binding 2,3-BPG: it shifts the sigmoidal binding curve to the right (see Fig. 2.38).

where it can be metabolized to 2,3-BPG by the pentose phosphate pathway (see Chapter 3).

Red cell glycolytic enzyme deficiencies

This group of inherited diseases occurs due to the deficiency of a glycolytic enzyme (e.g. hexokinase, phosphofructokinase, pyruvate kinase). The effect on both glycolysis and the concentration of 2,3-BPG depends on the site of the enzyme deficiency, i.e. either before or after the 2,3-BPG shunt, or a deficiency of one of the shunt enzymes. An abnormal concentration of 2,3-BPG affects the ability of the haemoglobin to transport and unload oxygen normally.

Causes of a raised concentration of 2,3-BPG

The main causes are:

- Long-term smoking, which is known to cause an increase in the concentration of 2,3-BPG. This partly compensates for a decreased oxygen supply caused by the exposure to carbon monoxide.

- Chronic anaemia, which results in a decrease in the number of erythrocytes or the amount of haemoglobin, leading to decreased oxygen supply to the tissues. A compensatory increase in 2,3-BPG allows for greater unloading of oxygen to the tissues.
- Altitude acclimatization (see above).

FRUCTOSE, GALACTOSE, ETHANOL AND SORBITOL

Fructose metabolism

The main dietary source of fructose is the disaccharide sucrose, which is hydrolysed by sucrase in the small intestine to fructose and glucose; fructose is also found in fruit and honey. Unlike glucose, fructose can enter cells without the help of insulin by using the (confusingly named) glucose transporter GLUT-5. There are two pathways for fructose metabolism, one in muscle, the other in liver, due to the presence of different enzymes in each tissue (see Fig. 2.39).

Fig. 2.39 The metabolism of fructose by liver and muscle cells leads to the production of intermediates that can then enter glycolysis.

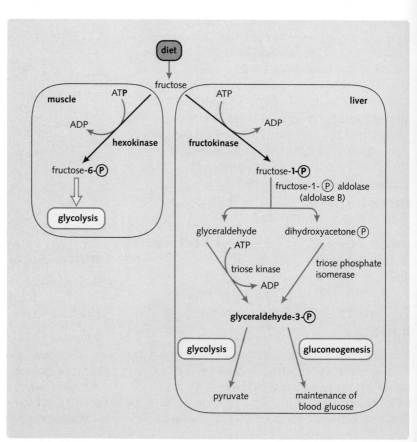

- In the liver, fructose is phosphorylated by the enzyme fructokinase to fructose-1-phosphate, which is then further metabolized to glyceraldehyde-3-phosphate to enter glycolysis or gluconeogenesis. Most dietary fructose is metabolized by the liver, such that little is left for metabolism by the muscle.
- In muscle, fructose is converted to fructose-6-phosphate by hexokinase to enter glycolysis after only one reaction.

Risks of excessive fructose ingestion

Fructose is metabolized rapidly compared with glucose. Intravenous fructose was once recommended for use in parenteral nutrition but no longer due to the following :

- The entry of fructose into the muscle uses GLUT-5, which is independent of insulin.
- Intravenous feeding with fructose depletes the cellular stores of phosphate thus lowering ATP concentration. Phosphofructokinase is disinhibited in muscle, and uncontrolled glycolysis from fructose 6-phosphate occurs, with lactic acid production.
- In the liver, fructose enters glycolysis as glyceraldehyde-3-phosphate or dihydroxyacetone phosphate, thus avoiding the rate-limiting step catalysed by phosphofructokinase, the key control point of glycolysis (see Fig. 2.2). Rapid infusion of fructose may cause a massive unregulated flux of glycolysis metabolites, leading to the production of large quantities of lactic acid and precipitating fatal lactic acidosis.

Errors of fructose metabolism

Errors of fructose metabolism are genetic (autosomal recessive) disorders that are due to a deficiency in one of the key enzymes involved in fructose metabolism; they are shown in Fig. 2.40.

Fructokinase deficiency: essential fructosuria

This is a benign, asymptomatic condition caused by an absence of fructokinase. Fructose is only metabolized by the hexokinase pathway, resulting in its much slower metabolism. This leads to a high concentration of fructose in the blood and urine.

Fructose-1-phosphate aldolase deficiency: hereditary fructose intolerance

Fructose-1-phosphate aldolase (aldolase B) cleaves fructose-1-phosphate to dihydroxyacetone phosphate and glyceraldehyde, allowing the entry of fructose into glycolysis or gluconeogenesis (see Fig. 2.40). Deficiency leads to the accumulation of fructose-1-phosphate and sequestration of intracellular phosphate in the tissues. This leads to the inhibition of both glycogen phosphorylase (glycogenolysis) and aldolase A (glycolysis and gluconeogenesis) because they are normally activated by phosphorylation. This causes the inhibition of glucose production, leading to hypoglycaemia.

Clinically, fructose-1-phosphate aldolase deficiency presents as soon as a baby is weaned on to fructose-containing foods. Features include hypoglycaemia, vomiting and eventually liver failure. Treatment is by the removal of fructose and sucrose from the diet.

Galactose metabolism

The major dietary source of galactose is lactose in milk and milk products. Lactose is hydrolysed by intestinal lactase into galactose and glucose. The entry of galactose into cells is independent of insulin.

Metabolism of galactose

The metabolism of galactose has four steps (Fig. 2.41):

1. Phosphorylation to galactose-1-phosphate by galactokinase.
2. Galactose-1-phosphate uridyl transferase catalyses the transfer of the uridyl group of UDP-glucose to galactose-1-phosphate to make UDP-galactose and glucose-1-phosphate.
3. Glucose-1-phosphate can be converted to the glycolytic intermediate glucose-6-phosphate and thus enter glycolysis.
4. UDP-galactose is converted back to UDP-glucose by UDP-hexose-4-epimerase.

Galactosaemia—an error of galactose metabolism

Galactosaemia is a rare, autosomal recessive disorder arising because of a deficiency in the enzyme galactose-1-phosphate uridyl transferase (see Fig. 2.41). Occasionally, it is caused by deficiency in galactokinase or UDP-hexose-4-epimerase. The

Fig. 2.40 Some errors of fructose metabolism.

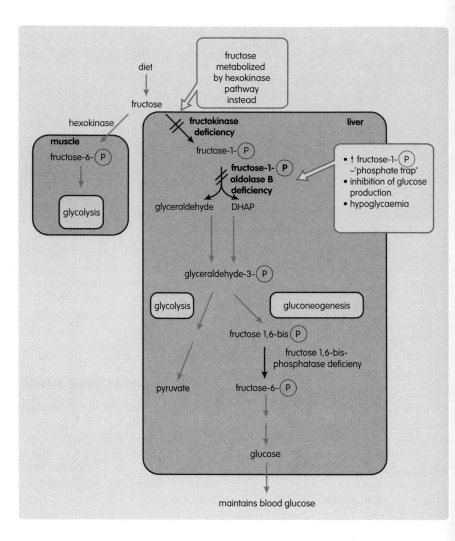

formation of UDP-galactose is prevented, meaning that galactose cannot be converted into glucose-6-phosphate.

The disease presents in neonates when lactose-containing milk feeds are introduced. As galactose cannot be converted into glucose, the babies become hypoglycaemic. This results in galactosaemia, galactosuria, and a build-up of toxic metabolic by-products. This can lead to a high concentration of galactose in the lens of the eye, where it is reduced by aldose reductase to galactitol, which is thought to facilitate cataract formation. An accumulation of galactitol also occurs in nerve tissue, liver and kidneys, leading to liver damage and mental retardation.

The clinical features are poor feeding, vomiting, jaundice, hypoglycaemia and hepatosplenomegaly.

Eventually, liver failure, cataracts and severe mental retardation occur if the condition is left untreated. The treatment is a lactose- and galactose-free diet.

Catabolism of ethanol

In the liver, three enzyme systems exist for the catabolism of ethanol (Fig. 2.42):

1. Cytosolic alcohol dehydrogenase pathway, probably the main route for the oxidation of ethanol. The activity of this enzyme is largely governed by the availability of NAD^+, which is required as a cofactor.
2. Microsomal ethanol oxidizing system (MEOS), which uses a cytochrome P450 enzyme system.
3. Peroxisomal oxidation of ethanol, which uses hydrogen peroxidase to oxidize ethanol.

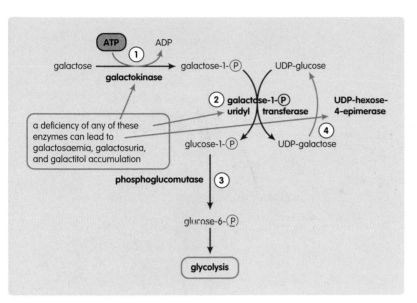

Fig. 2.41 The metabolism of galactose; a four-step pathway that converts galactose to glucose-6-phosphate. Glucose-6-phosphate then enters glycolysis. (Numbers refer to text.)

The product of all three systems is acetaldehyde, which then enters mitochondria for further oxidation by aldehyde dehydrogenase to acetate. Certain ethnic groups, in particular the Chinese, are genetically deficient in aldehyde dehydrogenase and consequently have a lower alcohol tolerance.

Metabolic effects of ethanol

The fate of acetate depends on the ratio of NADH to NAD^+. Both alcohol dehydrogenase and aldehyde dehydrogenase consume NAD^+, contributing to a high NADH:NAD^+ ratio resulting in:

- Inhibition of the TCA cycle. A high NADH:NAD^+ ratio prevents the oxidation of isocitrate to α-ketoglutarate, of α-ketoglutarate to succinyl CoA, and of malate to oxaloacetate (see Fig. 2.22).
- Inhibition of gluconeogenesis. A high NADH:NAD^+ ratio affects the dehydrogenase reactions, displacing the equilibrium in favour of the reduced compounds such that oxaloacetate is converted to malate and pyruvate to lactate (see Fig. 5.19). Therefore, less pyruvate and oxaloacetate (substrates) are available for gluconeogenesis by the liver.

Although acetate could, theoretically, be activated to acetyl CoA for oxidation by the TCA cycle, it is more likely that it is exported out of the liver for metabolism by other tissues.

The drug disulfiram (Antabuse) is used to discourage alcoholics from drinking. It inhibits aldehyde dehydrogenase, resulting in the accumulation of acetaldehyde if ethanol is consumed. This causes unpleasant effects such as nausea and flushing, which helps deter drinking.

Clinical significance of excessive ethanol ingestion

High levels of alcohol can lead to hyperlactataemia (i.e. because of the favoured conversion of pyruvate to lactate, see above). Since both lactate and urate share the same mechanism for renal tubular secretion, the more lactate produced the more urate will be retained. Urate may crystallize out in the joints, especially in the toes, leading to gout.

Hypoglycaemia can develop in malnourished or fasting individuals after a heavy drinking session. The inhibition of gluconeogenesis leads to this hypoglycaemia; medical students beware!

Alcohol can induce the cytochrome P450 enzymes that are responsible for the metabolism of many drugs, for example, barbiturates. Therefore, for an alcoholic patient on medication, the metabolism and effects of the drugs may be altered.

Fig. 2.42 The metabolism of ethanol. Three enzyme systems are responsible for the metabolism of ethanol in the liver: cytosolic alcohol dehydrogenase (main mechanism), microsomal ethanol oxidizing system (MEOS) in the smooth endoplasmic reticulum, and catalase in peroxisomes. The product, acetaldehyde, is then taken into the mitochondria for further metabolism to acetate. (Numbers refer to text.)

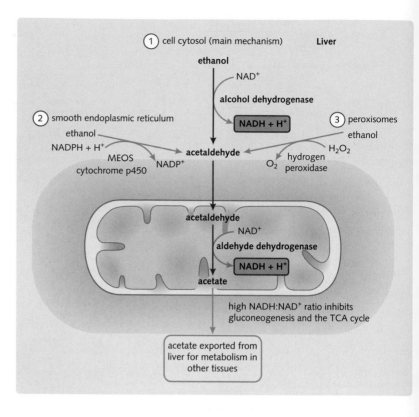

Sorbitol metabolism (polyol pathway)

Synthesis

Sorbitol is a sugar alcohol that can be synthesized endogenously from glucose by a number of tissues, such as the lens and retina of the eye, the liver, kidney and Schwann cells (the cells of the peripheral nervous system that make myelin).

Sorbitol synthesis requires the enzyme aldose reductase which reduces glucose to sorbitol.

Breakdown

Some tissues, especially the liver, contain sorbitol dehydrogenase, which oxidizes sorbitol to fructose (Fig. 2.43).

In the liver, this provides a way for dietary sorbitol to enter glycolysis or gluconeogenesis and be metabolized further (see Fig. 2.39).

This is also a useful pathway in sperm and in the seminal vesicles, where fructose is the preferred energy source.

Uses and complications of increased sorbitol

Sorbitol is used as a food sweetener in diabetic diets. It has about one-half the sweetness of sucrose but, more importantly, it is safe because it is absorbed slowly from the intestine and also transported slowly across cell membranes. Therefore at normal levels there is little chance of it accumulating.

Problems arise when the endogenous production of sorbitol increases. Since sorbitol does not cross cell membranes easily, it may remain trapped in the cells. Aldose reductase has a high K_m for glucose (about 60–70 mM). At normal blood glucose levels (3–5 mM), its activity is low, and the production of sorbitol is low. However, in poorly controlled diabetes, where blood glucose concentrations can reach sustained levels as high as 15–20 mM, there is an increased production of sorbitol, which may accumulate within cells. This causes the greatest problems in tissues that lack sorbitol dehydrogenase to break down the sorbitol. For example:

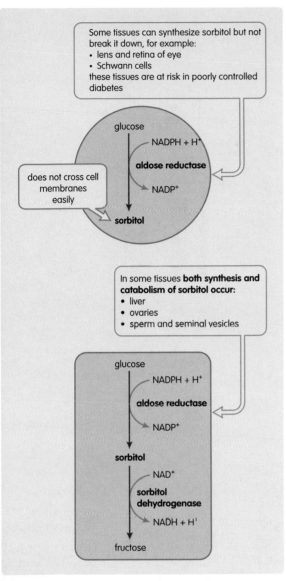

- In the lens and retina of the eye the increased sorbitol exerts a strong osmotic effect, causing water retention; the lens swells and becomes opaque, leading to cataract formation.
- In Schwann cells, the increased levels of sorbitol disrupt cell structure and function, causing demyelination of nerves and peripheral neuropathy.

Fig. 2.43 The metabolism of sorbitol from glucose by aldose reductase. Some tissues contain sorbitol dehydrogenase, which oxidizes sorbitol to fructose.

Production of NADPH

3

Objectives

You should be able to:

- Discuss the main functions of the pentose phosphate pathway.
- Understand the importance of the pyruvate–malate cycle.
- Describe the source and importance of NADPH.

PENTOSE PHOSPHATE PATHWAY AND PYRUVATE–MALATE CYCLE

Pentose phosphate pathway

The pentose phosphate pathway (PPP), also known as the hexose monophosphate shunt or the phosphogluconate pathway, provides an alternative route for the metabolism of glucose. Most of the pathways that have already been discussed are concerned with the generation of ATP. However, in the pentose phosphate pathway, no ATP is directly consumed or produced; instead, the pathway is important for the production of 'reducing power' in the form of NADPH.

Location
Mainly the liver, lactating mammary glands, adipose tissue, adrenal cortex and erythrocytes.

Site
Cell cytosol.

Main functions
The main functions of the pentose phosphate pathway are:

- Generation of NADPH necessary for reductive biosynthetic reactions; for example, biosynthesis of fatty acid and cholesterol.
- Production of ribose 5-phosphate (five-carbon sugar units) for biosynthesis of purines, pyrimidines, nucleotides and nucleic acids.
- In erythrocytes, NADPH is used to regenerate the antioxidant reduced glutathione, which protects the cells against damage from reactive oxygen intermediates.

Pathway

The pathway has two stages:

- An irreversible oxidative phase (Fig. 3.1), which consists of three irreversible reactions, resulting in the formation of ribulose-5-phosphate, CO_2 and two molecules of NADPH per molecule of glucose-6-phosphate oxidized.
- A reversible non-oxidative phase (Fig. 3.2) that consists of a series of five, reversible sugar phosphate interconversions, where ribulose-5-phosphate is converted either to ribose-5-phosphate for nucleotide synthesis or to intermediates of glycolysis such as glyceraldehyde-3-phosphate or fructose-6-phosphate. The pathway is therefore linked with the needs of glycolysis.

It is not necessary to know the names of all the intermediates of the reversible phase; just be aware that it involves the interconversion of three-, four-, five- and seven- carbon sugars, as shown in steps 1 to 5 in Fig. 3.2.

Fate of fructose-6-phosphate

The fate of fructose-6-phosphate formed in the pentose phosphate pathway depends on the specific needs of the tissue.

In the well-fed state in the liver and adipose tissue, glucose is phosphorylated to glucose-6-phosphate, which enters the pentose phosphate pathway to form fructose-6-phosphate. Accumulation of fructose-6-phosphate allosterically activates the rate-limiting enzyme of glycolysis, phosphofructokinase, and glycolysis results in increased formation of pyruvate.

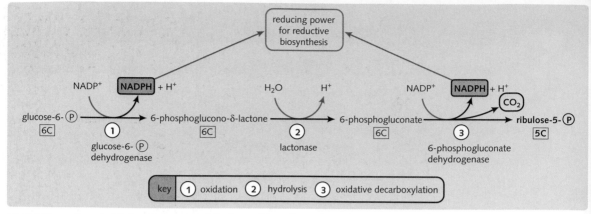

Fig. 3.1 The pentose phosphate pathway: phase I, the irreversible oxidative phase. Three irreversible reactions result in the production of two molecules of NADPH.

This is oxidatively decarboxylated to acetyl CoA, which can be used for fatty acid synthesis.

In erythrocytes, fructose-6-phosphate has a different fate. It is converted back to glucose-6-phosphate by the enzyme phosphoglucose isomerase to re-enter the pentose phosphate pathway, therefore creating a cycle and thus a continual supply of substrate for the pentose phosphate pathway. This allows the continued production of NADPH required for the regeneration of the antioxidant reduced glutathione to protect erythrocytes.

Control of the pentose phosphate pathway

The main control of the pathway is exerted at the first step; the irreversible glucose-6-phosphate dehydrogenase reaction. The controlling factor is the ratio of NADPH to NADP$^+$. As the cell uses up NADPH (e.g. during fatty acid synthesis) the concentration of NADP$^+$ increases, which activates the pentose phosphate pathway to increase NADPH formation. Therefore, the pentose phosphate pathway is activated by a low NADPH:NADP$^+$.

Control of the non-oxidative phase is by the requirement for products, namely ribose-5-phosphate and NADPH (see Fig. 3.2). The individual needs of the cell determine whether production of ribose-5-phosphate, or fructose-6-phosphate and glyceraldehyde-3-phosphate predominates. For example:

- If the NADPH requirement is greater than the ribose-5-phosphate requirement, for example in cells that take part in a lot of reductive synthetic reactions, all the ribose-5-phosphate formed is

converted to fructose-6-phosphate and glyceraldehyde-3-phosphate. These are converted back to glucose-6-phosphate to re-enter the pentose phosphate pathway and therefore generate more NADPH.

- If the ribose-5-phosphate requirement is greater than the need for NADPH, for example, in cells with a high rate of nucleic acid formation, fructose-6-phosphate and glyceraldehyde-3-phosphate are converted to ribose-5-phosphate by further sugar interconversions.

Pyruvate–malate cycle

The pyruvate–malate cycle (Fig. 3.3) has two functions:

- The production of NADPH in the reaction catalysed by the malic (malate dehydrogenase-decarboxylating) enzyme.
- The transport of acetyl CoA units from the mitochondria to the cytosol for fatty acid synthesis.

Fatty acid synthesis occurs in the cytosol. However, the carbon source, namely acetyl CoA, is produced by pyruvate dehydrogenase in the mitochondria. Thus, transport of acetyl CoA from the mitochondria into the cytosol requires the pyruvate–malate cycle (discussed further in chapter 4).

Sources of NADPH for fatty acid synthesis

The source of NADPH for fatty acid synthesis is the pentose phosphate pathway and the pyruvate–malate cycle.

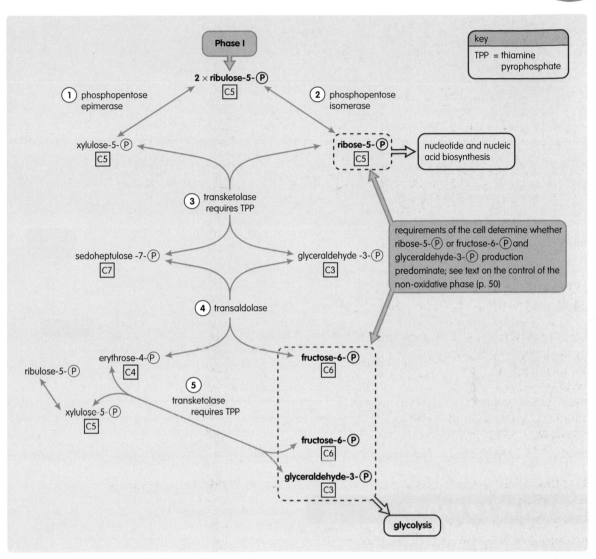

Fig. 3.2 The pentose phosphate pathway: phase II, the reversible non-oxidative phase.

The pentose phosphate pathway produces two molecules of NADPH for each molecule of glucose entering the pathway and contributes about 60% of the NADPH needed for fatty acid synthesis.

The pyruvate–malate cycle produces one molecule of NADPH for each acetyl CoA molecule transferred from the mitochondria to the cytosol and contributes about 40% of the NADPH needed.

The pyruvate–malate cycle shows an inter-relationship between glucose metabolism and fatty acid synthesis. When the need for ATP is low, the oxidation of acetyl CoA by the TCA cycle is minimal, thus providing acetyl CoA for fatty acid synthesis. Remember that these pathways are not all active at the same time.

Fig. 3.3 The pyruvate–malate cycle operates between the cell cytosol and mitochondria. The reaction sequence is as follows:

1. Oxaloacetate and acetyl CoA condense to form citrate, which leaves the mitochondria via the tricarboxylate carrier.
2. Citrate is cleaved in the cytosol by citrate lyase back to oxaloacetate and acetyl CoA.
3. Acetyl CoA can be used for fatty acid synthesis whereas oxaloacetate is reduced to malate.
4. Malate is oxidatively decarboxylated by the malic enzyme, re-forming pyruvate.
5. The reaction produces a significant amount of NADPH, which is used mainly for fatty acid synthesis.
6. Pyruvate is transported back into the mitochondria via a pyruvate carrier, where some of it is carboxylated to oxaloacetate and some converted to acetyl CoA.

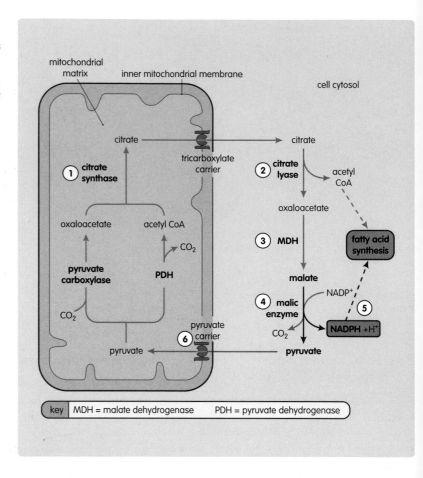

THE ROLES OF NADPH

NADPH in lipid biosynthesis

NADPH, like NADH, is a high-energy molecule, but its electrons, instead of being transferred to oxygen via the electron transport chain, are used for reductive biosyntheses, particularly for lipid synthesis. Each cycle of fatty acid synthesis, in which the growing fatty acid chain is lengthened by two carbon atoms, employs two reductions, each requiring NADPH as cofactor. Deficiency of NADPH leads to inhibition of fatty acid synthesis (see Chapter 4).

NADPH in the production of glutathione

Glutathione is a tripeptide formed from three amino acids; glutamate, cysteine and glycine. It exists in two forms: an active, reduced form and an inactive, oxidized form (Fig. 3.4). Reduced glutathione contains a reactive thiol group (–SH) on the cysteine residue, which can reduce hydrogen peroxide (H_2O_2) and other reactive oxygen intermediates (free radicals), hence detoxifying them. Thus, glutathione is an antioxidant which protects cells from damage.

Action of free radicals

Reactive oxygen intermediates are formed from molecular oxygen in most cells, as either by-products of aerobic metabolism or from exogenous sources; for example, smoking, radiation and the side effects of drugs and chemicals. They are highly reactive and attack cell components such as proteins, DNA and polyunsaturated fatty acids in cell membranes, resulting in disruption of membrane structure and cell integrity. Free radicals are thought to be partly responsible for the cell damage associated with inflammation, ageing and certain cancers. They are detoxified by two main mechanisms, which are outlined below.

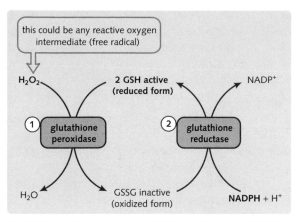

Fig. 3.4 The antioxidant action of glutathione. Glutathione (GSH) is an antioxidant. It reduces hydrogen peroxide and other reactive oxygen intermediates, inactivating them. In doing so it undergoes oxidation to its inactive, oxidized form (GSSG). NADPH is required for the regeneration of the active reduced form of glutathione by glutathione reductase, enabling it to continue its role as an antioxidant.

Superoxide dismutase exists in two forms: a copper- and zinc-containing cytoplasmic form and a manganese-containing mitochondrial form.

Non-enzymatic inactivation: dietary antioxidants
Vitamins A, C and E are antioxidants (see Chapter 8). However, there is no substantial evidence available to support the theory that increased dietary intake of these vitamins alone reduces the incidence of heart disease or cancer.

NADPH in the prevention of oxidation of haemoglobin

The oxidation of the iron (Fe^{2+}; ferrous form) in haemoglobin by H_2O_2 or other free radicals, yields methaemoglobin (Fe^{3+}; ferric form), which cannot transport oxygen effectively. Methaemoglobin is usually only present at low concentrations because erythrocytes possess an efficient enzyme system, NADH-dependent cytochrome b_5 reductase (methaemoglobin reductase), which catalyses the reduction of methaemoglobin to haemoglobin (Fig. 3.5).

Enzyme inactivation
Several enzymes are responsible for the inactivation of free radicals:

- Glutathione peroxidase (a selenium-containing enzyme) removes hydrogen peroxide (Fig. 3.4).
- Catalase (an iron-containing enzyme) removes hydrogen peroxide:
  $H_2O_2 \rightarrow H_2O + \frac{1}{2}O_2$.
- Superoxide dismutase detoxifies the superoxide radical ($O_2^{\bullet-}$):
  $2O_2^{\bullet-} + 2H^+ \rightarrow H_2O_2 + O_2$.

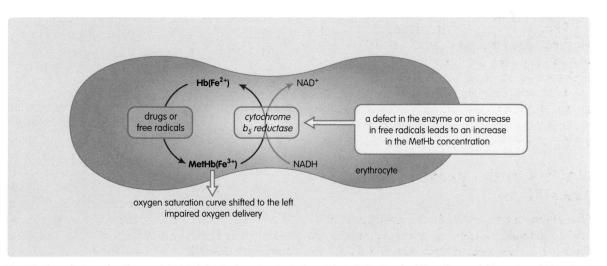

Fig. 3.5 The reduction of methaemoglobin. A defect in the enzyme cytochrome b_5 reductase can lead to methaemoglobinaemia and cyanosis.

The generation of excessive amount of free radicals and the action of certain drugs or toxins can result in the increased formation of methaemoglobin. In this scenario, the cytochrome b_5 reductase system cannot cope and the concentration of methaemoglobin in the blood rises, leading to methaemoglobinaemia. As methaemoglobin cannot transport oxygen effectively, this results in poor perfusion of tissues and cyanosis.

If adequate amounts of NADPH are present, the glutathione in erythrocytes can remove the excess free radicals and drugs, thus preventing oxidation of haemoglobin.

Newborn babies have only low concentrations of cytochrome b_5 reductase and are therefore susceptible to methaemoglobinaemia.

NADPH in drug metabolism

A continual supply of reduced glutathione is required in the liver for the conjugation and detoxification of certain drugs and steroid hormones, thus preventing accumulation and toxicity. NADPH is necessary to maintain a continuous supply of reduced glutathione, as already described.

Glucose-6-phosphate dehydrogenase deficiency

Glucose-6-phosphate dehydrogenase (G6PDH) controls the rate-limiting step of the pentose phosphate pathway (see Fig. 3.1). Although G6PDH deficiency is an uncommon cause of anaemia in the UK, it affects 130 million people worldwide, particularly in Africa, the Mediterranean and South-East Asia. The inheritance of G6PDH deficiency is sex-linked, affecting males and being carried by females. Carriers have about half the normal G6PDH activity, but have some degree of protection against *Plasmodium falciparum*, which causes malaria, giving carriers an evolutionary advantage. Over 400 different mutations have been identified in the gene coding for G6PDH, but only certain variants cause haemolytic anaemia.

Pathogenesis

A decrease in G6PDH activity leads to decreased NADPH formation and therefore decreased production of reduced glutathione (Fig. 3.6), with erythrocytes being very susceptible to oxidative damage.

The precipitating factors that cause oxidative stress and haemolysis are:

- Drugs: antibiotics (sulfamethoxazole), antimalarials (quinine, primaquine) and antipyretics (aspirin).
- Infection is the most common precipitating factor.
- Favism. Consumption of fava beans (broad beans) leads to haemolysis.
- Neonatal jaundice.

Treatment is to avoid precipitants and, in severe cases, consider a blood transfusion.

In an acute haemolysis due to G6PDH deficiency, the erythrocytes contain precipitates of oxidized denatured Hb (Heinz bodies) which attach to their cell membrane. These erythrocytes are recognized as abnormal by the spleen, resulting in the reticuloendothelial cells removing the precipitated Hb from the membrane. This results in the formation of microspherocytes and erythrocytes containing a membrane bleb or indentation (bite cells), which are the classic morphology seen in a blood smear.

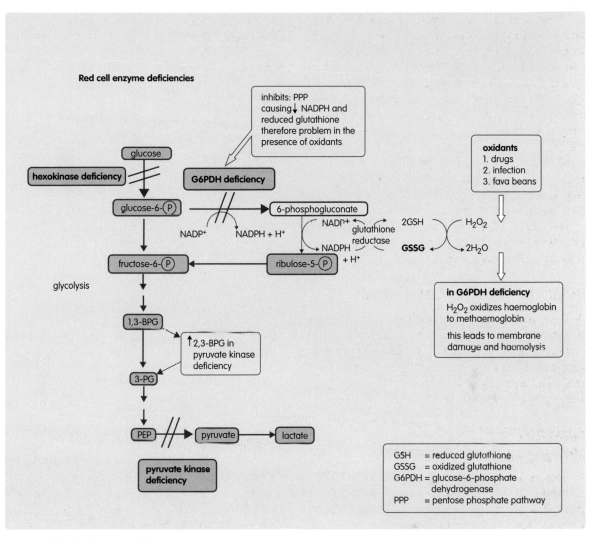

Fig 3.6 Red blood cell enzyme deficiencies.

Fatty acid metabolism and lipid transport

4

Objectives

You should be able to:

- Describe the process and regulation of fatty acid biosynthesis.
- Describe the process and regulation of lipid breakdown.
- Understand the importance of cholesterol in the body.
- Describe the pathways of lipid transport in blood.
- Discuss the roles of ketone bodies and its synthesis.

LIPID BIOSYNTHESIS

Fatty acids

Fatty acids are an essential fuel and major energy source. A lot of the fat used by the body comes from the diet, from either animal sources or plant sources. Fats obtained from animal sources include:

- tallow (beef fat).
- ghee (butter fat).
- lard (pork fat).
- chicken fat.
- blubber.
- fish oil (e.g cod liver oil).

Fat extracted from plant sources are known as vegetable oil. Common sources of vegetable oil include:

- sunflower.
- sesame seed.
- peanut.
- palm oil.
- walnut.

However, a number of tissues can also synthesize fatty acids *de novo* from acetyl CoA.

Fatty acid biosynthesis

Working definition

Fatty acid synthesis consists of a cyclical series of reactions in which a molecule of fatty acid is built from the sequential addition of two carbon units derived from acetyl CoA, to a growing fatty acid chain.

Fatty acid synthesis is not a reversal of the degradative pathway (known as β oxidation).

Location

Mainly in the liver, adipose tissue and lactating mammary glands; there is a small amount in the kidney.

Site

Cell cytosol.

Fig. 4.1 shows an overview of fatty acid biosynthesis and the main steps involved in the formation of the most common saturated fatty acid, palmitic acid. Construction of this 16-carbon fatty acid begins with the formation of acetyl CoA in the mitochondria. It is transported into the cell cytosol where it is carboxylated to malonyl CoA. It then undergoes a sequence of reactions catalysed by fatty acid synthase. It would be a good idea to have a look at this diagram now, before reading on.

NADPH necessary for fatty acid synthesis is generated by the pentose phosphate pathway and the pyruvate–malate cycle (about 60% from the pentose phosphate pathway and 40% via the malic enzyme; see Chapter 3). The steps of fatty acid synthesis are now considered in more detail.

Production of acetyl CoA

Pyruvate dehydrogenase (PDH) catalyses the irreversible, oxidative decarboxylation of pyruvate to acetyl CoA in the mitochondrial matrix (Fig. 4.2). Details of this reaction are covered in Chapter 2.

Fig. 4.1 An overview of fatty acid biosynthesis. The steps involved in the formation of palmitate:

1. Formation of the precursor, acetyl CoA from pyruvate in mitochondria.
2. Transport of acetyl CoA into the cytosol. Acetyl CoA combines with oxaloacetate to form citrate (citrate shuttle).
3. Carboxylation of acetyl CoA to malonyl CoA by acetyl CoA carboxylase.
4. Initiation of the synthesis of a new fatty acid molecule requires both acetyl CoA and malonyl CoA. They attach to the enzyme, fatty acid synthase, and condense to form acetoacetyl-ACP. This then undergoes a characteristic sequence of reactions catalysed by fatty acid synthase to make a four-carbon saturated fatty acid.
5. Fatty acid synthase also catalyses the sequential addition of a series of further two carbon units from malonyl CoA to the growing fatty acid chain.
6. Elongation by fatty acid synthase stops on formation of palmitate (C16).
7. Further elongation and insertion of double bonds are carried out by other enzymes.

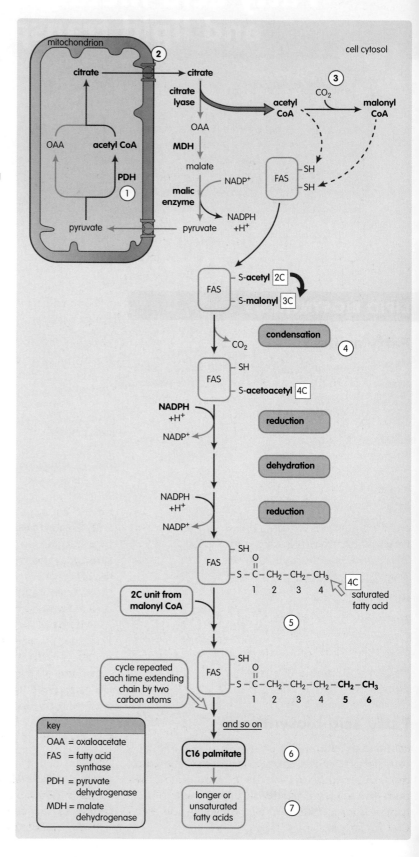

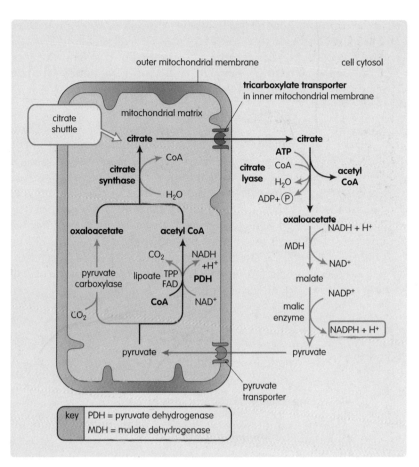

Fig. 4.2 Production of acetyl CoA and its transport by the citrate shuttle.

Acetyl CoA is also produced by the degradation of fatty acids, ketone bodies or amino acids.

Transport of acetyl CoA from mitochondria to the cytosol

The same pathway, namely the pyruvate–malate cycle, that produces NADPH for fatty acid synthesis also transports acetyl CoA from the mitochondria to the cell cytosol (see Fig. 4.2). The part of the cycle that transports acetyl CoA is called the citrate shuttle. Acetyl CoA is produced in the mitochondria but fatty acid synthesis occurs in the cytosol. The CoA portion of the acetyl CoA molecule cannot cross the mitochondrial membrane. Acetyl CoA condenses with oxaloacetate to form citrate, so that the acetyl group can be carried across by the tricarboxylate transporter. In the cytosol, citrate is cleaved by citrate lyase to release oxaloacetate for recycling and acetyl CoA for fatty acid synthesis.

Fate of acetyl CoA: the TCA cycle vs fatty acid synthesis

Normally in mitochondria, any citrate formed enters the TCA cycle for oxidation, leading to the generation of ATP. However, when the concentration of ATP is high, enzymes of the TCA cycle, especially isocitrate dehydrogenase, are inhibited because there is no need to generate further energy. The concentration of citrate rises, which activates the tricarboxylate transporter to transport citrate into the cytosol. As ATP is also needed for fatty acid synthesis, the high levels of both ATP and citrate favour lipogenesis.

Production of malonyl CoA from acetyl CoA

This is the irreversible, rate-limiting step of fatty acid synthesis (Fig. 4.3). The carboxylation of acetyl CoA is catalysed by acetyl CoA carboxylase. This reaction requires the vitamin biotin as a cofactor. Biotin is covalently attached to a lysine residue of the enzyme and takes part in the reaction. The biotin group of the enzyme is first carboxylated, creating an active carboxyl group for further transfer to acetyl CoA.

Biotin is therefore a carrier of activated carboxyl group, acting as a cofactor for other carboxylases, including pyruvate carboxylase (see Chapter 5).

Fatty acid synthase

Fatty acid synthesis requires several enzymes. In bacteria, these enzymes are all separate but in eukaryotes they are joined together, forming a multi-enzyme complex called fatty acid synthase. Fatty acid synthase is a dimer of two identical subunits. Each subunit consists of seven different enzymes which catalyse a different reaction in fatty acid synthesis. Each subunit also contains the acyl carrier protein.

Subunits of fatty acid synthase are folded into three domains joined by flexible regions. Both the acyl carrier protein and one of the enzymes, the condensing enzyme (β-ketoacyl synthase), contain important thiol (sulphydryl) groups (Fig. 4.4).

Function of the acyl carrier protein

The acyl carrier protein contains the vitamin pantothenic acid as a 4'-phosphopantetheine prosthetic group, which has a terminal thiol group. This is similar to the pantothenic acid group of coenzyme A (see Chapter 2). All the intermediates of fatty acid synthesis are joined to the acyl carrier protein. The phosphopantetheinyl group forms a long flexible arm that carries the growing acyl chain from one active site to the next within the fatty acid synthase complex. This enhances the efficiency of the overall synthetic process.

Fig. 4.3 Carboxylation of acetyl CoA to malonyl CoA by acetyl CoA carboxylase.

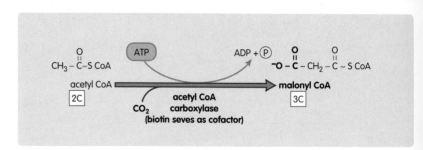

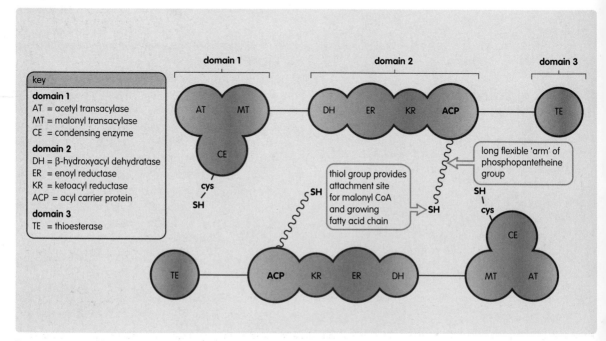

Fig. 4.4 Structure of fatty acid synthase: a dimer of two identical subunits, each folded into three domains.

Stages of fatty acid synthesis

Formation of saturated fatty acids

The stages of fatty acid synthesis are illustrated in Fig. 4.5.

1. Addition of acetyl and malonyl groups

Acetyl transacylase catalyses the transfer of the acetyl group from acetyl CoA to the thiol (–SH) group of the acyl carrier protein. It is then transferred to the thiol group of the β-ketoacyl synthase. Malonyl transacylase then transfers the malonyl group from malonyl CoA to the acyl carrier protein.

2. Condensation

β-Ketoacyl synthase catalyses the condensation of acetyl (2C) and malonyl (3C) groups to form acetoacetyl-ACP (4C). The reaction is driven by the loss of CO_2. The energy derived from ATP that was used to carboxylate acetyl CoA to malonyl CoA

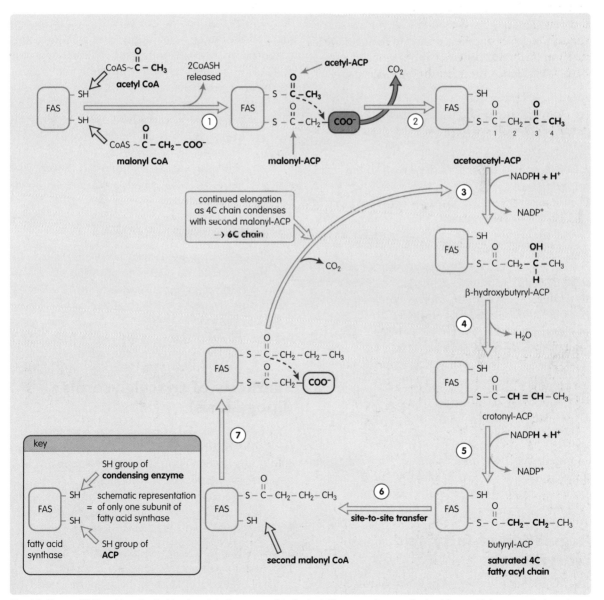

Fig. 4.5 Stages of fatty acid synthesis. Numbers 1 to 7 correspond to the text. The seven-stage synthesis of fatty acids has its cyclical part in steps 3–7, which add two carbons to the growing fatty acid chain for each cycle of the pathway.

(Fig. 4.3) had been contained in malonyl CoA; decarboxylation releases this energy and thus helps to drive elongation. The next three steps convert the acetoacetyl-ACP to a four-carbon, saturated acyl chain.

3. Reduction
The keto group at C3 (the β carbon) is reduced to an alcohol group by β-ketoacyl reductase. The reducing agent for this reaction is NADPH.

4. Dehydration
The removal of water by β-hydroxyacyl dehydratase introduces a double bond.

5. Reduction
Enoyl reductase catalyses the second reduction reaction, producing a saturated four-carbon fatty acyl chain. This completes the first elongation cycle.

6. Site-to-site transfer
The four-carbon chain is transferred to the thiol group of the cysteine residue of the β-ketoacyl synthase.

7. Addition of a second malonyl CoA to the acyl carrier protein
The four-carbon chain condenses with malonyl CoA and steps 2–6 are repeated to form a saturated six-carbon acyl chain.

The cycle is repeated a further six times until a 16-carbon chain, palmitate, is made, i.e. seven cycles altogether (Fig. 4.5). The enzyme thioesterase then catalyses the release of palmitate. Therefore, the synthesis of one molecule of palmitate uses one molecule of acetyl CoA and seven molecules of malonyl CoA. The overall reaction for the synthesis of palmitate is:

8 acetyl CoA + 14NADPH + 14H$^+$ + 7ATP → palmitate + 14NADP$^+$ + 8CoA + 7ADP + 7Pi + 7CO$_2$ + 7H$_2$O

Palmitate serves as the precursor for longer and unsaturated fatty acids. Remember, all the carbon atoms of fatty acids originally come from acetyl CoA.

Regulation of fatty acid biosynthesis

The main control point is the reaction catalysed by acetyl CoA carboxylase (Fig. 4.6). Control may be considered at two levels:

It is worth remembering the characteristic set of reactions, namely the reduction, dehydration, reduction motif of fatty acid synthesis. The opposite of these reactions is the oxidation, hydration and oxidation that occurs in the TCA cycle (Chapter 2) and fatty acid breakdown.

Allosteric regulation

Acetyl CoA carboxylase can exist in two forms: an inactive protomer or subunit form and an active polymer or filamentous form. Citrate activates acetyl CoA carboxylase by promoting the polymerization of protomers to active filaments. A rise in citrate concentration signals that acetyl CoA and ATP are available for fatty acid synthesis (since an increase in ATP inhibits enzymes of the TCA cycle leading to a build-up of citrate).

Acetyl CoA carboxylase is inhibited by the final product, palmitoyl CoA, which causes the depolymerization of its filaments.

Reversible phosphorylation

Acetyl CoA carboxylase is also controlled by hormone-dependent reversible phosphorylation in a way similar to glycogen synthase (see Chapter 2). Glucagon activates a cAMP-dependent protein kinase which phosphorylates acetyl CoA carboxylase, inactivating it. Insulin promotes dephosphorylation and activation of the enzyme and thus lipid synthesis.

Synthesis of triacylglycerols (lipogenesis)

Fatty acids are stored as triacylglycerol molecules in the cytosol of adipose cells. Please note that the term commonly used in clinical medicine is triglyceride, a synonym of triacylglycerol. Triacylglycerol consists of a glycerol backbone esterified with three fatty acids. Triacylglycerol formation can be thought of in three main stages (the numbers correspond to Fig. 4.7).

1. Formation of glycerol-3-phosphate
This occurs either by the phosphorylation of glycerol by glycerol kinase or by the reduction of the glycolytic intermediate, dihydroxyacetone phosphate, by glycerol-3-phosphate dehydrogenase.

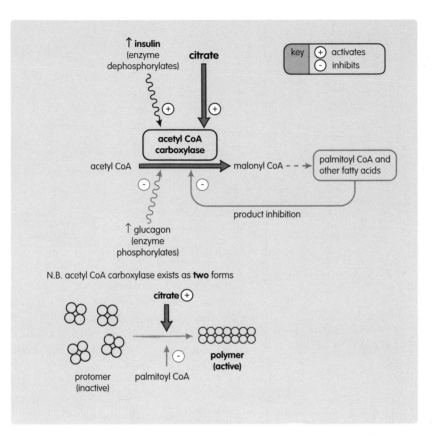

Fig. 4.6 Regulation of fatty acid biosynthesis. Insulin and glucagon control acetyl CoA carboxylase via reversible phosphorylation, whereas citrate and palmitoyl CoA allosterically regulate the enzyme.

2. Activation of fatty acids
Fatty acyl CoA synthetase activates the fatty acids by attaching them to CoA. The reaction requires ATP.

3. Esterification of glycerol-3-phosphate
Acyl transferase adds the activated fatty acids to glycerol-3-phosphate in stages.

During the synthesis of triacylglycerol, the intermediate phosphatidate formed can also be used for the synthesis of phospholipids (i.e. the addition of choline to form phosphatidyl choline, which is used for membrane biosynthesis).

Nomenclature of fatty acids

Fatty acids vary in chain length and in the degree of unsaturation. The configuration of the double bonds in most unsaturated fatty acids in animals is *cis* (*cis* refers to the orientation of the substituent groups, i.e. methyl groups to the double bond. *Cis* means that the methyl groups are on the same side of the double bond compared with *trans*, whereas with *trans* they are on opposite sides—remember 'A' level Chemistry!).

There are two ways of defining the position of a double bond: by counting from the carboxyl (–COOH) group and by counting from the end opposite to the carboxyl group (Fig. 4.8a and b).

Counting from the carboxyl group
Used by chemists; the position of the double bond is represented by the symbol Δ, followed by a number. For example, $\Delta 9,12$, 18:2, means an 18-carbon fatty acid containing two double bonds between the carbon atoms 9 and 10 and 12 and 13; that is, linoleic acid (Fig. 4.8a).

Counting from the end opposite to the carboxyl group
Used by biologists and more confusing! The symbol ω is used to depict the end opposite to the functional group (the methyl-terminal carbon). For example, $\omega 6,9$, 18:2 is an 18-carbon fatty acid

Fig. 4.7 Triacylglycerol synthesis consists of three distinct stages, as described in the text.

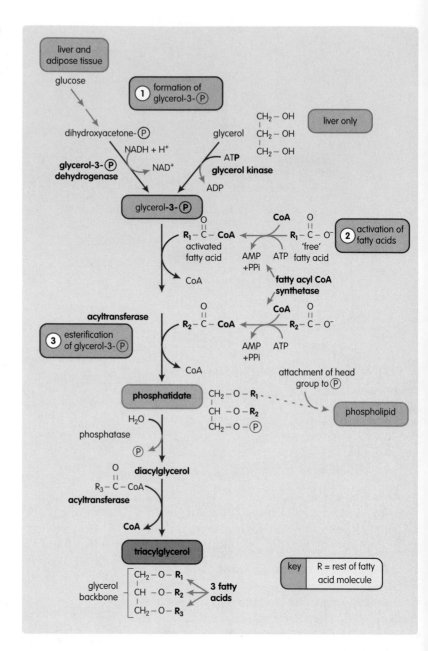

containing two double bonds between the carbon atoms 6 and 7 and 9 and 10. From Fig. 4.8b, it can be seen, however, that this is also linoleic acid.

Modification of fatty acids

Elongation of fatty acids

Fatty acid synthase only produces palmitate (C16) and a small amount of stearate (C18). Other enzymes are required to make longer fatty acids. These enzymes are found on the endoplasmic reticulum and in mitochondria.

Endoplasmic reticulum pathway

This pathway is similar to the normal pathway of fatty acid synthesis. However, there are three main differences:

• The enzymes are all separate and are located on the cytosolic surface of the smooth endoplasmic reticulum.

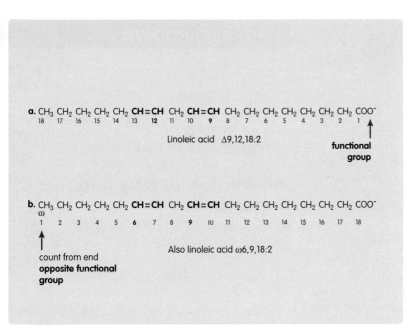

Fig. 4.8 The two ways of defining the position of a double bond:
a. By counting from the carboxyl group.
b. By counting from the end opposite (ω) the carboxyl group.

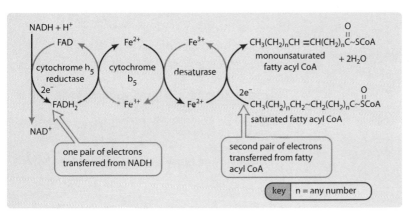

Fig. 4.9 Synthesis of unsaturated fatty acids. The desaturation pathway, located in the smooth endoplasmic reticulum, is responsible for the introduction of double bonds at positions $\Delta 4$, $\Delta 5$, $\Delta 6$ and $\Delta 9$.

- The intermediates for chain elongation are bound to CoA instead of an acyl carrier protein.
- The two-carbon donor is from malonyl CoA and not from malonyl-ACP.

Mitochondrial pathway

This pathway is basically a reversal of fatty acid breakdown (β oxidation), with one exception. The last step in elongation, the reaction catalysed by enoyl CoA reductase, requires NADPH for elongation, whereas the corresponding enzyme in β oxidation, acyl CoA dehydrogenase, requires FAD (see later). This pathway is important for the elongation of short-chain fatty acids, that is those containing 14 carbon atoms or less, and it takes place in the mitochondrial matrix.

Desaturation of fatty acids

This pathway is located in the membrane of the smooth endoplasmic reticulum (Fig. 4.9). The system is an electron transport chain consisting of three enzymes:

- NADH-cytochrome b_5 reductase.
- Cytochrome b_5.
- Fatty acyl CoA desaturase.

Two pairs of electrons are passed down the chain: one pair comes from the single bond of the fatty acid and one pair from NADH. Mammalian systems have four different desaturase enzymes capable of producing double bonds at positions $\Delta 4$, $\Delta 5$, $\Delta 6$ and $\Delta 9$. Unsaturated fatty acids are necessary for the synthesis of important membrane phospholipids and intracellular messengers (i.e prostaglandins).

Essential fatty acids

Mammals can only form double bonds at the positions $\Delta4$, $\Delta5$, $\Delta6$ and $\Delta9$, but lack the enzymes needed to create double bonds beyond the ninth carbon atom. Therefore, certain polyunsaturated fatty acids (PUFAs) that are vital for health, cannot be synthesized endogenously and must be taken in from the diet. The principal essential fatty acids are linoleic (C18:2) and α-linolenic (C18:3) acids, of the $\omega6$ and $\omega3$ series, respectively (see Fig. 4.10). From these, other important unsaturated fatty acids can be made. For example, arachidonic acid (C20:4) is synthesized from linolenic acid and is the precursor molecule for prostaglandins, leukotriene and thromboxane molecules. Fish oils are a particularly good source of the $\omega3$ series.

Evening primrose oil (EPO) and fish oil have been shown to have beneficial effects in the treatment of inflammatory diseases such as psoriasis and rheumatoid arthritis. EPO is rich in linolenic acid, a precursor of series 1 prostaglandin (PG) while fish oil is rich in omega-3 fatty acid eicosapentanoic acid, a precursor of series 3 PG. It is known that series 2 PG have the most potent inflammatory effect with pathological consequences. Dietary supplements of EPO and fish oil enhance production of series 1 and 3 PG, thus displacing the potent inflammatory effects of the 2 series.

Fig. 4.10 Essential fatty acids

ω series	No. of C atoms	No. of double bonds	Position of double bonds	Name
$\omega3$ series				
$\omega3, 6, 9$	18	3	cis $\Delta9,12, 15$	α-linolenic acid
$\omega6$ series				
$\omega6, 9$	18	2	cis $\Delta9, 12$	linoleic acid
$\omega6, 9, 12$	18	3	cis $\Delta6, 9, 12$	γ-linolenic acid (made from linolenic acid)
$\omega6, 9, 12, 15$	20	4	cis $\Delta5, 8, 11, 14$	arachidonic acid

LIPID BREAKDOWN

Triacylglycerol stores in adipose tissue serve as the body's major fuel reserve. Fatty acids are easily mobilized to provide energy during prolonged exercise or starvation. The oxidation of fat yields about 9 kcal/g (38.6 kJ) of energy compared with only 4 kcal/g (16.8 kJ) for protein and carbohydrate.

An overview of fatty acid breakdown

Working definition

Fatty acid breakdown is the process by which a molecule of fatty acid is degraded by the sequential removal of two carbon units, producing acetyl CoA which is then oxidized to CO_2 and H_2O by the TCA cycle.

Location

Many tissues, especially liver and muscle. Certain tissues are unable to oxidize fatty acids, namely the brain, erythrocytes and adrenal medulla, because they lack the necessary enzymes.

The four stages of lipid breakdown

Lipid breakdown can be conveniently divided into four main stages.

1. Hydrolysis of triacylglycerol by lipase: lipolysis

Lipolysis occurs in the cytosol of adipose cells. The hydrolysis of triacylglycerol produces glycerol and free fatty acids. Glycerol is phosphorylated and oxidized to dihydroxyacetone phosphate, which in turn is isomerized to glyceraldehyde-3-phosphate. This intermediate is in both the glycolytic and gluoneogenic pathways. It can therefore be converted into pyruvate or glucose in the liver. The free fatty acids travel in the blood bound to albumin and are taken up by muscle or liver cells for oxidation.

2. Activation of fatty acids

Before they can be oxidized, fatty acids are activated by attachment to CoA to form acyl CoA molecules; this takes place in the cell cytosol.

3. Transport into mitochondria

β Oxidation occurs in the mitochondrial matrix. The acyl CoA molecules are transported into the mitochondria by the carnitine shuttle.

4. β Oxidation

Fatty acids are degraded by a cyclical sequence of four reactions: oxidation, hydration, oxidation, and thiolysis. This results in the shortening of the fatty acid chain by two carbon atoms per sequence. The two carbon atoms are removed as acetyl CoA. For even-numbered saturated fatty acids this is straightforward, but other enzymes are necessary for the oxidation of unsaturated and odd-numbered fatty acids (see later).

These steps are now considered in more detail.

Lipolysis

The initial event in the breakdown of fat is the hydrolysis of triacylglycerol stores in adipose tissue. Triacylglycerol is converted into glycerol and three free fatty acids in two steps (Fig. 4.11):

1. A hormone-sensitive lipase hydrolyses triacylglycerol at the C1 and C3 positions to form monoacylglycerol.
2. A monoacylglycerol-specific lipase removes the remaining fatty acid.

The glycerol produced cannot be metabolized by adipose tissue because adipose tissue does not contain glycerol kinase. Glycerol is transported to the liver where it is phosphorylated, either to be used again to make triacylglycerol or to be converted to dihydroxyacetone phosphate, a glycolytic intermediate for gluconeogenesis. The free fatty acids produced are either re-esterified to triacyglycerol in the adipose tissue or travel in the blood to be taken up by the cells for oxidation.

Activation of fatty acids to fatty acyl CoA

Fatty acyl CoA synthetase (thiokinase) activates fatty acids by attaching them to CoA. The reaction occurs on the cytosolic face of the outer mitochondrial membrane and requires ATP, which is hydrolysed to AMP and pyrophosphate (PPi), breaking a high-energy phosphate bond. The reaction is made irreversible by the rapid hydrolysis of the pyrophosphate to two free inorganic phosphates by pyrophosphatase, consuming a second high-energy phosphate bond (Fig. 4.12). Therefore the activation of a fatty acid consumes 2 ATP equivalents. Fatty acids are non-polar molecules and can easily diffuse out of cells, but the attachment to a polar molecule such as CoA, 'traps' the fatty acid inside.

Transport of fatty acyl CoA molecules into mitochondria

The activation of fatty acids occurs in the cytosol but the enzymes for β oxidation are in the mitochondrial

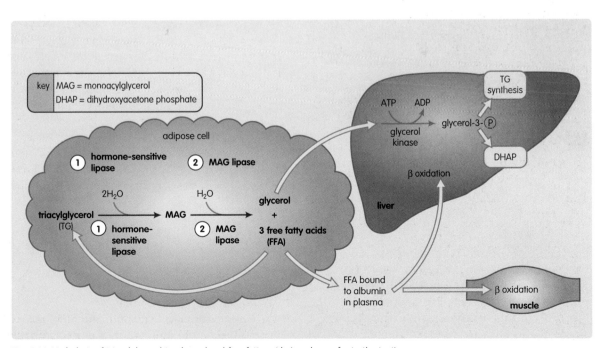

Fig. 4.11 Hydrolysis of triacylglycerol to glycerol and free fatty acids (numbers refer to the text).

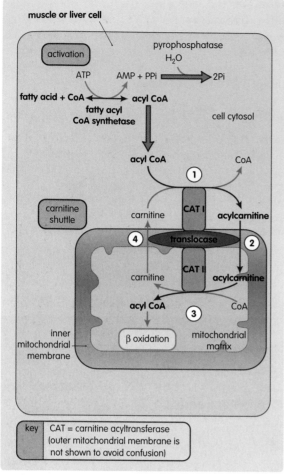

Fig. 4.12 Activation of fatty acids and their transport into mitochondria by the carnitine shuttle.
1. The acyl group is transferred from CoA to carnitine by carnitine acyl transferase I, an enzyme found on the cytosolic side of the inner mitochondrial membrane.
2. Acylcarnitine is transported across the membrane by the translocase to the mitochondrial matrix.
3. The acyl group is transferred back to CoA by carnitine acyl transferase II, located on the inner surface of the inner mitochondrial membrane.
4. Carnitine is returned to the cytosolic side in exchange for another molecule of acylcarnitine.

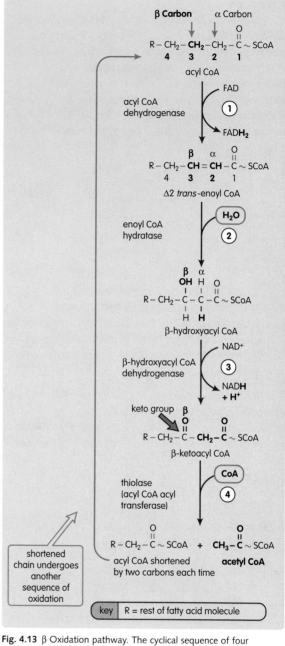

Fig. 4.13 β Oxidation pathway. The cyclical sequence of four reactions—oxidation, hydration, oxidation and thiolysis—shortens the fatty acid chain by two carbons each cycle. This continues until the fatty acid is completely oxidized to acetyl CoA.

matrix. The inner mitochondrial membrane is relatively impermeable to long-chain acyl CoA molecules, so a special transporter system, the carnitine shuttle, is required to carry the fatty acid across. The carnitine shuttle consists of three enzymes: a translocase and two carnitine acyl transferases, CAT I and II, as shown in Fig. 4.12.

β Oxidation

Acyl CoA molecules inside the mitochondrial matrix undergo β oxidation, in a cyclical sequence of four reactions (numbers refer to Fig. 4.13).

1. Oxidation
The oxidation of acyl CoA introduces a double bond between the C2 and C3 atoms. The $FADH_2$ formed enters the electron transport chain to produce 1.5 ATP (see Chapter 2). In the mitochondria there are three types of acyl CoA dehydrogenase, which act on long-, medium- and short-chain fatty acids. A deficiency in medium-chain acyl CoA dehydrogenase has been recognized (this is discussed further below).

2. Hydration
Hydration is the addition of water across the double bond between C2 and C3 by Δ2 enoyl-CoA hydratase.

3. Oxidation by NAD⁺
β-Hydroxyacyl CoA dehydrogenase converts the OH group at C3 (the β carbon) to a keto group. The NADH produced enters the electron transport chain to yield 2.5 ATP molecules. These three reactions of oxidation (dehydrogenation), hydration, and again oxidation resemble the last three reactions of the TCA cycle which convert succinate to oxaloacetate (see Chapter 2).

4. Thiolytic cleavage by CoA
Thiolase cleaves the molecule to release acetyl CoA, and acyl CoA is shortened by two carbon atoms. The shortened acyl CoA is ready to undergo another sequence of β oxidation. The four steps are repeated until the fatty acid is oxidized completely to acetyl CoA. The last round of oxidation produces two molecules of acetyl CoA.

ATP yield from the oxidation of the fatty acid palmitate

Each round of β oxidation produces one molecule each of $FADH_2$, NADH and acetyl CoA. The β oxidation of palmitate requires seven cycles, producing 7 $FADH_2$, 7 NADH and 8 acetyl CoA in total (see Fig. 2.21).

For even-numbered, saturated fatty acids, $(n/2) - 1$ cycles are required for complete oxidation, where n = the number of carbons of the fatty acid; e.g. C16 palmitate requires $(16/2) - 1 = 7$ cycles.

ATP yield
The activation of palmitate to palmitoyl CoA consumes 2 molecules of ATP. β oxidation generates:

- 7 $FADH_2$, which are oxidized by the electron transport chain to generate 10.5 ATP.
- 7 NADH, which are oxidized by the chain to generate 17.5 ATP.
- 8 acetyl CoA, which are oxidized by the TCA cycle to generate 80 ATP (remember, oxidation of each acetyl CoA by the TCA cycle yields 10 ATP).

Therefore the total energy generated from the oxidation of a molecule of palmitate is 106 ATP.

Oxidation of odd-numbered fatty acids

The oxidation of odd-numbered fatty acids (Fig. 4.14) is essentially the same as for even-numbered fatty acids, except that the last round of β oxidation produces one molecule of acetyl CoA and one molecule

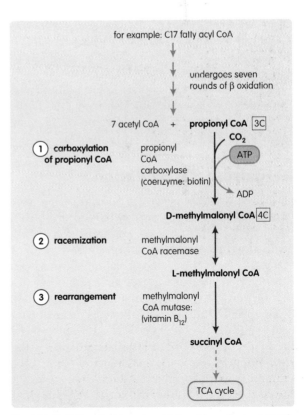

Fig. 4.14 Oxidation of odd-numbered fatty acids produces propionyl CoA, which is metabolized to succinyl CoA in three steps to enter the TCA cycle.

of propionyl CoA (3C), instead of two molecules of acetyl CoA. Propionyl CoA can either be carboxylated to succinyl CoA in a three-reaction sequence requiring biotin and vitamin B_{12}, which can then enter the TCA cycle, or can be used for gluconeogenesis.

Oxidation of unsaturated fatty acids

In the oxidation of unsaturated fatty acids, most of the reactions are the same as for saturated fatty acids except two additional enzymes are involved, enoyl CoA isomerase and 2,4-dienoyl reductase. Naturally occurring unsaturated fatty acids contain *cis* double bonds. The enzymes of β oxidation, particularly enoyl CoA hydratase, which is specific for the *trans* configuration of double bonds, do not metabolize these easily. Enoyl CoA isomerase converts a *cis* to a *trans* double bond, thus enabling β oxidation to proceed.

During the oxidation of some unsaturated fatty acids, for example, linoleic acid (*cis* Δ9,12, 18:2), the intermediate 2,4-dienoyl CoA is produced. This, again, is not a substrate for enoyl CoA hydratase. NADPH-dependent 2,4-dienoyl reductase reduces it to *trans* enoyl CoA, thus enabling β oxidation to continue.

The oxidation of unsaturated fatty acids is relatively slow compared with saturated fatty acids because the former is transported slowly into the mitochondria by the carnitine shuttle.

Peroxisomal β oxidation

Oxidation of fatty acids can also occur in peroxisomes, particularly in the kidney and liver. Approximately 5–10% of the total oxidation of fatty acids occurs in peroxisomes, with the rest in mitochondria. The pathway of β oxidation in mitochondria and peroxisomes is identical; it is the enzymes that are different. The enzymes of peroxisomes are more versatile and can oxidize a wider range of fatty acid analogues, including prostaglandins. However, the main function of peroxisomal oxidation is the shortening of very-long-chain fatty acids, for example those longer than 22–24 carbon atoms, in preparation for β oxidation by the mitochondrial system, as very-long-chain fatty acids cannot enter the mitochondria via the carnitine shuttle.

Different enzymes participate in peroxisomal β oxidation

Oxidation
The first oxidation step is catalysed by the FAD-containing enzyme acyl CoA oxidase, which passes its electrons directly to oxygen, so no ATP is formed. Energy is dissipated as heat instead.

Hydration and oxidation
These are performed by the bifunctional enzyme which has both enoyl CoA hydratase and 3-hydroxyacyl CoA dehydrogenase activity.

Thiolysis
Thiolase cleaves acyl CoA, releasing acetyl CoA and a shortened acyl chain.

Oxidation continues until acyl CoA molecules are fewer than 22 carbons in length, at which point they diffuse out of the peroxisomes, via a pore-forming protein in the peroxisomal membrane, for further oxidation in mitochondria.

Regulation of lipid breakdown

The control of lipid breakdown is exerted at three levels (Fig. 4.15): lipolysis, carnitine shuttle and β oxidation.

Control of lipolysis

Hormone-sensitive lipase (see Fig. 4.11) is regulated by reversible phosphorylation. Adrenaline during exercise, and glucagon and adrenocorticotrophic hormone (ACTH) during starvation, activate adenylate cyclase, which increases the levels of cAMP. This activates a cAMP-dependent protein kinase, which phosphorylates and activates lipase. The same cAMP-dependent protein kinase also phosphorylates and inhibits acetyl CoA carboxylase (see Fig. 4.6); that is, it stimulates lipolysis but inhibits fatty acid synthesis. This is similar to the reciprocal mechanism of control of glycogen phosphorylase and synthase by reversible phosphorylation (see Fig. 2.34). Insulin causes dephosphorylation of lipase, inhibiting lipolysis. As a long-term adaptation to prolonged starvation, cortisol stimulates the synthesis of lipase, thus increasing its concentration and activity for lipolysis.

Carnitine shuttle

Malonyl CoA inhibits carnitine acyl transferase I (CAT I), thus inhibiting the entry of acyl groups into

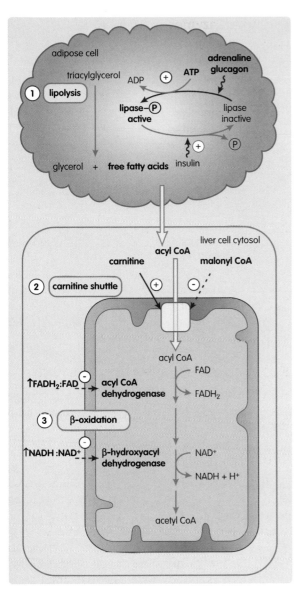

Fig. 4.15 Regulation of lipid breakdown. Control is exerted at three levels: **1.** lipolysis; **2.** the carnitine shuttle; **3.** β oxidation.

mitochondria. An increase in malonyl CoA is produced during fatty acid synthesis and ensures that newly synthesized fatty acids are not transported into mitochondria for oxidation as soon as they are made.

Inhibition of β oxidation by NADH and FADH$_2$

The oxidation reactions require a supply of FAD and NAD$^+$, which are regenerated via the electron transport chain. The enzymes of β oxidation compete with the dehydrogenase enzymes of the TCA cycle for

In exams you will often be asked to compare the processes of fatty acid synthesis and degradation. Fig. 4.16 should give you an idea of the main points to include.

NAD$^+$ and FAD because both pathways are usually active at the same time.

Errors of fatty acid metabolism

Medium-chain fatty acyl CoA dehydrogenase deficiency

Medium-chain fatty acyl CoA dehydrogenase deficiency has an incidence of 1/10 000 births. It is thought that the deficiency of this enzyme leads to a decreased oxidation of fatty acids and therefore an increase in, and a greater reliance on, glucose oxidation. When glycogen reserves become exhausted, severe hypoglycaemia occurs. It is believed that this is the cause of death in some cases of sudden infant death syndrome (cot death).

CHOLESTEROL METABOLISM

Role of cholesterol in the body

Cholesterol has many functions in the body, including being:

- An essential component of cell membranes, including myelin in the nervous system.
- A precursor of the five major classes of steroid hormones: progestagens, oestrogens, androgens, glucocorticoids and mineralocorticoids.
- A precursor of bile acids and vitamin D.

The body therefore requires a continuous supply of cholesterol.

Sources of cholesterol

Cholesterol can either be obtained from the diet or be synthesized endogenously by the body. Regulatory mechanisms exist which balance the amount of cholesterol made by the body daily with both the dietary intake and the amount excreted either in bile or as bile salts, to enable control of the plasma

Fig. 4.16 Comparison of fatty acid synthesis and degradation

	Synthesis	Degradation
Active	After meals: fed state	Fasting and prolonged exercise
Main tissues involved	Liver and adipose tissue	Muscle and liver
Site	Cytosol via citrate shuttle	Mitochondria via carnitine shuttle
2C donor/product	Acetyl CoA	Acetyl CoA
Active fatty acid carrier	Attached to ACP	Attached to CoA
Enzymes	FAS: enzymes all part of multienzyme complex	Probably not associated
Oxidant/reductant	NADPH	NAD^+ and FAD
Allosteric control	Citrate activates acetyl CoA carboxylase; palmitoyl CoA inhibits	Malonyl CoA inhibits CAT I
Hormonal control	Insulin activates acetyl CoA carboxylase; adrenaline and glucagon inhibit it	Adrenaline and glucagon activate lipase; insulin inhibits it
Product	Palmitate	Acetyl CoA

cholesterol level. Failure of this control may lead to high plasma cholesterol levels: this promotes atherosclerosis and consequently increases the risk of atherosclerosis-associated diseases—coronary heart disease, cerebrovascular disease and peripheral vascular disease.

Cholesterol synthesis

Cholesterol is a 27-carbon steroid molecule. All carbon atoms of cholesterol come from acetyl CoA. It is one of a large group of compounds derived from the five-carbon isoprene group (others include ubiquinone and the vitamins A, E and K). The easiest way to view cholesterol synthesis is to divide it into two stages (Fig. 4.17):

* Stage I: The formation of the isoprene unit, isopentenyl pyrophosphate (IPP). This is formed by the condensation of three molecules of acetyl CoA to 3-hydroxy-3-methylglutaryl CoA (HMG-CoA), followed by the loss of CO_2.
* Stage II: The progressive condensation of isoprene units to form cholesterol. Six isoprene (five-carbon) units link up to form squalene

(30 C atoms) which cyclizes to lanosterol, which in turn yields cholesterol.

Location
Cholesterol is made by most tissues (except erythrocytes) but the main site of synthesis is the liver.

Site
Cell cytosol, although some of the enzymes are found in the endoplasmic reticulum.

These stages are now considered in more detail and are clearly illustrated in Fig. 4.17.

Stage I: Formation of IPP

1. Formation of HMG-CoA from acetyl CoA
This occurs in two steps:

* Two molecules of acetyl CoA condense to form acetoacetyl CoA (4C).
* HMG-CoA synthase catalyses the addition of a third molecule of acetyl CoA to form HMG-CoA (6C).

HMG-CoA is also an intermediate in the synthesis of ketone bodies. However, ketone body formation

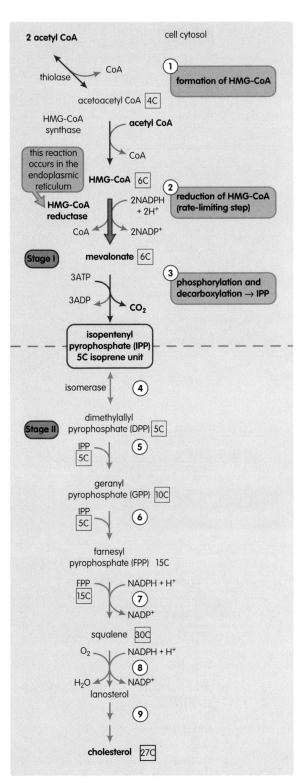

Fig. 4.17 Cholesterol synthesis. This multistep pathway is divided into two stages (numbers refer to the text).

occurs in the mitochondria whereas the reactions of cholesterol synthesis occur in the cell cytosol. The liver therefore contains two isoenzymes of HMG-CoA synthase: a cytosolic enzyme for cholesterol synthesis and a mitochondrial enzyme for ketone body formation.

2. Reduction of HMG-CoA to mevalonic acid (mevalonate)

This is the irreversible, rate-limiting step of cholesterol synthesis and thus the most important control site. The enzyme HMG-CoA reductase is found in the endoplasmic reticulum and requires NADPH as a reducing agent.

3. Phosphorylation and decarboxylation of mevalonate to IPP

Mevalonate is converted to IPP in three reactions requiring three molecules of ATP. The first two reactions are phosphorylations forming an intermediate (not shown in Fig. 4.17), which is then decarboxylated to form isopentenyl pyrophosphate (IPP).

Stage II: Progressive condensation of isoprene units to cholesterol

4. Isomerization of IPP to dimethylallyl pyrophosphate

The five-carbon isoprene units then link up in a stepwise fashion as shown in Fig. 4.17.

5. IPP and dimethylallyl pyrophosphate condense to form the 10-carbon, geranyl pyrophosphate

6. Another IPP condenses with geranyl pyrophosphate to form the 15-carbon, farnesyl pyrophosphate

7. Squalene synthase catalyses the reductive condensation of two molecules of farnesyl pyrophosphate, forming the 30-carbon molecule, squalene

All three condensation reactions (5, 6 and 7) release pyrophosphate which drives the reactions.

8. Cyclization of squalene to lanosterol (30C) by squalene monooxygenase

9. Conversion of lanosterol to cholesterol

The exact pathway is not known but it is thought to consist of about 20 steps! Basically, three methyl groups are removed to produce a 27-carbon molecule followed by the migration of the double bond to the Δ5 position to produce cholesterol (Fig. 4.18).

Regulation of cholesterol synthesis

Regulation is necessary in order to prevent high plasma cholesterol levels, which may lead to cholesterol deposition in arterial walls and formation of atherosclerotic plaques. The primary control site is the rate-limiting enzyme HMG-CoA reductase (Fig. 4.19).

Product inhibition

HMG-CoA reductase is allosterically inhibited by cholesterol. HMG-CoA reductase inhibition is the mechanism of action of drugs inhibiting cholesterol synthesis (statins).

Short-term hormonal regulation

- HMG-CoA reductase is also regulated by hormone-dependent reversible phosphorylation

by a similar mechanism to glycogen synthase (see Fig. 2.34) and acetyl CoA carboxylase.
- Glucagon activates a cAMP-dependent protein kinase that reversibly phosphorylates HMG-CoA

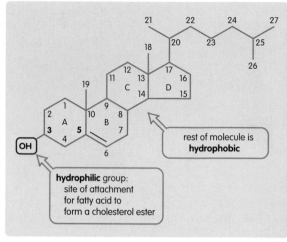

Fig. 4.18 Structure of cholesterol.

Fig. 4.19 Control of HMG-CoA reductase. This enzyme is not only affected by cholesterol as its product in an allosteric fashion but also because cholesterol actually down-regulates the transcription of HMG-CoA reductase which catalyses the rate-limiting step of cholesterol synthesis.

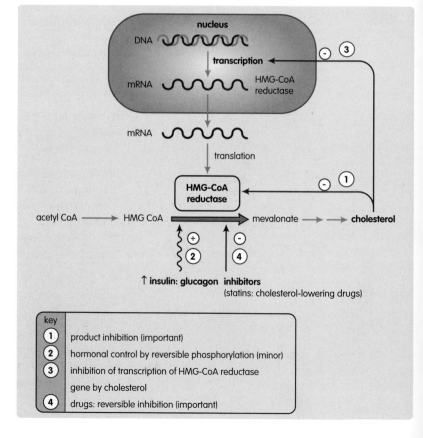

reductase, inhibiting it and therefore decreasing the rate of cholesterol synthesis.

- Insulin dephosphorylates the enzyme, leading to its activation and an increase in cholesterol synthesis.

Long-term regulation of HMG-CoA reductase

- This is the most important control mechanism.
- The amount of cholesterol, both dietary and endogenous, taken up by cells affects the amount of HMG-CoA reductase synthesized.
- A high intracellular cholesterol level causes a decrease in the rate of transcription of the HMG-CoA reductase gene, inhibiting it and leading to a reduction in cholesterol synthesis.

High intracellular cholesterol concentrations also suppress the synthesis of low-density lipoprotein (LDL) receptors, resulting in a decrease in the up-take of these lipoproteins (and thus cholesterol) by the cell. A low intracellular cholesterol concentration stimulates receptor synthesis. This is the most important mechanism that regulates plasma cholesterol concentration.

Packaging of cholesterol

Most of the cholesterol in the blood is in the form of cholesterol esters, formed by the addition of a fatty acid to the C3-hydroxyl group (see Fig. 4.18). Esterification makes the cholesterol more hydrophobic, enabling it to be packaged, stored and transported more easily. Two enzyme systems are responsible for the esterification of cholesterol (numbers refer to Fig. 4.20):

1. In cells:
   - If the cholesterol taken up or synthesized by cells is not immediately required, then it is esterified by acyl CoA:cholesterol acyl transferase (ACAT).
   - ACAT transfers a fatty acid from a fatty acyl CoA to cholesterol, forming a cholesterol ester that can be stored in the cell.
2. In the high-density lipoproteins:
   - A similar enzyme, known as lecithin:cholesterol acyl transferase (LCAT), is found associated with high-density lipoproteins (HDL).
   - HDL is responsible for picking up free cholesterol from peripheral tissues and transporting it to the liver: it acts as a cholesterol scavenger.

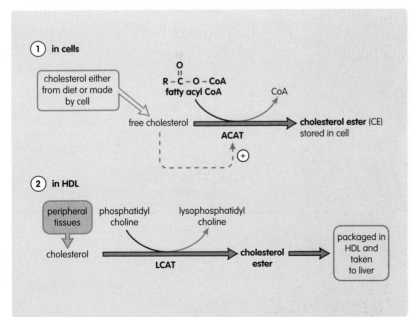

Fig. 4.20 Two enzyme systems are responsible for the esterification of cholesterol—acyl CoA:cholesterol acyl transferase in cells, and lecithin:cholesterol acyl transferase in HDL.

In patients with high plasma cholesterol, the treatment of choice is statins. Statins act by competitively inhibiting HMG-CoA reductase. This results in the lowering of intracellular cholesterol concentration and consequently, upregulation of expression of the LDL receptors. The cells increase LDL uptake, leading to their increased clearance from the bloodstream.

- LCAT catalyses the transfer of a fatty acid from the phospholipid, phosphatidylcholine, to cholesterol.
- HDL then carries cholesterol esters to the liver, either to be reused or excreted.

TRANSPORT OF LIPIDS

Lipoproteins

Lipids are insoluble in aqueous solution and are transported in plasma in association with proteins (apolipoproteins) in the form of lipoproteins (Fig. 4.21). Lipoproteins solubilize the lipids and provide an efficient transport system for them. If the

system fails, the plasma lipid concentration will increase. In the long term, a high plasma cholesterol level is associated with an increased risk of atherosclerosis.

Some apolipoproteins are only weakly associated with lipoprotein complexes and can be transferred easily between them. They have a number of functions, including acting:

- As recognition sites or ligands for receptors.
- As structural components.
- As activators or coenzymes for enzymes involved in lipid metabolism.

The functions of the major apolipoproteins are summarized in Fig. 4.22.

Classes of lipoprotein

There are five main classes of lipoproteins: chylomicrons (CM), very-low-density lipoproteins (VLDL), intermediate-density lipoproteins (IDL, also known as lipoprotein remnants, low-density lipoproteins (LDL) and high-density lipoproteins (HDL). They are classified according to increasing density, with CMs having the lowest density and HDLs the highest. As protein is denser than lipid, HDL, which has the highest density, contain the most protein. Lipoproteins differ in composition, size, function, and the apolipoproteins present on their surface. These properties are summarized in Fig. 4.23.

Fig. 4.21 Basic structure of a lipoprotein particle consists of a non-polar lipid core containing triacylglycerol (TG) and cholesterol esters surrounded by a polar outer coat of phospholipids and free cholesterol, which also contains proteins known as apolipoproteins.

Fig. 4.22 Functions of major apolipoproteins	
Apolipoprotein	**Function**
A-I	Activates lecithin: cholesterol acyl transferase
A-II	Activates hepatic lipase
B-48	Structural chylomicrons (CM)
B-100	Structural; binds to the apoB/E (LDL) receptor. Increases cholesterol uptake
C-I	Cofactor for lecithin: cholesterol acyl transferase
C-II	Activates lipoprotein lipase
C-III	Inhibits lipoprotein lipase?
E	Binds to apo B/E (LDL) receptor and increases uptake of LDL and remnant particles including CM remnants

Fig. 4.23 Classification and properties of lipoproteins

Class	Main composition	Diameter (nm)	Source and function	Major apolipoproteins
CM	90% triacylglycerol	500	Transport of **dietary** triacylglycerol	A-I, II, B-48, C-I, II, III, E
VLDL	65% triacylglycerol	43	Transport of **endogenously** synthesized triacylglycerol from the liver to peripheral tissues	B-100, C-I, II, III, E
IDL	35% phospholipid 25% cholesterol	27	Formed by partial hydrolysis of VLDL, precursor of LDL	B-100, C-III, E
LDL	50% cholesterol 25% protein	22	Formed by hydrolysis of IDL; carries cholesterol to peripheral tissues	B-100
HDL	55% protein 25% phospholipid	8	Formed in the liver and intestine; 2 main functions: • reverse cholesterol transport removes cholesterol from tissues and takes it to liver; 'cholesterol scavenger' • exchanges apolipoproteins and cholesterol esters with chylomicrons and VLDL	A-I, II, C-I, II, III, D, E

Pathways of lipid transport

Lipids can either be obtained from the diet (exogenous lipids) or synthesized by the body (endogenous lipids). There are two different pathways for lipid transport in the body:

- Exogenous pathway: CM transport dietary lipid absorbed from the intestine to the tissues (Fig. 4.24).
- Endogenous pathway: VLDLs, IDLs and LDLs form a continuous cascade. The VLDLs transport endogenously synthesized triacylglycerol from the liver to the tissues (Fig. 4.25).

These pathways can now be considered in more detail.

Exogenous pathway (numbers refer to Fig. 4.24)

1. CM formation

Triacylglycerols in the diet are digested in the stomach and small intestine by lipases to form free fatty acids and 2-monoacylglycerols. These products are absorbed and assembled by the intestinal epithelial cells into chylomicrons, a triacylglycerol-rich plasma lipoprotein with some cholesterol and apolipoprotein B-48. These newly formed chylomicrons are referred to as nascent CM.

2. Circulation of chylomicrons

Nascent CM travel in the lymphatic system and enter the blood via the thoracic duct. When they reach the blood they acquire apolipoprotein C-II and E from HDL.

3. Hydrolysis of triacylglycerol

CM are carried in the blood to tissues (i.e adipose tissue and muscle). As they pass through the capillaries of tissues, the enzyme lipoprotein lipase, found on the luminal surface of the capillary endothelium, is activated by apolipoprotein C-II on the surface of the CM. Lipoprotein lipase hydrolyses a large part of the CM triacylglycerol to glycerol and free fatty acids. The fatty acids are taken up by cells, either for oxidation or re-synthesis to triacylglycerol.

Fig. 4.24 Exogenous pathway of lipid transport (numbers refer to the text below).

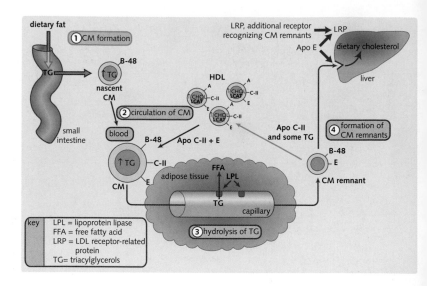

4. Formation of CM remnants

The removal of triacylglycerol leaves behind a much smaller CM remnant particle. Apolipoprotein C-II is returned to HDL. Apolipoproteins B-48 and E are recognized by remnant receptors on liver cells and the CM remnants are taken up by the liver and degraded.

Endogenous pathway (numbers refer to Fig. 4.25)

The liver is the main site of lipid synthesis.

1. Assembly of VLDL

VLDLs are synthesized in the liver, mostly from triacylglycerol, and are released as nascent VLDL particles containing surface apolipoprotein B-100. Like CMs, VLDLs acquire apolipoprotein C-II and E from HDL. VLDLs transport endogenous triacylglycerol from the liver to peripheral tissues.

2. Hydrolysis by lipoprotein lipase (LPL) in tissues

Lipoprotein lipase removes triacylglycerol in the same way as for CMs. VLDLs become smaller in size and more dense (VLDL remnants, particles practically identical to IDL). Cholesterol released from the remnants contributes to the inhibition of HMG-CoA reductase, resulting in a decrease in the endogenous synthesis of cholesterol by the liver (see Fig. 4.19).

3. Formation of IDL and LDL

Some triacylglycerols, phospholipids and apolipoprotein C-II are transferred to HDL. Cholesterol ester transfer protein (CETP) transfers cholesterol esters in exchange for triacylglycerol and phospholipids, from HDL to IDL. Some of the IDLs are taken up by the liver via receptors that recognize both apolipoprotein B-100 and apolipoprotein E on their surface (not shown in Fig. 4.25); but the rest forms LDL (note that the well-known LDL-receptor is in fact an apoB-100/E receptor).

4. LDL provides cholesterol for peripheral tissues

LDL binds to LDL receptors on cell membranes and is internalized by receptor-mediated endocytosis. Lysosomal enzymes hydrolyse LDL, releasing free cholesterol into the cell.

5. HDL metabolism

HDL is made in the liver and has two main functions:

- It accepts the free cholesterol from peripheral tissues and lipoproteins and esterifies it by the action of LCAT (see Fig. 4.20). The cholesterol esters formed are either transferred to VLDL or IDL, or are carried back to the liver by 'reverse cholesterol transport'.
- HDL exchanges apolipoproteins, cholesterol esters and triglycerides with other lipoproteins (CM and VLDL) as already described.

Effects of cholesterol inside cells

Cholesterol inhibits HMG-CoA reductase activity and therefore cholesterol synthesis. It does this by product inhibition and by inhibition of the transcription of the HMG-CoA reductase gene (see Fig. 4.19). Cholesterol also inhibits LDL receptor

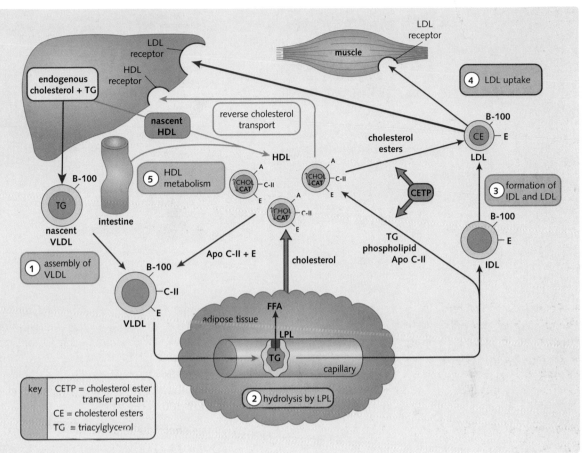

Fig. 4.25 Endogenous pathway of lipid transport (numbers refer to the text below).

synthesis. An increased cholesterol concentration in the cell down-regulates the synthesis of LDL receptors by decreasing the rate of transcription of the LDL receptor gene. This limits the uptake of cholesterol.

Whereas an increase in LDL-cholesterol is harmful, an increase in HDL-cholesterol has a protective effect because it removes cholesterol from tissues and takes it to the liver for degradation and excretion. It is known that one to two glasses of red wine each day increases the levels of HDL. Unfortunately, this beneficial effect is limited to one to two glasses of wine daily – also, exercise is probably a better way to raise one's HDL.

If cholesterol is not immediately required by the cell, the enzyme ACAT esterifies cholesterol for storage in cells (see Fig. 4.20).

Disorders of lipid metabolism and transport

The dyslipidaemias are a group of disorders caused by a defect in lipoprotein formation, transport or degradation (Fig. 4.26). They describe the accumulation of lipids in the blood and, in most cases, an increased risk of atherosclerosis. Thus dyslipidaemias occur as a result of a deficiency in either:

- An enzyme; for example, LPL deficiency.
- An apolipoprotein; for example, apolipoprotein C-II deficiency.
- A receptor; for example, LDL receptor.

Dyslipidaemias used to be classified according to the Fredrickson classification but this is now rarely

Fig. 4.26 Disorders of lipid metabolism: dyslipidaemias (hyperlipidaemias)

Name	Cause	Effect on lipoproteins
Familial LPL deficiency or apo C-II deficiency, autosomal recessive	Decreased or absent LPL activity	Increased CM cause a milky serum Increased triacylglycerol may cause acute pancreatitis
Familial hypercholesterolaemia, autosomal dominant (1/500)	Defect or total absence of LDL receptors (occasionally caused by a defect in apolipoprotein B-100)	Decreased uptake of LDL by tissues and increased plasma cholesterol concentration Homozygotes have no receptors Increased risk of atherosclerosis
Familial combined hyperlipidaemia, autosomal dominant	Overproduction of apo B by liver	Increased VLDL secretion leads to increased LDL; (increased plasma cholesterol and triacylglycerol) Increased risk of atherosclerosis
Familial dysbetalipoproteinaemia	Abnormal apolipoprotein E decrease in remnant clearance by liver	Increased remnant particles (IDL) Increased risk of atherosclerosis
Familial hypertriglyceridaemia	Overproduction of VLDL by the liver	Increased VLDL; Increased risk of atherosclerosis

used. Instead, they are clinically divided into hypercholesterolaemia, hypertriglyceridaemia and mixed disorders. There are two complementary approaches to the treatment of dyslipidaemias: diet and/or drugs. The main drugs used to control lipid metabolism are listed in Fig. 4.27.

The main clinical features of the more important dyslipidaemias are now considered.

Familial lipoprotein lipase or apolipoprotein C-II deficiency

This is a rare, autosomal recessive disorder due to either a deficiency of the enzyme lipoprotein lipase (LPL), or apolipoprotein C-II required for the activation of LPL. Since it results in a failure of the clearance of chylomicrons from the bloodstream, it is also called familial chylomicronaemia.

Familial hypercholesterolaemia (FH)

Familial hypercholesterolaemia is the most common and the most important inherited lipid disorder. It is an autosomal dominant disease with a prevalence of 1/500 (0.2%) for heterozygotes and 1/100 000 for homozygotes. The cause in the majority of patients (95%) is a defect in the LDL receptor: either a decrease in the actual number of receptors or malfunctioning receptors (i.e a mutation in the apoB-100 binding site). A smaller number of patients (5%) have a defective apoB-100 molecule. For all patients, there is a defect in the uptake of LDL, leading to an increase in plasma LDL concentration. In homozygotes, no LDL receptors are present, leading to grossly elevated plasma cholesterol levels, as high as 20 mmol/L. This causes a massive deposition of cholesterol in the arterial walls and skin. These patients

Fig. 4.27 Main drugs used to control lipid metabolism

Drug	Mechanism of action
Statins: simvastatin, lovastatin, atorvastatin, rosuvastatin	Inhibit **HMG-CoA reductase**, decreasing cholesterol synthesis; cell compensates for lower intracellular cholesterol by increasing LDL receptor synthesis, resulting in increased cholesterol uptake thus leading to decreased plasma cholesterol
Fibrates: bezafibrate, gemfibrozil	Activate LPL (main effect), thus lowering plasma TG; slightly suppress HMG-CoA reductase, decrease the synthesis of apo B and increase apo A
Anion exchange resins: cholestyramine, colestipol	Bind bile acids in gastrointestinal tract preventing their reabsorption and therefore decrease plasma LDL levels
Nicotinic acid	Decreases VLDL production by liver and thus LDL; increases LPL activity, leading to decreased triacylglycerol
Fish oils	Reduce VLDL synthesis in the liver

Fig. 4.28 The clinical features of familial hypercholesterolaemia

Clinical Features	Diagnosis and Management
Homozygotes: tendon xanthomata: thickening of Achilles tendon and xanthomata over extensor tendons of fingers xanthelasma: yellowish fatty deposits in skin of eyelid (non-diagnostic) premature arcus senilis: thin white rim around iris of eye	**Diagnosis:** fasting cholesterol usually > 16 mmol/L **Management:** • diet: very low in cholesterol and saturated fat • drugs: statins, cholesterol binding resins, nicotinic acid (see Fig. 4.27) • low-density lipoprotein removal by plasmapheresis • liver transplant • gene therapy: trials are under way
Heterozygotes: • as above but not as severe • may have no physical signs	**Diagnosis:** fasting cholesterol, usually > 8 mmol/L **Management:** • diet • cholesterol-lowering drugs

usually develop coronary heart disease in childhood and, if untreated, rarely survive to adult life.

The clinical features, diagnosis and management of familial hypercholesterolaemia are discussed in Fig. 4.28. The prognosis for homozygotes is poor. Plasmapheresis, if used regularly, is successful in the short term. Liver transplantation offers the possibility of a cure. For heterozygotes, the prognosis is reasonable; nevertheless these patients tend to develop coronary heart disease earlier than the normal population and therefore require lipid-lowering treatment.

Do not confuse familial hypercholesterolaemia with the polygenic form, common hypercholesterolaemia.

Familial combined hyperlipidaemia

Familial combined hyperlipidaemia is relatively common, with a prevalence of 1/300. The genetic basis is unclear, but it is probably autosomal dominant. The abnormality is an overproduction of apolipoprotein B, leading to an increased VLDL secretion from the liver, which results in an increased plasma LDL.

Familial dysbetalipoproteinaemia

Familial dysbetalipoproteinaemia is rare, with a prevalence of 1/10 000. It occurs due to inheritance of an abnormal apolipoprotein E molecule. It results in the increased accumulation of IDL (remnants) in the blood. Patients have an increased risk of coronary heart disease.

The clinical features are palmar xanthomas and tuberous xanthomas over the knees and elbows.

Familial hypertriglyceridaemia

It is an autosomal dominant disorder caused by an increased synthesis of VLDL by the liver, leading to a raised plasma VLDL. Other risk factors such as obesity and alcohol are also implicated in its aetiology, leading to an increase in plasma VLDL and chylomicrons. Plasma triacylglycerol is very high and consequently there is usually high plasma cholesterol.

The increased triacylglycerol concentration is associated with an increased risk of pancreatitis. Patients may present with eruptive xanthomas and lipaemia retinalis.

Common hypercholesterolaemia

This includes patients who have a raised serum cholesterol but do not have familial hypercholesterolaemia. Its inheritance is polygenic: that is, it is influenced by several genes. The plasma cholesterol is not as high as in familial hypercholesterolaemia and is influenced by the environment (e.g. diet). Dietary treatment alone is often successful.

KETONE BODIES AND KETOGENESIS

The roles of the ketone bodies

Ketone bodies, acetoacetic acid, 3-hydroxybutyric acid and acetone, provide an alternative fuel for cells and are produced at low levels at all times. They are only produced in significant quantities during states such as starvation, prolonged intense exercise or uncontrolled diabetes. A large increase in ketone bodies decreases blood pH (acidaemia), leading to ketoacidosis.

Starvation

In the fed state, the brain uses only glucose as its energy source, since fatty acids do not cross the blood–brain barrier. During starvation, the brain adapts to using ketone bodies as its major fuel because they are soluble and therefore can cross the barrier. This reduces the need for glucose when glycogen reserves are depleted. In such starved state, glucose comes from the breakdown of muscle protein into amino acids, which are then oxidized to glucose by gluconeogenesis. Therefore, the use of ketone bodies as a fuel spares glucose and preserves muscle protein. In starvation the production of ketone bodies is usually equal to their rate of use. This prevents their accumulation and the decrease in blood pH.

Diabetes

In well-controlled diabetes, tissues receive an adequate glucose supply, and ketone body production is minimal. Poorly controlled diabetes leads to the massive production of acidic ketone bodies, to the point where the rate of formation is far greater than the rate of use. This, as the accumulation of hydrogen ions exceeds the buffering capacity of the blood, can lead to life-threatening ketoacidosis..

Synthesis of ketone bodies

Ketone bodies are formed from acetyl CoA arising mainly from the β oxidation of fatty acids (Fig. 4.29).

Location
Liver mitochondria.

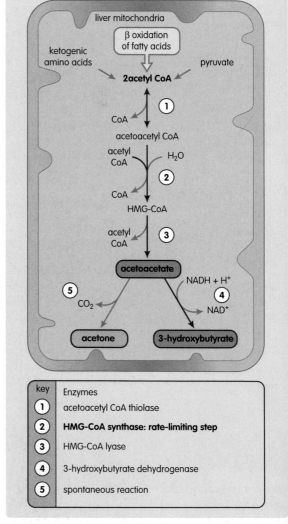

Fig. 4.29 Synthesis of ketone bodies. The five-step pathway to synthesize ketone bodies takes place in liver mitochondria; the first two steps are the same as for cholesterol synthesis.

Pathway

The synthesis of ketone bodies (ketogenesis) is a five-step pathway and is illustrated in Fig. 4.29. Three molecules of acetyl CoA condense to form HMG-CoA, which is then cleaved to acetoacetate. The first two reactions are the same as for cholesterol synthesis, but ketone bodies are formed in the mitochondria, whereas cholesterol is synthesized in the cytosol (see Fig. 4.17).

3-Hydroxybutyrate is formed by the reduction of acetoacetate. The ratio of 3-hydroxybutyrate to acetoacetate formed depends on the availability of NADH.

Spontaneous decarboxylation of acetoacetate forms acetone, but usually only a small amount is made. Acetone can be smelt on the breath when the concentration of ketone bodies is high, especially in people with poorly controlled diabetes.

Control of the pathway

Acetyl CoA formed by β oxidation of fatty acids usually enters the TCA cycle. During starvation or diabetes, the oxaloacetate necessary for acetyl CoA to combine with, to form citrate, is directed to gluconeogenesis to help maintain the blood glucose. Therefore, acetyl CoA is used to form ketone bodies instead.

Use of ketone bodies

Ketone bodies are carried in the blood to various tissues, mainly the heart, muscle and the brain, where they are oxidized in mitochondria to acetyl CoA, which can enter the TCA cycle (Fig. 4.30). Ketone bodies are important sources of energy for these tissues. In fact, the heart uses ketone bodies as a fuel in preference to glucose. The liver cannot use ketone bodies as a fuel source despite being the site of their synthesis because it lacks 3-ketoacyl CoA transferase. Erythrocytes cannot metabolize ketone bodies because they have no mitochondria.

Metabolic adaptation to starvation, exercise and diabetes are very common topics for exam questions. The use of ketone bodies as fuel is just one of the adaptation mechanisms. You must know which fuels are used and why.

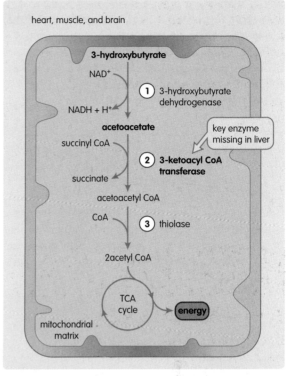

Fig. 4.30 Oxidation and utilization of ketone bodies. The pathway includes three reactions:
1. The oxidation of 3-hydroxybutyrate back to acetoacetate.
2. The activation of acetoacetate, which involves the transfer of CoA from succinyl CoA, catalysed by 3-ketoacyl CoA transferase. Therefore, only tissues with this enzyme can oxidize ketone bodies (it cannot take place in the liver).
3. Thiolase cleaves acetoacetyl CoA to produce two molecules of acetyl CoA, which enter the TCA cycle for oxidation and ATP production.

During starvation, the advantage of switching to ketone bodies as the source of energy is that it decreases the need for endogenous glucose production (gluconeogenesis) that uses muscle proteins and eventually leads to muscle wasting. This 'glucose-sparing' effect of ketone bodies is an important adaptation to starvation.

ATP yield from the oxidation of ketone bodies

The oxidation of 3-hydroxybutyrate produces two molecules of acetyl CoA. The oxidation of each acetyl CoA by the TCA cycle yields 10 molecules of ATP. There is no net formation of NADH (the NADH formed in the breakdown of 3-hydroxybutyrate is used in its synthesis). So, the oxidation of 3-hydroxybutyrate produces 20 molecules of ATP. However, in order to calculate the true, total ATP yield from the oxidation of a ketone body, it is necessary to take into account the origin of the acetyl CoA. For example, if the acetyl CoA used in the synthesis of 3-hydroxybutyrate arose from the oxidation of a fatty acid, a total of 26 molecules of ATP would be generated (Fig. 4.31). The ATP yield from the oxidation of a glucose molecule is 32 ATP (see Fig. 2.20). Therefore, the ATP yield from the oxidation of a ketone body is comparable with that of glucose, showing that ketone bodies are an excellent energy source and substitute for glucose during states such as starvation.

Fig. 4.31 ATP yield from the oxidation of 3-hydroxybutyrate if the acetyl CoA from which it was synthesized was derived from a fatty acid

	ATP yield
Two ATP required to activate fatty acid → acyl CoA	−2

To form two acetyl CoA, fatty acid undergoes two rounds of β oxidation
    release two NADH → electron transport chain
    release two $FADH_2$ → electron transport chain
	5
	
	3

Oxidation of two molecules acetyl CoA by TCA cycle	20
Total	26 ATP

Protein metabolism

Objectives

You should be able to:

- Define essential and non-essential amino acids.
- Contrast the two main pathways of protein degradation.
- Describe the urea cycle, its regulation and function.
- Describe the process and regulation of gluconeogenesis.
- Compare and contrast amino acid metabolism in the absorptive and post-absorptive state.

BIOSYNTHESIS OF NON-ESSENTIAL AMINO ACIDS

Essential amino acids

In the body there are 20 amino acids, nine of which are essential; the other 11 are non-essential. The essential amino acids cannot be synthesized by the body and have to be obtained from the diet.

These nine essential amino acids are:

- Phenylalanine (Phe).
- Valine (Val).
- Tryptophan (Trp).
- Threonine (Thr).
- Isoleucine (Ile).
- Methionine (Met).
- Histidine (His).
- Lysine (Lys).
- Leucine (Leu).

Non-essential amino acids

These 11 amino acids can be synthesized by the body from intermediates of the TCA cycle and other metabolic pathways. They are:

A good mnemonic for remembering the essential amino acids is 'Private Tim Hill', abbreviated as: PVT TIM HiLL

- Tyrosine (Tyr).
- Glycine (Gly).
- Alanine (Ala).
- Cysteine (Cys).
- Serine (Ser).
- Aspartate (Asp).
- Asparagine (Asn).
- Glutamate (Glu).
- Glutamine (Gln).
- Arginine (Arg).
- Proline (Pro).

Although arginine is synthesized by the body, the rate of synthesis is insufficient to meet the needs during periods of rapid cell growth (infancy, childhood or illness); thus it is considered as an essential amino acid during such periods.

The pathways for the synthesis of non-essential amino acids will be considered in this chapter.

Key reactions of amino acid metabolism

There are two main reactions essential to amino acid metabolism: transamination and oxidative deamination.

Transamination: means of conversion of one amino acid into another

Working definition

Aminotransferases (or transaminases) catalyse the transfer of the α-amino group (NH_3^+) from an amino acid to an α-ketoacid (either pyruvate, oxaloacetate or, most often, α-ketoglutarate) (Fig. 5.1). A new amino acid and a new keto acid are formed. If the acceptor is α-ketoglutarate, then glutamate is produced. All transamination reactions are fully reversible. Remember, the amino group is not released.

Site

Aminotransferases are found in both the cytosol and the mitochondria.

Mechanism

Aminotransferases require pyridoxal phosphate (PLP), a vitamin B_6 derivative, as a cofactor.

Pyridoxal phosphate is covalently linked to a lysine residue in the active site of the enzyme and takes part in the reaction. The two most important aminotransferases are alanine aminotransferase (ALT) and aspartate aminotransferase (AST).

Aminotransferases are central to amino acid metabolism. They are used for the synthesis and breakdown of amino acids. During breakdown, all amino groups are ultimately transferred to α-ketoglutarate because only glutamate can undergo oxidative deamination.

Transamination involving essential amino acids is normally unidirectional since the body cannot synthesize the equivalent α-keto acid.

Oxidative deamination: removal of the amino group

Glutamate dehydrogenase removes the amino group from glutamate, leaving behind the carbon skeleton (Fig. 5.2). The ammonia formed enters the urea cycle (see later) and the carbon skeletons (α-keto acids) are all glycolytic and TCA cycle intermediates. Glutamate dehydrogenase is specific for glutamate and it can use either NAD^+ or $NADP^+$ as a cofactor.

Site

Mitochondria.

Control

The reaction is reversible. ATP and GTP allosterically inhibit the enzyme; GDP and ADP activate it. When energy levels are low, amino acids are deaminated to produce α-ketoglutarate for the TCA cycle to generate energy. Deamination can also be achieved by other minor enzymes (see later).

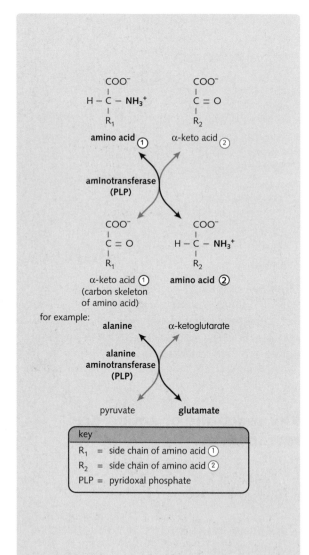

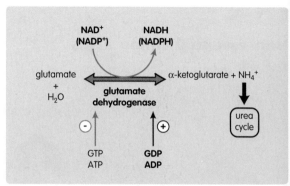

Fig. 5.1 Transamination reaction. Aminotransferases (or transaminases) catalyse the transfer of the α-amino group (NH_3^+), from an amino acid to an α-ketoacid (either pyruvate, oxaloacetate or, most often, α-ketoglutarate).

Fig. 5.2 Oxidative deamination of glutamate. Glutamate dehydrogenase removes the amino group from glutamate, leaving behind the carbon skeleton, α-ketoglutarate.

Biosynthetic pathways of non-essential amino acids

Tyrosine

Tyrosine is formed from the hydroxylation of the essential amino acid phenylalanine by phenylalanine hydroxylase (Fig. 5.3). This is an irreversible reaction; therefore phenylalanine cannot be made from tyrosine. The enzyme requires the cofactor tetrahydrobiopterin, which takes part in the hydroxylation. The genetic deficiency of phenylalanine hydroxylase leads to phenylketonuria, a disease characterized by an accumulation of phenylalanine (this is discussed fully below). Tyrosine is a precursor in the synthesis of catecholamines (dopamine, adrenaline and noradrenaline), the pigment melanin and the hormone thyroxine. Its synthesis is regulated by the demand for these molecules.

Serine, glycine and cysteine

These three amino acids are all formed from glycolytic intermediates. Both glycine and cysteine can be formed from serine.

Serine synthesis

There are a number of possible pathways for the synthesis of serine (letters refer to Fig. 5.4).

a. The main pathway takes place in the cytosol. Serine is formed from the glycolytic intermediate 3-phosphoglycerate in three steps: oxidation, transamination to 3-phosphoserine, and hydrolysis to serine.
b. Serine can also be synthesized from glycine in mitochondria. Serine hydroxymethyl transferase transfers a hydroxymethyl group to glycine. The

reaction is reversible; glycine and serine are interconvertible. The enzyme requires pyridoxal phosphate as a cofactor.

Glycine synthesis

c. Glycine synthesis takes place via two main pathways, both of which occur in mitochondria (see Fig. 5.4):
  - Glycine can be formed from CO_2, NH_4^+, and N^5N^{10}-methylene tetrahydrofolate (THF) (a donor of one-carbon units, see Chapter 6) in a reaction catalysed by glycine synthase

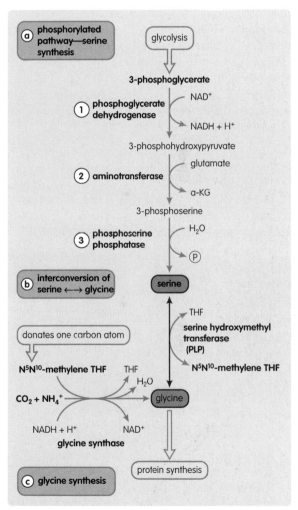

Fig. 5.4 Serine and glycine synthesis. A number of pathways are available to synthesize serine:
a. The main pathway occurs in the cell cytosol.
b. Serine is also synthesized from glycine in mitochondria by serine hydroxymethyl transferase. This is a reversible reaction and therefore is also a pathway for glycine synthesis.
c. Glycine can also be formed from CO_2, NH_4^+ and N^5N^{10}-methylene-THF in mitochondria.

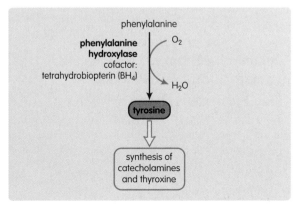

Fig. 5.3 Tyrosine synthesis. Tyrosine is formed by the hydroxylation of the essential amino acid phenylalanine by phenylalanine hydroxylase.

(glycine cleavage enzyme). This is probably the main pathway.

- From serine, by way of serine hydroxymethyl transferase (this is merely a reversal of serine synthesis).

Glycine has many functions in the body:

- It is a component of proteins, especially collagen, and is also used in the synthesis of glutathione, creatine, porphyrins and purine.
- It participates in the metabolism and excretion of drugs.
- It acts as an inhibitory neurotransmitter in the brain.

Cysteine synthesis

Cysteine is formed from serine and the essential amino acid methionine in the cytosol (Fig. 5.5). Cysteine synthesis is dependent on an adequate supply of methionine in the diet. A large number of steps are involved and only the main ones are shown (numbers refer to Fig. 5.5):

1. Activation of methionine and formation of homocysteine (details of this reaction are in Fig. 6.2).
2. Condensation of serine with homocysteine to form cystathionine.
3. Hydrolysis by cystathionase to form cysteine and homoserine.

Alanine

Alanine is formed by a simple one-step transamination of pyruvate (Fig. 5.6). The formation depends on the energy status of the cell and the demand for glycolysis.

Aspartate and asparagine synthesis

Asparagine is a derivative of the acid aspartate (Fig. 5.7).

1. Aspartate is formed by the transamination of oxaloacetate (a TCA cycle intermediate). Aspartate is an important amino acid in metabolism because of its role as an amino group donor in the urea cycle and in purine and pyrimidine synthesis.
2. Asparagine is formed by the transfer of an amide group from glutamine to aspartate. The reaction requires ATP and the equilibrium is in favour of asparagine synthesis.

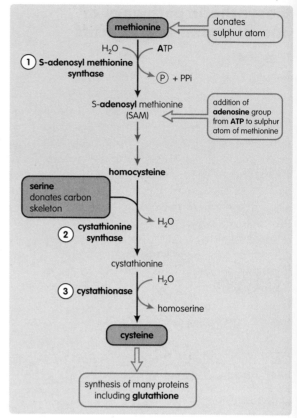

Fig. 5.5 Synthesis of cysteine. Cysteine is formed from serine and the essential amino acid methionine in the cell cytosol. Some of the steps have been omitted.

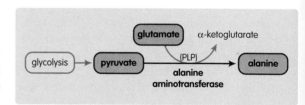

Fig. 5.6 Transamination of pyruvate to form alanine. Alanine is formed by a simple one-step transamination of pyruvate. The formation depends on the demand for glycolysis and energy status of the cell.

Glutamate, glutamine, proline and arginine

These amino acids are grouped together because glutamate is the precursor of the other three. They are all formed from α-ketoglutarate (numbers refer to Fig. 5.8).

1. Glutamate is formed during the reductive amination of α-ketoglutarate by glutamate dehydrogenase. Glutamate plays a key role in amino acid metabolism, since it is the only

amino acid that can undergo oxidative deamination (see Fig. 5.2). Glutamate is also formed by transamination of most other amino acids.

2. Glutamine is formed from the amidation of glutamate by glutamine synthetase (like asparagine). Glutamine is used for purine and pyrimidine synthesis. As well as producing glutamine for protein synthesis, the reaction serves as a pathway for the removal of ammonia in the liver and the kidney.

3. Proline is synthesized from glutamate in three steps: reduction of glutamate to glutamate γ-semialdehyde, spontaneous cyclization to pyrroline-5-carboxylate and reduction to proline.

4. Arginine is formed from the reduction of glutamate to glutamate γ-semialdehyde, which is transaminated to ornithine. Ornithine is metabolized in the urea cycle to form arginine (discussed later in this chapter).

Biological derivatives of amino acids

Amino acids also act as precursors for the biosynthesis of:

- Purines and pyrimidines (see Chapter 6).
- Porphyrins (see Chapter 6).
- Neurotransmitters (i.e serotonin, dopamine, adrenaline, noradrenaline).
- Hormones (i.e thyroxine, melatonin).

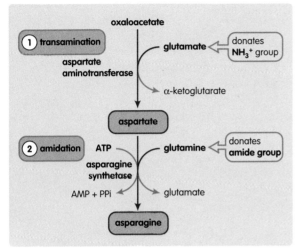

Fig. 5.7 Synthesis of aspartate and asparagine. Aspartate is formed by the transamination of oxaloacetate (1). Asparagine is formed by transfer of an amide group from glutamine to aspartate (2) (refer to text).

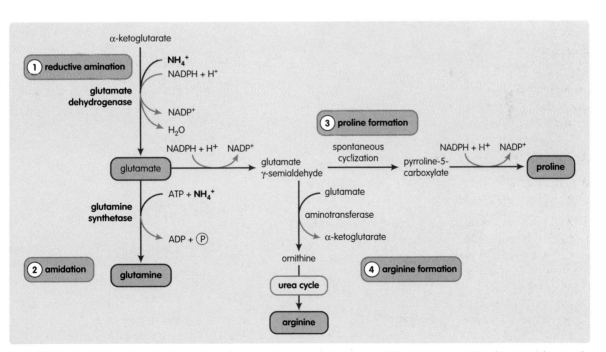

Fig. 5.8 Synthesis of glutamate, glutamine, proline and arginine. Glutamate is the precursor of the other amino acids in this group. They are all formed from α-ketoglutarate (numbers refer to text).

Serotonin (5-hydroxytryptamine) is formed from the hydroxylation of tryptophan by tryptophan hydroxylase, a tetrahydrobiopterin-dependent enzyme, followed by decarboxylation by a pyridoxal phosphate-containing enzyme. It is a neurotransmitter in the brain and causes contraction of smooth muscle of arterioles and bronchioles (Fig. 5.9).

The neurotransmitters dopamine, adrenaline and noradrenaline are derivatives of the amino acid tyrosine (Fig. 5.10). Tyrosine hydroxylase, which requires tetrahydrobiopterin as a cofactor, acts on tyrosine to produce dihydroxyphenylalanine (DOPA). DOPA then undergoes decarboxylation by DOPA decarboxylase, with pyridoxal phosphate as cofactor, to form dopamine. The adrenal medulla converts dopamine to noradrenaline by the enzyme dopamine-β-hydroxylase. Noradrenaline is further converted to adrenaline by the enzyme phenylethanolamine N-methyltransferase.

Tyrosine is also a precursor of the thyroid hormones, thyroxine (T_4) and triiodothyronine (T_3). The uptake of iodine by the thyroid gland is incorporated into tyrosine residues on the thyroglobulin protein. The tyrosines are iodinated at one (monoiodotyrosine) or two (diiodotyrosine) sites and then coupled to form the active hormones (diiodotyrosine + diiodotyrosine → tetraiodothyronine (thyroxine, T_4); diiodotyrosine + monoiodotyrosine → triiodothyronine (T_3)).

The hormone melatonin (N-acetyl-5-methoxytryptamine) is a sleep-inducing molecule. It is formed from serotonin through the actions of arylalkylamine N-acetyltransferase (AANAT) and hydroxyindole-O-methyltransferase (Fig. 5.9); both enzymes are present in the pineal gland and retina. Melatonin is involved in the regulation of the circadian rhythm and is mainly synthesized at night.

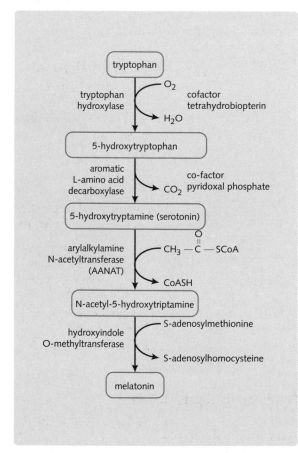

Fig. 5.9 Synthesis of serotonin and melatonin from trypothan.

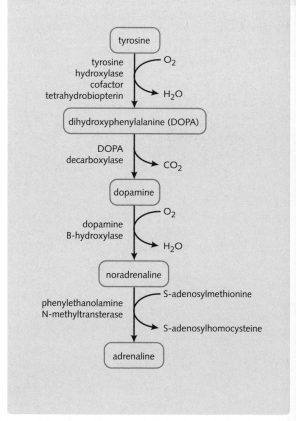

Fig. 5.10 Synthesis of dopamine, noradrenaline and adrenaline from tyrosine.

It has been proposed that brain concentration of neurotransmitters is associated with mood disorders. In depression, there is insufficient serotonin present for neurotransmission, resulting in depressed brain function. This has led to the use of selective-serotonin reuptake inhibitors, SSRIs (e.g. Prozac), which increases synaptic concentrations of serotonin, as a treatment for depression.

The amino acid pool can be thought of in terms of a sink without a plug, therefore requiring a continual daily input to keep it topped up, because protein is not stored.

It is not necessary to learn these pathways in detail; a basic outline is all you need. Fig. 5.11 is an overview of amino acid synthesis. If all fails just learn that!

PROTEIN BREAKDOWN AND THE DISPOSAL OF NITROGEN

Protein turnover

There is a continual turnover of protein: proteins in the body are constantly being synthesized from amino acids and degraded back to them.

Amino acid pool

There is a pool of amino acids present in the body which remains in equilibrium with tissue protein (Fig. 5.12). Amino acids are continually taken from the pool for protein synthesis and replaced through the hydrolysis of dietary and tissue protein. Any amino acids not immediately used are lost, since protein cannot be stored. In a healthy adult, the total amount of protein in the body is constant; because the rate of protein synthesis is equal to the rate of protein breakdown. In an average 70 kg person, about 300 g of protein is synthesized each day and 300 g is degraded. Fig. 5.13 shows how this protein is used.

Nitrogen balance

The breakdown of protein leads to a net daily loss of nitrogen (as urea) from the body, which corresponds to about 35–55 g protein lost. Therefore, a diet must provide at least 35–55 g of protein daily.

Because under these conditions, dietary intake is equal to the loss, the body is said to be in nitrogen balance.

Positive nitrogen balance

This occurs when nitrogen intake is greater than nitrogen loss. Conditions associated with this are:

- Growth.
- Pregnancy.
- Convalescence.

Negative nitrogen balance

This occurs when nitrogen intake is less than nitrogen loss from the body. Conditions associated with this are:

- Malnutrition.
- Starvation.
- Cachexia (seen in advanced stages of cancer).
- Post-traumatic state (surgery, severe burns or sepsis).
- Lack of an essential amino acid (remember, all 20 are needed for protein synthesis).
  This is discussed further in Chapter 8.

Rate of protein turnover

Between 1% to 2% of the total body protein is turned over daily. The rate of turnover varies for individual proteins:

- Regulatory proteins (i.e. digestive enzymes, lactate dehydrogenase or RNA polymerase) have short half-lives (minutes to hours).
- Structural proteins (i.e. collagen) usually have long half-lives : they last for years.
- Haemoglobin has an intermediate half-life of about 120 days.

Protein degradation

There are two possible pathways for protein degradation; both resulting in the breakdown of proteins to their constituent amino acids by proteases.

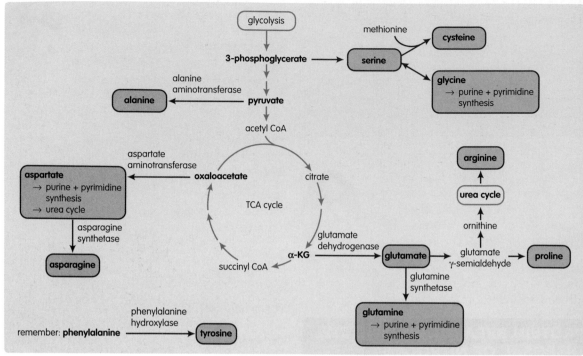

Fig. 5.11 Overview of the biosynthesis of non-essential amino acids. If all else fails, just learn this!

Fig. 5.12 Amino acid pool in the body is in dynamic equilibrium with tissue proteins.

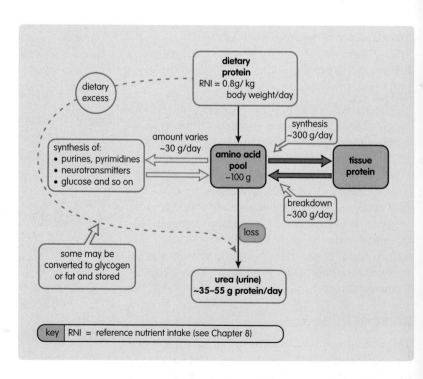

Fig. 5.13 Daily turnover of tissue proteins. In an average 70 kg person the daily turnover of protein is about 300 g/day

Amount	Use
70 g	Turnover of digestive enzymes and gut cells
20 g	Synthesis of plasma proteins
8 g	Synthesis of haemoglobin
20 g	White blood cell turnover
75–100 g	Turnover of muscle cells
80–100 g	Various synthetic pathways
	N.B. under certain conditions (e.g. stress, infection or pregnancy) the synthesis of certain proteins may increase

Ubiquitin pathway

The ubiquitin pathway degrades abnormal proteins and short-lived cytosolic proteins; it is ATP-dependent and is located in the cytosol (Fig. 5.14).

Structure of ubiquitin

Ubiquitin is a small, basic protein that binds to proteins to be targeted for degradation. It is a 'tagging' system. At the carboxyl terminal, ubiquitin, has a glycine residue that attaches to lysine residues on target proteins to form: ubiquitin-C-glycine–lysine-target protein complex.

The sequence of events

The ubiquitin pathway consists of four stages (steps below refer to Fig. 5.14): the enzymes E1, E2 and E3 participate in the pathway.

1. The activation of ubiquitin by attachment to E1, the ubiquitin activating enzyme. The reaction is driven by the hydrolysis of ATP.
2. The transfer of activated ubiquitin to E2, the ubiquitin carrier molecule.
3. E3 transfers ubiquitin to the target protein. The E3 enzyme 'reads' the N-terminal amino acid on proteins to determine whether a protein may be tagged with ubiquitin (see below).
4. The degradation of the tagged protein by 26S protease complex (endopeptidase also called megapain) to peptides.

Lysosomal pathway

The second pathway of protein degradation is the lysosomal pathway. It degrades long-lived membrane or extracellular proteins, and cellular organelles (i.e mitochondria). It is ATP-independent and is located

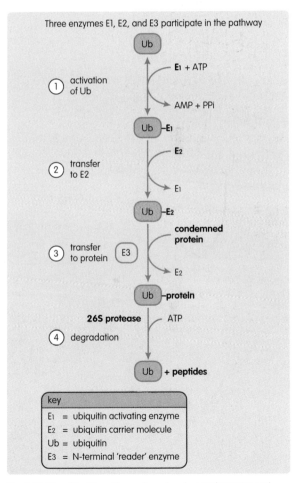

Fig. 5.14 The ubiquitin pathway degrades abnormal proteins and short-lived cytosolic proteins; it is ATP-dependent and is located in the cytosol (numbers refer to text).

in lysosomes (Fig. 5.15). The proteins, to be degraded, must enter lysosomes, and there are two processes by which they can do this:

- Endocytosis; the internalization of extracellular proteins for degradation in lysosomes.
- Autophagy, where intracellular proteins or organelles are engulfed by the plasma membrane or endoplasmic reticulum to form autophagosomes.

Both results in the degradation of proteins by lysosomal proteases (cathepsins).

Lysosomal activity, and therefore protein degradation, increases in starvation (increased protein breakdown provides substrates for gluconeogenesis) and in many disease states, including diabetes, hyperthyroidism and chronic inflammatory diseases.

Signals for degradation

Protein degradation is not random but is affected by structural characteristics of the protein.

N-end rule

Proteins are divided into short- and long-lived by the nature of their amino-terminal (N-terminal) amino acid. It is the E3 enzyme that reads the N-terminal residues.

- Methionine, glycine, alanine and serine stabilize the N-terminal. These amino acids are not easily tagged by ubiquitin, and proteins containing them have long half-lives.
- Phenylalanine, tryptophan, aspartate, arginine and lysine destabilize the N-terminal and are signals for rapid ubiquitin tagging.

PEST region

Proteins containing PEST regions (–Pro–Glu–Ser–Thr; named according to the one-letter nomenclature for amino acids) are rapidly degraded and have short half-lives. An example is cAMP-dependent protein kinase.

Conformational changes

The binding of ligands to receptors often causes a conformational change that may expose a PEST region or a region susceptible to protease action.

Disposal of protein nitrogen and the urea cycle

An overview

Any amino acids surplus to the body's requirements are degraded. The amino group is removed, forming ammonia. Because ammonia is extremely toxic, it is

Fig. 5.15 The lysosomal pathway degrades long-lived, membrane or extracellular proteins and organelles, for example mitochondria. Extracellular proteins enter cells by endocytosis where, as intracellular proteins, they are engulfed by the endoplasmic reticulum to form autophagosomes.

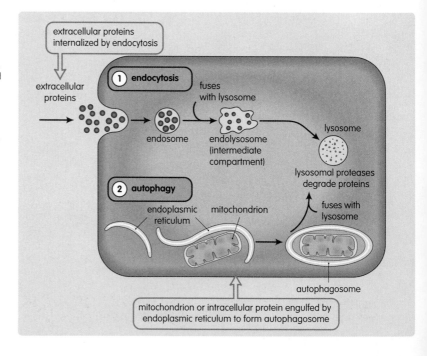

converted into non-toxic urea, by the urea cycle, for excretion in the urine. A small amount of ammonia can also be incorporated into glutamine (see Fig. 5.8). The removal of the amino group from amino acids leaves behind the carbon skeletons (α-keto acids). Their metabolism is discussed later in this chapter.

The major site of amino acid degradation is the liver. Nitrogen disposal can be divided into two main stages:

- The removal of the amino group from amino acids.
- The formation of urea via the ornithine cycle.

These two stages are now considered in more detail.

Removal of amino group

There are two possible routes for the removal of the amino group.

Transdeamination

This route consists of an initial transamination in the cytosol, followed by oxidative deamination in mitochondria (see Figs 5.1 and 5.2):

- α-ketoglutarate accepts an amino group from donor amino acids to form glutamate in a cytosolic reaction catalysed by aminotransferase.
- The glutamate is then transported by the glutamate carrier into the mitochondria where it is oxidatively deaminated by glutamate dehydrogenase to form α-ketoglutarate and ammonium ions.

Transamination

This involves two transamination reactions (numbers refer to Fig. 5.16):

1. The first reaction transfers the amino group to α-ketoglutarate, forming glutamate.
2. The second reaction, catalysed by aspartate aminotransferases, transfers the amino group from glutamate to oxaloacetate, forming aspartate.

Aspartate then enters the urea cycle by condensing with citrulline. Thus, a second amino group enters the urea cycle, providing a second nitrogen atom to form urea.

Deamination can also be achieved by other enzymes, but these are only minor pathways. For example, there is a non-specific L-amino acid oxidase, but it is not very important physiologically. There are also specific enzymes such as serine and threonine dehydratases, which deaminate serine and threonine respectively, by removal of H_2O and NH_4^+, and cysteine desulphydrase, which deaminates cysteine and produces hydrogen sulphide as a by-product.

Formation of urea by the ornithine cycle

The urea cycle consists of five reactions (described below) that synthesize the organic compound urea from two inorganic compounds, CO_2 and NH_4^+ (Fig. 5.17). Urea (NH_2–CO–NH_2) contains two nitrogen atoms: one nitrogen is supplied by ammonia formed by the transdeamination of amino acids; the other derives from aspartate. The cycle uses a carrier molecule, ornithine, which is regenerated (this is similar to the way the TCA cycle uses oxaloacetate).

Location

Liver hepatocytes, mainly the periportal cells.

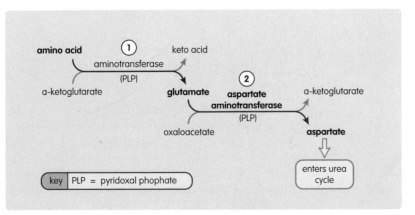

Fig. 5.16 The transamination route involves two transamination reactions.

Fig. 5.17 The urea cycle consists of five reactions that yield the organic compound urea from two inorganic compounds: CO_2 and NH_4.

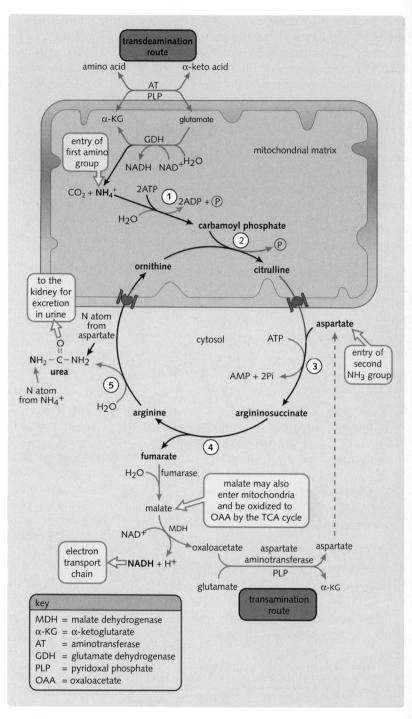

Site

The first two reactions occur in mitochondria, the last three in the cytosol.

Urea cycle

Numbers refer to Fig. 5.17.

1. Formation of carbamoyl phosphate

This is the irreversible, rate-limiting step of the pathway, catalysed by carbamoyl phosphate synthase I (CPS I). The reaction consumes two molecules of ATP. (There is also a carbamoyl phosphate synthase II enzyme in the cytosol but this is only involved in pyrimidine synthesis [see Chapter 6].)

2. Formation of citrulline

The carbamoyl group is transferred to ornithine by ornithine transcarbamoylase to form citrulline. Specific transporters for citrulline and ornithine are present in the inner mitochondrial membrane.

3. Synthesis of argininosuccinate

Argininosuccinate synthase catalyses the condensation of citrulline with aspartate. The reaction is driven by the cleavage of ATP to AMP and pyrophosphate, which in turn is rapidly hydrolysed to two inorganic phosphates. Therefore the reaction consumes two ATP equivalents.

4. Cleavage of argininosuccinate to fumarate and arginine by argininosuccinate lyase

5. Cleavage of arginine to ornithine and urea by arginase

Arginase is specific to the liver; therefore only the liver can produce urea. The urea formed is transported in the blood to the kidneys for excretion in urine.

Fate of fumarate

The fumarate formed is converted to malate by fumarase. Malate can either be converted to oxaloacetate and then aspartate in the cytosol as shown in Fig. 5.17, or it can be transported into mitochondria and enter the TCA cycle. Either way, the NADH formed can be oxidized by the electron transport chain to produce 2.5 molecules of ATP.

The ATP balance in the urea cycle

In the overall reactions:

- Four ATP equivalents are consumed for every molecule of urea formed (reactions 1 and 3).
- The conversion of fumarate to oxaloacetate produces NADH, which is oxidized by the electron transport chain to generate 2.5 ATP.

Therefore, overall 1.5 ATP are consumed for every molecule of urea formed by the cycle; energy is required, not generated.

Control of the urea cycle

Control can be considered at two levels:

Short-term allosteric control

The main control of the urea cycle is by N-acetyl glutamate (formed from acetyl CoA and glutamate), which allosterically activates carbamoyl phosphate synthase I (CPS I), the enzyme which catalyses the rate-limiting step of the urea cycle. The sequence of events is as follows: following a protein-rich meal, the excess amino acids are deaminated, resulting in an increased concentration of glutamate and consequently, N-acetyl glutamate. N-acetyl glutamate activates CPS I, and thus the urea cycle, which is then able to cope with the extra nitrogen load.

Long-term regulation

Changes in the diet are thought to induce or repress transcription of the urea cycle enzymes. For example, in starvation, the increased breakdown of tissue protein induces the synthesis of enzymes to cope with the extra load of ammonia.

Why is it beneficial to form urea?

Ammonia is toxic. By conversion to urea (a nontoxic, organic compound), it can be easily excreted by the kidneys. Urea possesses a number of characteristics which makes it an efficient nitrogen-eliminating molecule:

- It is a small, uncharged and water-soluble molecule. It can diffuse across membranes easily and be excreted in the urine.
- Nearly 50% of its weight is nitrogen, making it a very efficient nitrogen carrier.
- Relatively little energy is required for its synthesis—only 1.5 ATP are required for every mole of urea formed.

A normal diet produces 35–55 g of urea each day. In birds, ammonia is converted to uric acid for excretion, which is quite insoluble.

Ammonia toxicity

Ammonia is one of the most toxic compounds produced by the body. Elevated levels (hyperammonaemia) can cause symptoms of ammonia intoxication: tremors, slurred speech and blurred vision. At very high concentrations, ammonia causes irreversible brain damage, coma and death. It is therefore essential that ammonia is detoxified rapidly to urea by the liver.

Proposed mechanisms of ammonia toxicity

Ammonia toxicity affects the brain and central nervous system. Whereas the effects of ammonia toxicity are well-known, its mechanism of action is still unclear. An increase in the concentration of ammonia causes a shift in the equilibrium of the

A genetic deficiency in each of the urea cycle enzymes has been identified; all are rare, the most common being ornithine transcarbamoylase deficiency. These deficiencies result in a failure to synthesize urea, leading to hyperammonaemia and irreversible mental retardation from ammonia toxicity. Ammonia toxicity is also seen in patients with liver damage due to cirrhosis.

glutamate dehydrogenase reaction towards glutamate formation (Fig. 5.18). This leads to a depletion of α-ketoglutarate, which results in a decrease in TCA cycle activity and therefore ATP production. Shifting the equilibrium of the reaction also leads to an increase in the ratio of NAD$^+$ to NADH, which also results in a decrease in ATP levels. The brain and nervous system require large amounts of energy and are particularly susceptible to ammonia toxicity.

High levels of ammonia may also react with glutamate, forming glutamine, which may damage the brain directly. Decreasing levels of glutamate (a neurotransmitter) in the brain can also cause problems.

FORMATION OF GLUCOSE FROM NON-CARBOHYDRATE SOURCES

Proteins as an energy source

Fed state

In the fed state, proteins undergo digestion in the stomach and small intestine to release amino acids,

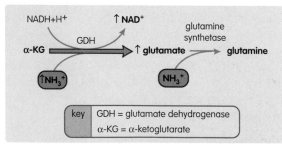

Fig. 5.18 Mechanisms of ammonia toxicity. An increase in the concentration of ammonia causes a shift in the equilibrium of the glutamate dehydrogenase reaction towards glutamate formation, which leads to the depletion of α-ketoglutarate, a substrate of the TCA cycle.

which are taken up by cells and used for the synthesis of body's own proteins and other molecules. However, if amino acids are surplus to the body's requirements, they would either be used directly as a fuel to produce ATP, or converted to glycogen or fat and stored in this form for later use. Amino acids are never stored as protein.

Starvation

During prolonged exercise or starvation, the body has to rely on its energy stores for fuel. Glycogen reserves only last between 12 and 24 hours. The main concern in these states is how to maintain the blood glucose concentration and provide fuel for the brain and erythrocytes. Fat, as has already been shown, cannot be converted to glucose (see Fig. 2.15). In prolonged starvation the brain adapts to using ketone bodies as its main fuel, although some glucose is still required. This is complicated by the fact that the erythrocytes cannot metabolize ketone bodies because they have no mitochondria (see Chapter 4). Therefore, a pathway to maintain constant glucose production is required. Gluconeogenesis is such a pathway and its substrates are the 'alternative' sources of glucose. Lactate and glycerol provide some glucose, but the majority is obtained from the amino acids released during breakdown of muscle protein. Amino acids produced from muscle protein are transaminated to alanine and glutamine, which are then released into the blood. Alanine is taken up by the liver for gluconeogenesis. Glutamine is used as a fuel by the small intestine and is a gluconeogenic substrate in the kidney (the only other organ capable of gluconeogenesis).

Gluconeogenesis

Gluconeogenesis is the production of glucose from non-carbohydrate source. Gluconeogenesis is the process in which glucose is produced from:

- Glycerol (released by triacylglycerol hydrolysis) (see Fig. 4.11).
- Lactate (from anaerobic glycolysis in erythrocytes and active skeletal muscle).
- Amino acids (from the breakdown of muscle protein).

Location

Liver (in prolonged starvation it can also occur in the kidney cortex).

Site

Cell cytosol—except for the first step, the carboxylation of pyruvate, which occurs in mitochondria.

Pathway

Gluconeogenesis is not just a reversal of glycolysis. Although some of the reactions of glycolysis are reversible and are common to both glycolytic and gluconeogenic pathways, the three irreversible reactions of glycolysis, those catalysed by hexokinase, phosphofructokinase-1 (PFK-1) and pyruvate kinase, have to be bypassed. How this is achieved is shown in Fig. 5.19, and explained in stages 1–3 below.

1. Conversion of pyruvate to phosphoenolpyruvate (PEP)

This occurs via two reactions:

a. The carboxylation of pyruvate to oxaloacetate. Pyruvate carboxylase is found in the mitochondria. The oxaloacetate formed cannot cross the inner mitochondrial membrane; therefore it is reduced to malate, which is transported into the cytosol where it is re-oxidized. Pyruvate carboxylase requires the vitamin biotin as a cofactor and its mechanism of action is similar to acetyl CoA carboxylase (see Chapter 4).

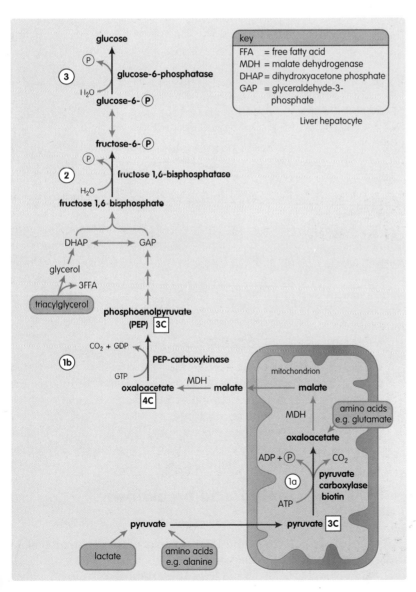

Fig. 5.19 Gluconeogenesis is not simply a reversal of glycolysis. The three essentially irreversible reactions of glycolysis have to be bypassed. The first reaction, the carboxylation of pyruvate to oxaloacetate, occurs in the mitochondrial matrix. The rest of the reactions occur in the cell cytosol. Details of the individual reactions 1 to 3 are found in the text.

b. The decarboxylation and phosphorylation of oxaloacetate by PEP-carboxykinase. The PEP-carboxykinase and the other enzymes involved are in the cytosol.

2. Hydrolysis of fructose 1,6-bisphosphate

The hydrolysis of fructose 1,6-bisphosphate by fructose 1,6-bisphosphatase bypasses the PFK reaction (rate-limiting step of glycolysis).

3. Hydrolysis of glucose-6-phosphate

The hydrolysis of glucose-6-phosphate by glucose-6-phosphatase bypasses the irreversible hexokinase reaction to form free glucose. Glucose-6-phosphatase is unique to the liver.

Regulation of gluconeogenesis

Gluconeogenesis is active during fasting and starvation (Fig. 5.20).

Hormonal control

In starvation, the levels of glucagon, cortisol and adrenocorticotrophic hormone (ACTH) are high, which activates gluconeogenesis and inhibits glycolysis. The actions of glucagon are:

- It activates a cAMP-dependent protein kinase, which causes phosphorylation and inactivation of pyruvate kinase in the glycolytic pathway (see Fig. 2.10).
- Through phosphorylation of a bifunctional enzyme, 6-phosphofructo-2-kinase/fructose 2,6-bisphosphatase, it decreases the concentration of fructose 2,6-bisphosphate, the allosteric activator of phosphofructokinase-1 (glycolytic enzyme) but inhibitor of fructose 1,6-bisphosphatase (gluconeogenic enzyme). Thus it decreases the rate of glycolysis and increases gluconeogenesis.
- It increases the rate of transcription of PEP-carboxykinase gene.
- It inhibits the rate of transcription of pyruvate kinase gene.

Allosteric activation by acetyl CoA

During starvation, the rate of lipolysis and β oxidation is high, leading to a large increase in the amount of acetyl CoA. Acetyl CoA allosterically activates pyruvate carboxylase, stimulating gluconeogenesis. It has an opposite, inhibitory effect on pyruvate dehydrogenase. Therefore, the formed

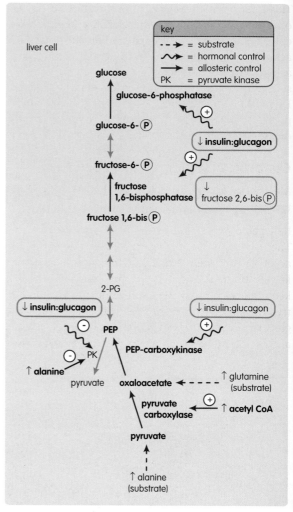

Fig. 5.20 Regulation of gluconeogenesis: fasting and starved state. Control is at two levels. Hormonal control: glucagon activates gluconeogenesis. Allosteric control: acetyl CoA activates pyruvate carboxylase. An increased supply of amino acids, alanine and glutamine activate gluconeogenesis.

pyruvate will be channelled into gluconeogenesis rather than into the TCA cycle.

An increased supply of substrates, particularly of the amino acids alanine and glutamine, favours gluconeogenesis. A high concentration of cortisol favours mobilization of amino acids from muscle.

Amino acid breakdown

Amino acid breakdown involves two stages:

- The removal of amino groups by transamination and oxidative deamination (see Figs 5.1 and 5.2).
- The catabolism of the carbon skeletons.

The carbon skeletons of amino acids can be metabolized to intermediates of the TCA cycle and glycolytic pathway. The breakdown of all 20 amino acids converges to yield seven products: pyruvate, acetyl CoA, acetoacetyl CoA, α-ketoglutarate, succinyl CoA, fumarate and oxaloacetate (Fig. 5.21). Depending on the energy status of the cell, these products can either be oxidized to generate energy or used to synthesize glycogen or fat.

Concepts of amino acid catabolism

Metabolically, amino acids can be classified into two types: ketogenic and glucogenic.

Ketogenic amino acids

These are amino acids that are broken down to either acetyl CoA or acetoacetyl CoA; they are able to form ketone bodies. Only leucine and lysine are purely ketogenic (see Fig. 5.21). Isoleucine, phenylalanine, tryptophan and tyrosine are both ketogenic and glucogenic; their breakdown yields both acetyl CoA and acetoacetyl CoA and some precursors of glucose.

Glucogenic amino acids

These are amino acids that can be broken down to either pyruvate or one of the intermediates of the TCA cycle. They are then channelled into gluconeogenesis for glucose synthesis (glucogenic).

Pathways of amino acid catabolism

Amino acids can be divided into seven groups based on their breakdown product. Several breakdown pathways are possible for each amino acid, but only the main ones are discussed here:

- Five amino acids form pyruvate: alanine, serine, glycine, cysteine and threonine (Fig. 5.22). Note that hydroxyproline can also be converted to pyruvate.
- Two amino acids form oxaloacetate:
  - Aspartate: by its transamination by aspartate aminotransferase.
  - Asparagine: its hydrolysis by asparaginase releases ammonia and yields aspartate, which undergoes transamination to oxaloacetate.

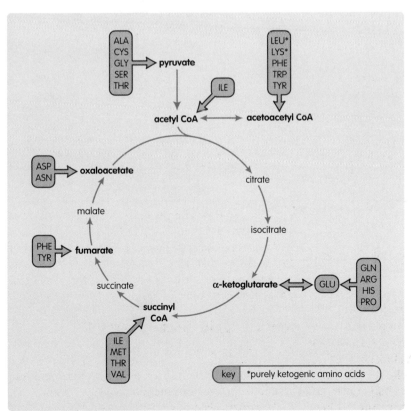

Fig. 5.21 Entry points of amino acid carbon skeletons into the TCA cycle and glycolytic pathways. The breakdown of all 20 amino acids converges to yield seven products: pyruvate, acetyl CoA, acetoacetyl CoA, α-ketoglutarate, succinyl CoA, fumarate and oxaloacetate. These products, depending on the energy status of the cell, can either be oxidized to generate energy or used to synthesize glycogen or fat.

- Five amino acids form glutamate and α-ketoglutarate (Fig. 5.23).
- Four amino acids form succinyl CoA (Fig. 5.24).
- Phenylalanine and tyrosine form fumarate. The hydroxylation of phenylalanine by phenylalanine hydroxylase produces tyrosine (a reversal of its synthesis – see Fig. 5.3). Tyrosine is then transaminated and undergoes a series of reactions to form fumarate. Since acetoacetyl CoA is also produced, they are both ketogenic and glucogenic amino acids.

- Isoleucine forms acetyl CoA: its breakdown produces both acetyl CoA and succinyl CoA (see Fig. 5.24).
- Leucine, lysine and tryptophan form acetoacetyl CoA (phenylalanine and tyrosine can also produce acetoacetyl CoA). Leucine is a branched-chain amino acid and its breakdown is discussed below.

Lysine undergoes a number of reactions: a reduction to saccharopine, two oxidations to form amino-

Fig. 5.22 Breakdown of amino acids to pyruvate. Six amino acids form pyruvate

Amino acid	Important reactions	Enzymes involved	Product
Alanine	Transamination	Alanine aminotransferase	Pyruvate
Serine	Deamination and dehydration	Serine dehydratase	Pyruvate
Glycine	Methylation to serine followed by dehydration	Serine hydroxymethyl transferase Serine dehydratase	Pyruvate
Cysteine	Two main steps: • oxidation to cysteine sulphinate • transamination	Cysteine dioxygenase Cysteine aminotransferase	Pyruvate
Threonine	Aminoacetone pathway	Threonine dehydrogenase	Pyruvate

Fig. 5.23 Breakdown of amino acids to glutamate and α-ketoglutarate. Five amino acids form glutamate and α-ketoglutarate

Amino acid	Important reactions	Enzymes involved	Product
Glutamine	Hydrolysis	Glutaminase	Glutamate
Glutamate	Oxidative deamination	Glutamate dehydrogenase	α-ketoglutarate
Proline	Two main steps: • oxidation → pyrroline-5-carboxylate • oxidation → glutamate	Proline oxygenase Dehydrogenase	Glutamate
Arginine	Two steps: • cleaved to ornithine (part of urea cycle) • transamination	Arginase Aminotransferase	Glutamate
Histidine	Two main steps: • deamination and hydrolysis to N-formiminoglutamate (FIGlu) • transfer of formimino group to THF	Histidase Glutamate formiminotransferase	Glutamate

Fig. 5.24 Breakdown of amino acids to succinyl CoA. Four amino acids form succinyl CoA (only the important reactions are shown). (SAM, S-adenosylmethionine; BCAA, branched-chain amino acids)

Amino acid	Key reactions	Enzymes involved	Product
Isoleucine (BCAA)	Three reactions: • transamination • oxidative decarboxylation • dehydrogenation	BCAA aminotransferase BCAA α-ketoacid dehydrogenase	Succinyl CoA and acetyl CoA
Valine (BCAA)	All BCAAs have a similar breakdown pathway	As above	Succinyl CoA
Methionine	Condensation with ATP to form SAM hydrolysis to homocysteine	SAM synthase	Succinyl CoA
Threonine	Dehydration to α-ketobutyrate	Threonine dehydratase	Succinyl CoA

adipate, transamination to α-ketoadipate, and then further reactions to eventually form acetoacetyl CoA (it is not necessary to know this in detail). The breakdown of tryptophan is even more complicated!

Branched-chain amino acids (BCAA)

The BCAAs are isoleucine, leucine and valine; these are degraded by a common pathway of three reactions:

- Transamination: a branched-chain amino acid aminotransferase transaminates all three amino acids.
- Oxidative decarboxylation: by a branched-chain α-ketoacid dehydrogenase, which requires thiamine pyrophosphate as a cofactor. A deficiency of this enzyme causes an accumulation of the keto acids derived from BCAAs in the urine; this is called maple syrup urine disease (see below).
- Dehydrogenation.

Not all tissues can oxidize BCAAs: the liver has limited ability for this because it lacks the branched-chain amino acid aminotransferase. BCAAs are mainly oxidized by peripheral tissues, particularly muscle.

DISORDERS OF AMINO ACID METABOLISM

Disorders of amino acid metabolism are very rare inborn errors of metabolism that result in severe developmental abnormalities if untreated. They include phenylketonuria, albinism, alkaptonuria, maple syrup urine disease and histidinaemia.

Phenylketonuria

Phenylketonuria (PKU) is an autosomal recessive disorder resulting from deficiency of the enzyme phenylalanine hydroxylase. In some patients it may be due to a deficiency in the enzymes that synthesize its cofactor tetrahydrobiopterin (see Fig. 5.3). The disease is characterized by an increased plasma phenylalanine level. It has a prevalence of 1:10 000–20 000 live births.

Mechanism

Normally, phenylalanine hydroxylase catalyses the hydroxylation of phenylalanine to tyrosine. Tyrosine is an important amino acid: it is the precursor of dopamine, catecholamines and melanin. In PKU, phenylalanine accumulates in the plasma and tissues and is converted into phenylketones (phenylpyruvate, phenyllactate and phenylacetate), which are not normally produced in significant

You are not going to be asked to discuss the different degradation pathways of the amino acids. Know about transamination and deamination reactions, and where the amino acid carbon skeletons feed into the TCA cycle; learn Fig. 5.21.

Fig. 5.25 Diagnosis and clinical features of phenylketonuria

Clinical features	Diagnosis and management
Central nervous system involvement: untreated, presents at 6–12 months with development delay, failure to thrive and seizures **Hypopigmentation**: many affected infants are fair-haired, blue eyed and pale, since phenylalanine inhibits tyrosinase which converts tyrosine to melanin	All neonates are screened for raised phenylalanine levels at 5–7 days, when milk feeding is established (so the phenylalanine levels are adequate); part of Guthrie test **Management**: • restriction of dietary phenylalanine • blood phenylalanine levels are monitored regularly and maintained in the normal range to allow normal growth and development

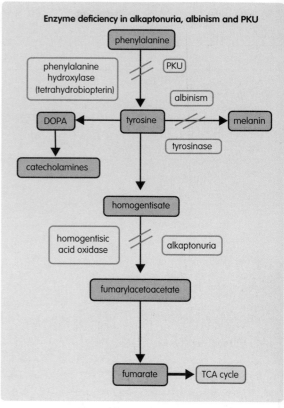

Fig. 5.26 Enzyme deficiencies in alkaptonuria, albinism and phenylketonuria (PKU).

amounts. High levels of phenylalanine may impair development and in the long-term can cause mental retardation (Fig. 5.25).

Treatment of phenylketonuria is by restriction of dietary phenylalanine. However, phenylalanine is an essential amino acid, therefore too much dietary restriction can also cause poor growth and neurological symptoms. Patients with PKU cannot make tyrosine and it becomes an essential amino acid.

Pregnancy
In PKU patients, the restriction of dietary phenylalanine is for life. It is particularly important during pregnancy when hyperphenylalaninaemia in the mother may damage the fetus, causing microcephaly, mental retardation and heart defects.

Alkaptonuria
Alkaptonuria is a rare, autosomal recessive disorder with a prevalence of 1:100 000. It is caused by a deficiency of the enzyme homogentisic acid oxidase, normally involved in the breakdown of tyrosine to

In the UK, all newborn babies (at the age of 5–10 days) are screened for phenylketonuria (PKU), congenital hypothyroidism and cystic fibrosis, using what is known as the Guthrie test. This involves obtaining a small sample of blood from a heel prick and placing the droplets of blood on a collection card. The card is then sent to the laboratory for testing.

fumarate (Fig. 5.26). Unlike other amino acid disorders, it does not produce serious effects until adult life.

Mechanism
Enzyme deficiency leads to an accumulation of homogentisate, which polymerizes to produce a black–brown pigment that is deposited in cartilage and other connective tissue. This process is called ochronosis.

Clinical features
Joint damage and arthritis. Homogentisate is excreted in the urine; on standing, the urine turns black because of the formation of alkapton. Sweat may also be black. There is no specific treatment.

Albinism
Albinism is a deficiency of the enzyme tyrosinase which converts tyrosine into melanin. The incidence is 1:13 000. The clinical features and management of albinism are discussed in Fig. 5.27.

Fig. 5.27 Clinical features and management of albinism

Clinical features	Management
Amelanosis: • whitish hair, pale skin, and grey–blue eyes • low pigment in iris and retina leads to failure to develop fixation reflex; resulting in nystagmus, photophobia and constant frowning • pale skin leads to sunburn and skin cancer	Tinted contact lenses from early infancy may allow development of normal fixation in some patients High sun protection In the long term, results in severe visual impairment

Disorders of amino acid metabolism are all rare autosomal recessive disorders, which usually present in neonates with failure to thrive and developmental delay; the treatment is dietary restrictions.

Histidinaemia, homocystinuria and maple syrup urine disease

These three diseases are described in Fig. 5.28.

AMINO ACID METABOLISM IN INDIVIDUAL TISSUES

Amino acid transport

Several transporters carry amino acids across the cell membrane. The concentration of free amino acids outside the cell is much lower than the concentration inside. Therefore most amino acid transporters function as active transport systems in which the movement of amino acids into cells, against their concentration gradient, is driven by the hydrolysis of ATP.

Five main transport systems exist, based on the specificity of the transporter for the side chain of the amino acid (Fig. 5.29).

The γ-glutamyl cycle

Unlike the specific transport systems described in Fig. 5.29, the γ-glutamyl cycle transports a wide range of amino acids into cells, and is particularly active for neutral amino acids.

Function

The γ-glutamyl cycle is responsible for the active transport of amino acids into cells via the synthesis and breakdown of a glutathione carrier (Fig. 5.30). Three molecules of ATP are required for the trans-

Fig. 5.28 Genetically determined amino acid disorders

Disorder	Enzyme defect	Biochemical feature	Clinical features
Histidinaemia 1:10 000	Histidase	↑ histidine in blood and urine	Mental retardation
Homocystinuria (rare)	Cystathionine synthase (see Fig. 5.5)	↑ homocysteine in urine ↑ methionine in blood	Failure to thrive, progressive mental retardation, and dislocation of lens in eye
Maple syrup urine disease 1:200 000 (very rare)	Branched-chain α-ketoacid dehydrogenase	↑ excretion of branched-chain amino acids, valine, leucine and isoleucine and their α-ketoacids in plasma and urine; compounds smell like maple syrup	Neonates present with metabolic acidosis, hypoglycaemia, and seizures Delay in diagnosis leads to neurological problems

port of one amino acid molecule into the cell and the regeneration of glutathione.

Location/site

Kidney renal tubular cells and the endoplasmic reticulum of hepatocytes and brain cells.

Amino acid specificity	Transported amino acids	Diseases resulting from a defect of the carrier system
Small neutral amino acids	Alanine, serine, threonine	Non-specific
Large, neutral and aromatic amino acids	Isoleucine, leucine, valine, tyrosine, tryptophan phenylalanine	Hartnup's disease: a defect in the intestinal and renal transporter for neutral amino acids
Basic amino acids	Arginine, lysine, cysteine, ornithine	Cystinuria: a defect in kidney tubular reabsorption of all four basic amino acids
Proline and glycine	Proline, glycine	Glycinuria
Acidic amino acids	Glutamate, aspartate	Non-specific

Fig. 5.29 Specific transport systems for amino acids

Amino acid metabolism

Amino acids are taken up into tissues by active transport and are used for protein synthesis. Excess amino acids are not stored by the body: those not immediately required are degraded. The role of protein as an energy source has already been mentioned. Here we consider amino acid metabolism in individual tissues during the absorptive (fed) state and post-absorptive (fasting) state.

Absorptive (fed) state

A summary of amino acid metabolism in tissues during the fed state is given in Fig. 5.31.

Small intestine

After a protein-rich meal, protein digestion takes place in the small intestine. The amino acids released are absorbed by intestinal epithelial cells. A large proportion of amino acids are transaminated to alanine, which is released into the portal vein and taken to the liver. Therefore, alanine is the major amino acid secreted by the gut and the principal carrier of nitrogen in the plasma.

Liver

Alanine and other diet-derived amino acids delivered from the small intestine follow a number of possible pathways:

Fig. 5.30 γ-Glutamyl cycle for amino acid transport.

1. Glutathione is formed in the cell and transported to the external surface of the plasma membrane.
2. The enzyme, γ-glutamyl transpeptidase, catalyses the transfer of a γ-glutamyl group from glutathione to the amino acid. This enables uptake of the γ-glutamyl amino acid by the cell (or the cells of other organs if it travels in the blood first).
3. γ-Glutamyl cyclotransferase releases the amino acid for use by the cell.
4. The glutathione is reformed by the action of oxoprolinase, γ-glutamyl-cysteinyl synthetase and glutathione synthetase, in three ATP-dependent reactions.

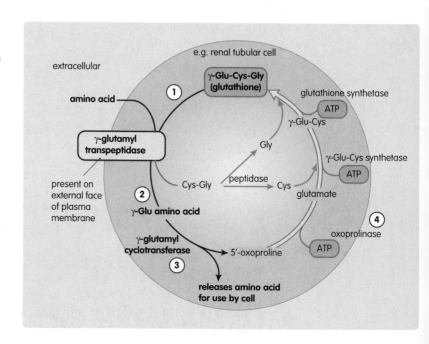

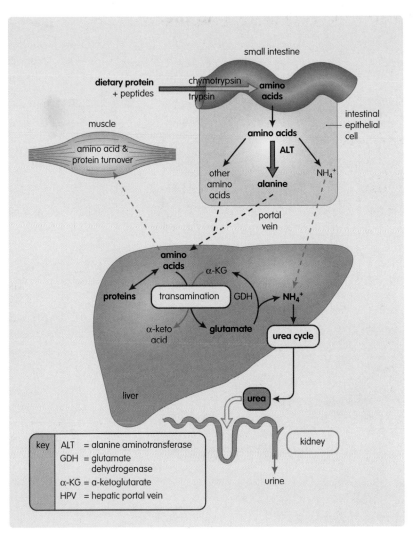

Fig. 5.31 Summary of amino acid metabolism in tissues during the absorptive state.

- Protein synthesis.
- Transamination to glutamate, which may be oxidatively deaminated to produce NH_4^+, which in turn enters the urea cycle (some NH_4^+ comes from the hydrolysis of glutamine in the small intestine). The urea formed is taken to the kidneys for excretion. Some of the glutamate formed may also be used for protein synthesis.

Post-absorptive (fasting) state

The fasting state is the period of 4 to 8 hours after a meal when there is no dietary supply of amino acids. A summary of amino acid metabolism in tissues in the fasting state is given in Fig. 5.32.

Muscle

The breakdown of muscle protein releases amino acids, which are transaminated to alanine and glutamate. Glutamine is formed by amidation of glutamate. Nucleic acid turnover provides the NH_4^+ for this reaction. Glutamine is taken up by the intestine and the kidney. The formed alanine goes to the liver. The breakdown of muscle protein also releases branched-chain amino acids, which are taken up primarily by the brain.

Intestine

The fate of glutamine depends on the energy status of the cell:

Fig. 5.32 Summary of amino acid metabolism in tissues in the post-absorptive state (refer to text for explanation).

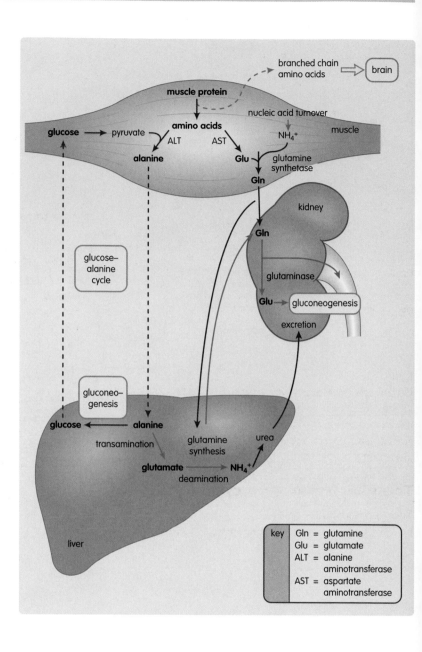

- It can be used for nucleotide synthesis to compensate for the very high turnover rate of intestinal cells (see Chapter 6).
- It undergoes hydrolysis to glutamate to release NH_4^+, which travels to the liver to enter the urea cycle.

The formed glutamate is transaminated either to alanine or citrulline (a urea cycle intermediate), both of which are taken to the liver.

Liver

In the liver, alanine is either:

- Converted to pyruvate and then to glucose by gluconeogenesis, providing an energy source for the muscle. Together, these reactions constitute the glucose–alanine cycle (Fig. 5.33).

Or

- Transaminated to glutamate. Glutamate can be deaminated to form NH_4^+, which enters the urea cycle.

The balance between these two processes depends on the energy state of the cell.

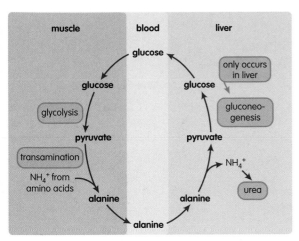

Fig. 5.33 The glucose–alanine cycle shows how carbon skeletons alternate between protein and glucose. Alanine released by muscle is converted back to glucose in the liver by gluconeogenesis. The glucose formed is taken back to the muscle for use.

Kidney

Glutamine released from muscle is taken up by kidney cells. It is hydrolysed by glutaminase to release ammonia which is excreted in urine. In starvation, glutamate serves as a substrate for gluconeogenesis (see Fig. 5.19).

The glucose–alanine cycle

The glucose–alanine cycle (see Fig. 5.33) shifts carbon skeletons between protein and glucose. Alanine from muscle is converted back to glucose in the liver by gluconeogenesis—glucose is, in turn, used by muscle. This is very similar to the Cori cycle where lactate formed by active skeletal muscle is taken to the liver to be converted back to pyruvate and then to glucose by gluconeogenesis. Glucose formed is then taken back to muscle (see Chapter 7).

Glycoproteins

Glycoproteins are complex molecules which are produced through the glycosylation of proteins in the endoplasmic reticulum or in the Golgi apparatus. The addition of sugar residues can occur either at asparagine (N-glycosylation) or at hydroxylysine, hydroxyproline, serine or threonine (O-glycosylation) residues. Glycosylation alters the properties of proteins, changing their stability, solubility and physical bulk. The sugar chains can also act as recognition signals that direct protein targeting and influence cell–cell interations. Examples of glycoproteins are:

- Antibodies (immunoglobulins) which interact with antigens.
- Major histocompatibility complex (MHC) proteins, which are expressed on the surface of cells and interact with T-cells as part of the adaptive immune response.
- Hormones (follicle-stimulating hormone, luteinizing hormone and thyroid-stimulating hormone).

Purines, pyrimidines and haem

Objectives

You should be able to:

- Discuss the roles of one-carbon units in amino acid synthesis.
- Describe the processes involved in purine and pyrimidine metabolism.
- Discuss the clinical features, causes and management of gout.
- Discuss the main features of haem and bilirubin metabolism.

ONE-CARBON POOL

One-carbon units

Single carbon units exist in a number of oxidation states; for example methane, formaldehyde and methanol. They are used in the synthesis and elongation of many organic compounds. To do this, carbon units require a carrier to activate them and to enable their transfer to the molecule being synthesized. The main carriers used are folate and S-adenosyl methionine. The one-carbon pool refers to single carbon units attached to these carriers.

S-adenosyl methionine

S-adenosyl methionine (SAM) is a high-energy compound formed by the condensation of the amino acid methionine with ATP. It contains an activated methyl group, which can be transferred easily to a variety of molecules. SAM is the major donor of methyl groups for biosynthetic reactions; for example, the methylation of noradrenaline to adrenaline.

Folate

The active form of folate is 5,6,7,8-tetrahydrofolate (THF). THF is a carrier of one-carbon units, which bind to its nitrogen atoms at positions N^5, N^{10} or both, to form the compounds shown in Fig. 6.1. THF receives these one-carbon fragments from donor molecules such as serine, glycine or histidine, and transfers them to intermediates in the synthesis of other amino acids, purines and thymidine. These THF compounds are all interconvertible except the N^5-methyl group.

Fig. 6.1 Compounds formed by the binding of THF to various one-carbon compounds

One-carbon unit	Compound
—CH=NH	N^5-formimino THF
—CHO	N^5-formyl THF
—CHO	N^{10}-formyl THF
=CH—	N^5, N^{10}-methenyl THF
—CH$_2$—	N^5, N^{10}-methylene THF
—CH$_3$	N^5-methyl THF

Students always tend to find the concept of the one-carbon pool confusing. All you need to realize is that THF and SAM are just carriers of one-carbon groups which are used in the synthesis of a range of molecules, mainly amino acids, purines and pyrimidines.

Folate metabolism

Formation of THF

THF is formed by the two-step reduction of folate by dihydrofolate reductase (DHFR) (Fig. 6.2). DHRF is competitively inhibited by methotrexate, a folic acid analogue used in the treatment of certain cancers. By inhibiting folate synthesis, methotrexate decreases the amount of THF available for purine and pyrimidine formation, thus decreasing DNA and RNA synthesis in cells.

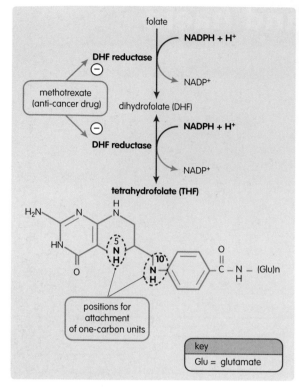

Fig. 6.2 Formation of tetrahydrofolate (THF). THF is formed by the two-step reduction of folate by dihydrofolate (DHF) reductase.

Methotrexate is used in the treatment of cancer and autoimmune diseases. The affinity of methotrexate for DHFR is about 1000-fold higher than that of folate. It also has a greater negative effect on rapidly dividing cells (such as malignant and myeloid cells), which rapidly replicate their DNA, thus inhibiting growth and proliferation of these cancer cells. However, it is also toxic to the rapidly dividing cells of bone marrow and gastrointestinal mucosa, causing anaemia, neutropenia and nausea.

Methyl-folate trap (Fig. 6.3)

Reactions involving transfer of methyl groups result in the formation of N^5-methyl THF. Unlike other THF compounds, N^5-methyl THF is not interconvertible further, therefore THF cannot be released and remains trapped as N^5-methyl THF. However, the methionine salvage pathway is present. Methionine is formed by methylation of homocysteine using N^5-methyl THF as the methyl group donor, thus

In vitamin B_{12} deficiency, the methionine salvage pathway is inhibited and THF remains as N^5-methyl THF. Eventually, all the body's folate becomes trapped, resulting in folate deficiency secondary to B_{12} deficiency (see Chapter 8). This results in decreased nucleotide synthesis and DNA and RNA formation. As blood cells require high levels of nucleotides for their turnover, they are particularly sensitive to folate deficiency, leading to megaloblastic anaemia.

releasing THF. This reaction is catalysed by homocysteine methyltransferase and requires vitamin B_{12} as an essential cofactor (methyl-cobalamin).

Amino acids and the one-carbon pool

The synthesis and breakdown of certain amino acids produce THF carriers that can be used in the synthesis of other amino acids and nucleotides. The following reactions demonstrate the use of the one-carbon pool.

Formation of SAM from methionine (numbers refer to Fig. 6.3)

1. Condensation of ATP and methionine to form SAM.
2. SAM contains an activated methyl group that can be donated to a number of acceptor molecules, forming S-adenosyl homocysteine.
3. Hydrolysis of S-adenosyl homocysteine releases adenosine to form homocysteine.
4. Homocysteine can be used either for the synthesis of the amino acid cysteine (see Chapter 5), or for
5. Regeneration of methionine in the methionine salvage pathway.

PURINE METABOLISM

Structure and function of purines

Purines are the nitrogenous bases adenine, guanine and hypoxanthine. They have a double-ring structure, consisting of a six-carbon ring and a five-carbon ring. They can either exist as free bases or with a pentose sugar (5C), usually ribose or deoxyribose,

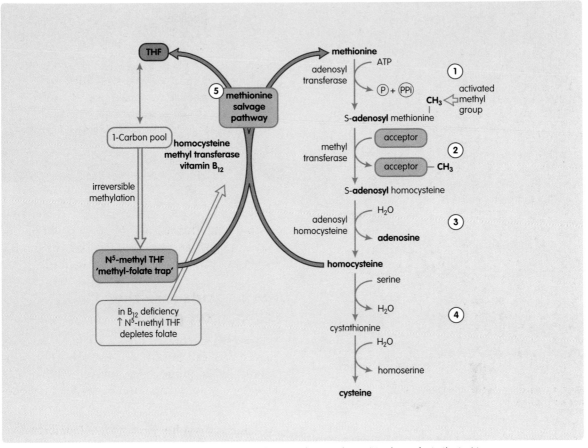

Fig. 6.3 Formation of S-adenosyl methionine (SAM) and the methionine salvage pathway. (Numbers refer to the text.)

attached at the N9 position to form a nucleoside (i.e adenosine). Phosphorylation of the sugar at the C5 position leads to the formation of mono-, di- and tri-nucleotides as shown in Fig. 6.4. The phosphate groups cause these molecules to be negatively charged. The main functions of purines are listed in Fig. 6.5.

An overview of purine metabolism

Diet provides negligible amounts of purines because they are broken down in the gut to form uric acid. Two pathways are concerned with the formation of purine nucleotides (Fig. 6.6).

I. De novo synthesis of purines

The purine ring is assembled on a molecule of ribose-5-phosphate; therefore, the purines are synthesized as mononucleotides instead of as free bases. This process occurs in the cytosol of hepatocytes and there are two stages:

- Formation of inosine monophosphate. Eleven reactions are necessary to form inosine monophosphate (IMP), the nucleotide of hypoxanthine. In the first reaction, 5-phosphoribosyl-1-pyrophosphate (PRPP) catalyses the phosphorylation of ribose-5-phosphate at the C1 position, forming 5-phosphoribosyl-1-pyrophosphate. In the second reaction, PRPP amidotransferase catalyses the synthesis of 5-phosphoribosylamine, which is an irreversible rate-limiting step of the pathway. The rest of the reactions are concerned with the construction of the purine ring by the addition of five carbon and four nitrogen atoms from amino acids (aspartate, glycine and glutamine), CO_2 and THF derivatives.

113

Fig. 6.4 Structure of purines, nucleosides and nucleotides.

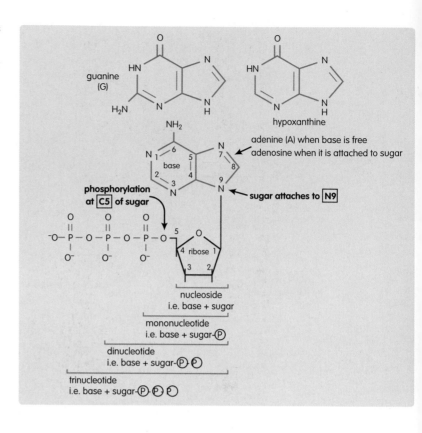

Fig. 6.5 Main functions of purines	
Functions	**Examples**
Building blocks of DNA and RNA	Adenine and guanine
Components of cofactors, particularly adenine	NAD^+, FAD, CoA
Components of high-energy compounds in cell	ATP, GTP, AMP, etc
Components of regulatory compounds	ATP, ADP, NAD^+, etc
Components of signalling molecules	cAMP, cGMP, GTP, G-proteins
Components of neurotransmitters	cGMP

• Conversion of IMP to AMP (adenosine monophosphate) and guanosine monophosphate (GMP) (Fig. 6.7).

II. Salvage pathways

When nucleic acids and nucleotides are broken down, free bases are released. The salvage pathway recycles these free bases by re-attaching ribose-5-phosphate to them (Fig. 6.8). It is a one-step pathway where the ribose-5-phosphate is transferred to the free bases from PRPP. The release of pyrophosphate makes the reactions irreversible. Only two enzymes are necessary: adenine phosphoribosyl transferase (APRT) and hypoxanthine guanine phosphoribosyl transferase (HGPRT). The pathway is simple and requires much less ATP than *de novo* synthesis because the bases do not have to be made first.

Regulation of purine biosynthesis

Purine synthesis is controlled allosterically by feedback inhibition at four major control sites:

• PRPP synthetase. This is inhibited by the end products GMP and AMP. As PRPP is also an intermediate in both the salvage pathway and pyrimidine synthesis (discussed later in this chapter), this is not the major control site.
• PRPP amidotransferase. This irreversible, rate-limiting reaction is unique to purine synthesis. It is allosterically inhibited by the end products IMP, AMP and GMP.

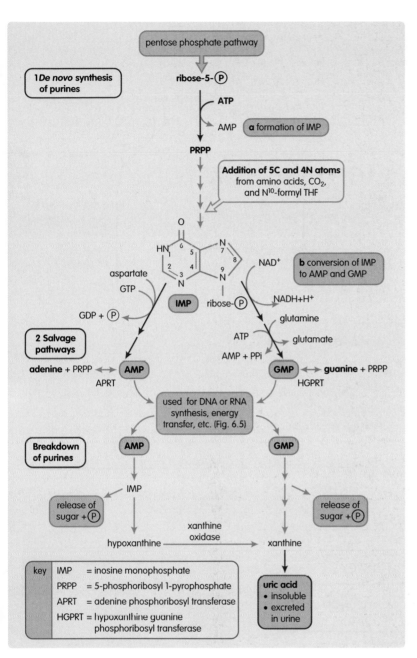

Fig. 6.6 Overview of purine metabolism. Two pathways are concerned with the formation of purine nucleotides:
1. *De novo* synthesis of purines, where the purine ring is assembled on a molecule of ribose-5-phosphate. The pathway consists of two stages:
   a. Formation of IMP, which occurs in 11 reactions. The purine ring is constructed by addition of C and N atoms from a number of sources: amino acids, CO_2 and THF derivatives.
   b. IMP is then converted to either GMP or AMP.
2. Salvage pathways 'recycle' free purines released during nucleic acid turnover by re-attaching a sugar phosphate unit to them.

There is only one pathway for purine breakdown, which converts the purines to the free bases hypoxanthine and xanthine; these are then oxidized to uric acid for excretion by the kidney.

- Adenylsuccinate synthase. This is inhibited by the end product AMP.
- IMP dehydrogenase. This is inhibited by the end product GMP.

If regulation is lost because of a defect in one of these four regulatory enzymes, this may lead to the overproduction of AMP and GMP, in excess of the requirements for nucleic acid synthesis and other functions. The excess purines are broken down to uric acid, which may become deposited in tissues, leading to symptoms of gout.

Lesch–Nyhan syndrome

Lesch–Nyhan syndrome is a very rare, X-linked disorder caused by an almost complete absence of the salvage enzyme hypoxanthine guanine phosphoribosyl transferase (HGPRT). HGPRT catalyses the addition of 5-phosphoribosyl-1-pyrophosphate

Fig. 6.7 Conversion of inosine monophosphate (IMP) to AMP and GMP. Both conversions involve two steps. Conversion of IMP to GMP involves:
1. Oxidation at the C2 position by IMP dehydrogenase, forming xanthosine monophosphate.
2. The amino group of glutamine is then inserted at the C2 position by GMP synthase to form GMP. This reaction requires ATP.

Conversion of IMP to AMP involves:
1. Addition of aspartate at the C6 position to form adenylsuccinate. This reaction requires GTP.
2. Adenylsuccinate lyase then eliminates the C-skeleton of aspartate as fumarate, leaving behind the amino group at C6 to form AMP.

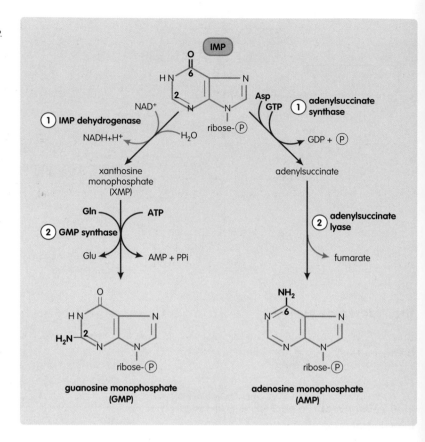

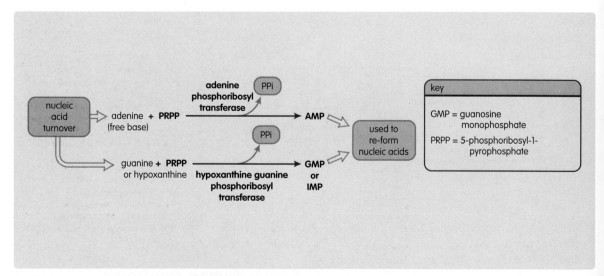

Fig. 6.8 Salvage pathways. When nucleic acids and nucleotides are broken down, free bases are released. The salvage pathway recycles these free bases by re-attaching ribose-5-phosphate to them by transfer from PRPP.

(PRPP) to the purine bases, guanine and hypoxanthine, in the salvage pathway (see Fig. 6.8). In Lesch–Nyhan syndrome a decreased level of HGPRT results in:

- Increased guanine and hypoxanthine in excess of their requirements, which are broken down to form large amounts of uric acid, leading to severe hyperuricaemia and gout.
- Increased levels of PRPP, which is therefore used for the *de novo* synthesis of purines, leading to purine overproduction and severe neurological disturbances.

The prognosis is very poor; sufferers usually die by the age of 5 years. The clinical features and diagnosis of Lesch–Nyhan syndrome are discussed in Fig. 6.9.

Breakdown of purines

Breakdown of purines occurs in two stages: the breakdown of the nucleotide to a free base hypoxanthine or xanthine, and the formation of uric acid (Fig. 6.10).

1. Breakdown of the nucleotide to a free base: hypoxanthine or xanthine

Three reactions are necessary (numbers and letters refer to Fig. 6.10):

a. Removal of the phosphate group by a nucleotidase.
b. Removal of ribose as ribose-1-phosphate by nucleoside phosphorylase.
c. Release of the amino group.

Fig. 6.9 Clinical features and treatment of Lesch–Nyhan syndrome

Clinical features	Diagnosis and treatment
Hyperuricaemia causing: • kidney stones • arthritis • gout Severe neurological disturbances: • spasticity and mental retardation • self-mutilation (bite fingers and lips to the bone) Symptoms begin at about 3 months	**Diagnosis:** • orange nappy (urine) • hypoxanthine guanine phosphoribosyl transferase activity • symptoms **Treatment:** • allopurinol lowers uric acid levels and helps to control gout and arthritis • with time, high purine levels result in worsening of neurological symptoms because no treatment is possible • boys usually die from kidney failure because of high sodium urate deposits causing kidney stones

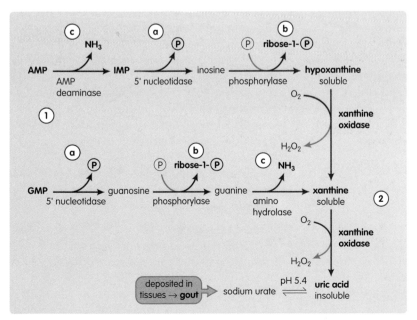

Fig. 6.10 Breakdown of purines. Breakdown of purines occurs in two stages:
1. The breakdown of the nucleotide to a free base, hypoxanthine or xanthine. For both AMP and GMP, three reactions are necessary, although the order differs:
   a. removal of the phosphate group;
   b. removal of ribose as ribose-1-phosphate;
   c. release of amino group.
2. Formation of uric acid by the oxidation of hypoxanthine and xanthine by xanthine oxidase.

AMP and GMP are degraded by the same three reactions; only the order differs (Fig. 6.10). AMP and IMP form hypoxanthine and GMP forms xanthine.

2. Formation of uric acid

Uric acid formation requires two steps, which are both catalysed by the enzyme xanthine oxidase (see Fig. 6.10):

a. Oxidation of hypoxanthine to xanthine.
b. Oxidation of xanthine to uric acid.

Xanthine oxidase is the key enzyme involved in purine degradation. It is unusual because it is a molybdenum- and iron-containing flavoprotein that uses molecular oxygen as an oxidizing agent.

In humans, the uric acid formed is excreted in the urine. Uric acid is insoluble. The acidic pH of urine allows it to precipitate out at high concentrations as sodium urate. Hyperuricaemia, that is, high serum levels of uric acid may lead to gout (see below).

Xanthine oxidase inhibitors

Xanthine oxidase is the key enzyme involved in controlling the amount of uric acid produced. Treatment with xanthine oxidase inhibitors decreases the amount of uric acid formed and increases the amounts of the soluble precursors hypoxanthine and xanthine, which are easily excreted in the urine. Allopurinol, an analogue of hypoxanthine, is the most commonly used xanthine oxidase inhibitor. It has a number of actions:

- It is a competitive inhibitor of xanthine oxidase.
- The salvage enzyme can catalyse addition of ribose-5-phosphate to allopurinol, forming allopurinol ribonucleotide. This can inhibit the rate-limiting enzyme of *de novo* purine synthesis, namely by PRPP amidotransferase, leading to a decrease in the level of purines and also of the PRPP pool.
- Allopurinol can be metabolized by xanthine oxidase to oxypurinol, an even stronger inhibitor of xanthine oxidase.

Gout

The prevalence of gout varies from about 0.1–0.2% in Europe to as high as 10% in the Maori population of New Zealand. It is caused by an abnormality of uric acid metabolism, resulting in hyperuricaemia and the deposition of sodium urate crystals in joints, soft tissues and the kidney (Fig. 6.11).

Fig. 6.11 Clinical features and diagnosis of gout

Clinical features	Diagnosis
Hyperuricaemia	Synoval fluid examination: affected joint is aspirated and fluid examined under microscope for long, needle shaped, negatively birefringent crystals
Recurrent attacks of acute arthritis caused by deposition of sodium urate crystals in joints; usually only one joint is affected (big toe > 90%)	
	Hyperuricaemia does not necessarily cause gout
Kidney stones and ↑ risk of renal disease	
Tophi under skin and around joints	

Gout predominantly affects men in middle life. It does not occur before puberty (unless it is part of Lesch–Nyhan syndrome). In women, it only occurs after menopause (the male to female ratio is 8:1). It is an inherited condition in some families.

Causes of gout

Genetic

- Decreased HGPRT levels; to 2–5% of normal. Similar to Lesch–Nyhan syndrome but not as severe.
- Overactive PRPP synthetase, involved in the regulation of purine biosynthesis (see above). Overactivity causes release from normal control, leading to increased rates of *de novo* synthesis of purines.
- Insensitive PRPP amidotransferase, the rate-controlling enzyme of purine synthesis. A mutant form has full activity but no regulatory sites, therefore feedback control is lost, causing overproduction of purines.
- The excess purines produced in these conditions are broken down to uric acid, leading to hyperuricaemia and gout.

Secondary causes

- Increased purine turnover, for example in leukaemia, myeloproliferative disorders, and due to the use of cytotoxic drugs in the treatment of cancers.

> Aspirin is contraindicated in gout because it impairs the excretion of uric acid by the renal tubules, thus aggravating hyperuricaemia.

- Decreased excretion of uric acid, for example drug therapy (thiazides, aspirin), lead toxicity, excess alcohol.

Treatment of gout

Acute attacks are treated with anti-inflammatory drugs: colchicine or non-steroidal anti-inflammatory drugs (e.g. indometacin) provide relief within 24–48 hours.

Long-term prevention is aimed at decreasing uric acid levels.

- Simple measures are weight reduction, decreased alcohol intake and withdrawal of drugs such as salicylates and thiazides.
- Allopurinol, a xanthine oxidase inhibitor, is the main drug used for the prevention of gout (see above).
- Probenecid, a uricosuric drug, is an alternative to allopurinol. It has a direct action on the renal tubule, preventing the reabsorption of uric acid in the kidney, causing it to be excreted.

PYRIMIDINE METABOLISM

Structure and function of pyrimidines

Structure

There are three main pyrimidines: thymine, cytosine and uracil. Like purines, the pyrimidines are mostly found associated with a five-carbon sugar attached at N1 to form the nucleosides thymidine, cytidine and uridine (Fig. 6.12). The sugar may be mono-, di- or tri-phosphorylated to form the corresponding nucleotides.

Functions

Pyrimidines are the building blocks of DNA and RNA: thymine and cytosine are present in DNA and cytosine and uracil are present in RNA.

Nucleotide derivatives are activated intermediates in a number of synthetic reactions; for example, UDP-glucose, the precursor of glycogen (see Chapter 2).

Biosynthesis of pyrimidines

There are three main stages in the biosynthesis of pyrimidines (Figs. 6.13 and 6.15). All of the three stages take place in the cell cytosol.

a. Construction of the pyrimidine ring to form uridine monophosphate (UMP). Unlike purine synthesis, the pyrimidine ring is synthesized before attachment to ribose-5-phosphate, that is, it is formed as a free base. The ring is derived

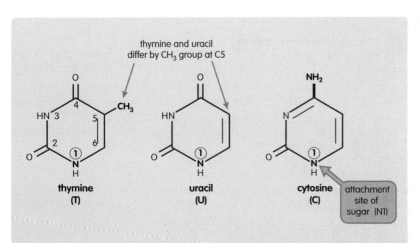

Fig. 6.12 Structure of pyrimidines. Like purines, the pyrimidines are mostly found associated with a five-carbon sugar attached at N1 to form nucleosides.

from glutamine, aspartate and CO_2 (Fig. 6.14). There are six steps in the reaction sequence (refer to Fig. 6.13). In the first three steps, the enzymes involved are present as a single polypeptide chain, forming a multi-functional enzyme (CAD), which consists of carbamoyl phosphate synthase II, aspartate *trans*-carbamoylase and dihydroorotase. In a way similar to fatty acid synthase, the enzymes are linked together to minimize side reactions and loss of substrate.

b. Conversion of UMP to uridine triphosphate (UTP) and cytidine triphosphate (CTP), the ribonucleotides found in RNA. UMP is phosphorylated to UDP and UTP as shown in Fig. 6.13. CTP is formed from UTP by amination, that is, the addition of an NH_2 group from glutamine to position 4 of the pyrimidine ring. Both UTP and CTP are used for RNA synthesis.

c. Formation of the deoxyribonucleotides dCTP and dTTP found in DNA (Fig. 6.15).

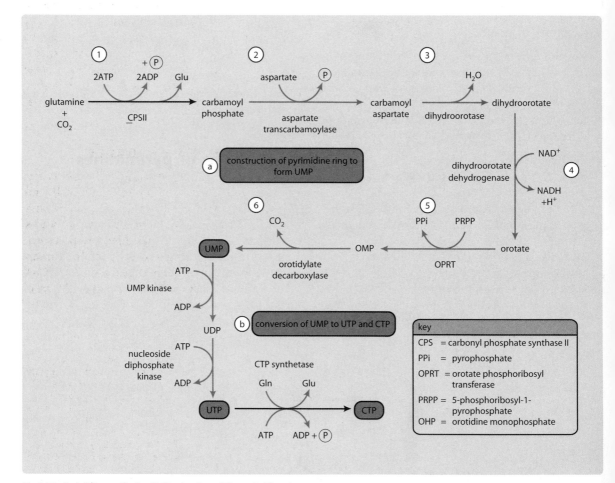

Fig 6.13. Pyrimidine synthesis. A) Construction of the pyrimidine ring.

1. Synthesis of carbamoyl phosphate by carbamoyl phosphate synthase II (CPSII). This is the rate-limiting step. Carbamoyl phosphate is also the precursor of urea; however, urea is formed by the mitochondrial enzyme, carbamoyl phosphate synthase I.
2. Addition of aspartate.
3. Closure of the ring by dihydroorotase.
4. Oxidation of dihydroorotate to orotate using NAD^+.
5. Conversion of the free pyrimidine to a nucleotide by the addition of ribose-5-phosphate from PRPP. This is catalysed by orotate phosphoribosyl transferase (OPRT) and is driven by the hydrolysis of pyrophosphate to two free molecules of inorganic phosphate. PRPP is thus required for the synthesis of both purines and pyrimidines.
6. Decarboxylation of orotidine monophosphate (OMP) to UMP by orotidylate decarboxylase. Both OPRT and orotidylate decarboxylase are also found together as a single polypeptide.

Regulation of pyrimidine synthesis

The rate-limiting step is the formation of carbamoyl phosphate by carbamoyl phosphate synthase II. CPSII is inhibited by the end products of pyrimidine synthesis, namely UDP and UTP. The reaction is activated by ATP and PRPP.

Regulation of deoxyribonucleotide synthesis

Ribonucleotide reductase catalyses the irreversible reduction of all four nucleoside diphosphates (ADP, GDP, CDP and UDP) to their corresponding deoxy forms and is therefore subject to regulation. The

enzyme has four subunits (two B1 and two B2). Each B1 subunit has two allosteric sites distinct from the active site: an activity site and a substrate specificity site. The binding of the product dATP to the activity site inhibits the enzyme. The binding of the substrate, a ribonucleotide, e.g. ATP, to the substrate specificity site, activates the enzyme.

Salvage pathways

The salvage pathways for pyrimidines are similar to those for purines (Fig. 6.16). The breakdown of nucleotides releases free pyrimidines, thymine and uracil. These pyrimidines are salvaged by the enzyme uracil/thymine phosphoribosyl transferase (UTPRT), which transfers a ribose-5-phosphate from PRPP to the free pyrimidines to re-form the mononucleotides. However, the enzyme UTPRT cannot salvage cytosine. Therefore cytidine (nucleoside) is deaminated to uridine; this is then converted to uracil, which can be salvaged.

Breakdown of pyrimidines

Purines are excreted with their ring still intact as uric acid. The pyrimidine ring, however, can be split and broken down to soluble structures. Uracil and cytosine are broken down to β-alanine, which forms acetyl CoA. Thymine is degraded to β-amino-isobutyrate, which forms succinyl CoA. The carbon skeletons of the pyrimidines, namely acetyl CoA and succinyl CoA, can be oxidized by the TCA cycle.

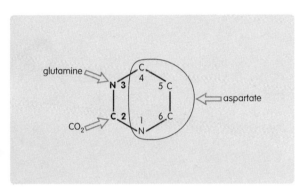

Fig. 6.14 The pyrimidine ring. The ring is derived from glutamine, aspartate and CO_2.

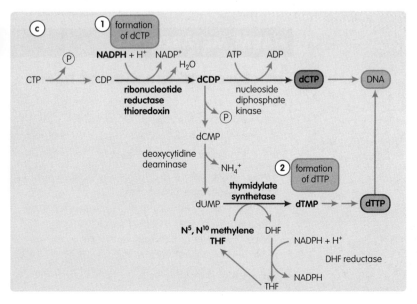

Fig. 6.15 Third stage of pyrimidine synthesis: the formation of deoxyribonucleotides.
1. Ribonucleotide reductase reduces CDP to deoxyCDP by removal of the C2 hydroxyl group on ribose, converting it to deoxyribose. The dCDP formed is phosphorylated to dCTP.
2. dTTP is formed by the methylation of dUMP. Thymidylate synthetase transfers a methyl group from N^5,N^{10}-methylene THF to position 5 of the pyrimidine ring, forming dTMP, which can be phosphorylated to dTTP (numbers refer to text below). DHF, dihydrofolate; THF, tetrahydrofolate.

Fig. 6.16 Salvage pathway.

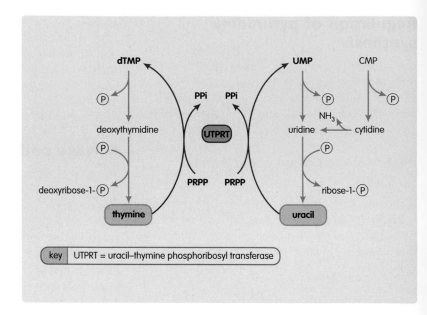

key | UTPRT = uracil–thymine phosphoribosyl transferase

Anti-cancer drugs

These drugs inhibit the formation of nucleotides, leading to a decrease in DNA synthesis and cell growth. Cancer cells divide rapidly and have an increased demand for DNA synthesis. These drugs help to slow down the growth of cancer cells. However, they also affect normal cell replication, leading to serious side effects (Fig. 6.17).

Most anti-cancer drugs affect normal cell replication and proliferation, especially cells of the bone marrow, gastrointestinal tract, gonads, skin and hair follicles. This results in severe side effects such as anaemia, neutropenia (making patients susceptibile to infection), hair loss, vomiting, infertility, impaired wound healing and stunting of growth.

Fig. 6.17 Action of anti-cancer drugs

Drugs	Action	Effects on pyrimidine and purine synthesis
Glutamine antagonists: azaserine, diazo-oxo-norleucine	Analogues of glutamine: competitively inhibit enzymes that use glutamine as substrate	↓ pyrimidine synthesis: inhibits CPS II ↓ purine synthesis: inhibits PRPP amidotransferase and reaction 5 (Fig. 6.13)
Folate antagonists: methotrexate	Inhibits DHF reductase leading to decreased available THF for transfer of one-carbon units	Inhibits methylation of dUMP to dTMP causing ↓ dTMP synthesis ↓ pyrimidine synthesis (Fig. 6.15)
5-fluorouracil	Analogue of dUMP: irreversibly inhibits thymidylate synthetase	Inhibits synthesis of dTMP; no effect on purine synthesis

HAEM METABOLISM

Structure and function of haem

Structure

Haem is a complex structure containing an iron atom (as Fe^{2+}) placed in the centre of a tetrapyrrole ring of protoporphyrin IX (Fig. 6.18).

- The basic structure is a four-ringed cyclic structure called a porphyrin.
- Each ring is called a pyrrole ring and the rings are linked together via methenyl bridges.
- Three types of side chains can be attached to the pyrrole ring—methyl, vinyl or propionyl—and the arrangement of these is important to the activity.

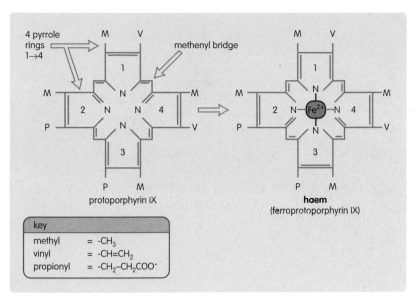

Fig. 6.18 Structure of haem. Haem consists of an Fe^{2+} atom placed in the centre of protoporphyrin IX.

key
methyl	= -CH$_3$
vinyl	= -CH=CH$_2$
propionyl	= -CH$_2$-CH$_2$COO$^-$

- Porphyrins bind metal ions to form metalloporphyrins.

Functions

Haem is the prosthetic group found in a number of proteins. The function of haem in each group can vary (Fig. 6.19). The Fe^{2+} atom (ferrous form) at the centre of the haem structure can undergo oxidation to Fe^{3+} (ferric form); this is important for its function in cytochromes and enzymes, enabling it to act as a recyclable electron carrier. However, in haemoglobin and myoglobin, Fe^{3+} cannot bind oxygen, and its function as an oxygen transporter is impaired (it forms methaemoglobin, see Chapter 3).

Haem biosynthesis

The main locations of haem biosynthesis are:

- Bone marrow erythroid cells, where haem is used to form haemoglobin.
- Hepatocytes, where haem is used for cytochrome synthesis, particularly cytochrome P450 which is involved in drug metabolism.

The human body makes 40–50 mg/day of haem, about 80–85% of which is used for haemoglobin synthesis. Mature erythrocytes lack mitochondria and therefore they cannot make haem.

Site

Haem biosynthesis is partitioned between mitochondria and the cytosol (Fig. 6.20).

Fig. 6.19 Functions of haem in different proteins

Protein	Function of haem
Haemoglobin and myoglobin	Reversibly binds O_2 for transport
Peroxidases and catalase	Forms part of the active site of enzyme
Cytochromes (a, b, c, and P450)	Electron carrier: continually oxidized and reduced, enhancing electron flow

An overview of the pathway (Fig. 6.20)

- There are eight reactions; the first and last three occur in the mitochondria, the rest are in the cytosol.
- Protoporphyrin IX is derived from glycine and succinyl CoA.
- Eight moles of each are required to form eight moles of δ-aminolevulinic acid (ALA), which condenses to form four moles of porphobilinogen (PBG). These, in turn, condense to form one mole of uroporphyrinogen I (UROgen I).
- The rest of the reactions modify the side chains.
- If the side chains on porphyrins are arranged symmetrically, then the molecules are physiologically inactive. When the side chains are arranged asymmetrically, the molecules are active.

Fig. 6.20 Haem synthesis.
1. The synthesis of ALA. ALA synthase catalyses the condensation of glycine and succinyl CoA in the mitochondria. The reaction requires pyridoxal phosphate (PLP) as a cofactor. This is the irreversible, rate-limiting step of haem synthesis.
2. The formation of porphobilinogen (PBG). ALA dehydrase catalyses the dehydration of two molecules of ALA to form PBG. The enzyme is inhibited by heavy metals such as lead.
3. Formation of uroporphyrinogen I (UROgen I). UROgen I synthase catalyses the condensation of four molecules of PBG to form UROgen I (inactive).
4. UROgen III cosynthase produces the asymmetrical active uroporphyrinogen III (UROgen III). The rest of the reactions alter the side chains and the degree of unsaturation of the porphyrin ring.
5. The first decarboxylation results in the formation of coproporphyrinogen III.
6. The second decarboxylation forms protoporphyrinogen IX in the mitochondria.
7. Oxidation to protoporphyrin IX.
8. Ferrochelatase inserts the Fe^{2+} ion into the ring to form haem.

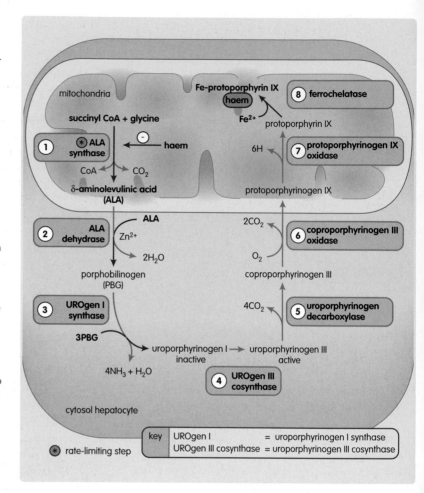

Protoporphyrinogen IX is a colourless, unstable, easily oxidized precursor of porphyrin. Porphyrins are highly coloured (red), stable compounds that characteristically absorb ultraviolet light at a wavelength of 400 nm.

Lead poisoning

The human body contains about 120 mg of lead. Excessive ingestion or inhalation can result from contaminated food, water or air. In the UK, the common sources are old lead piping and petrol. Lead inhibits three key enzymes of haem synthesis, resulting in the accumulation of intermediates:

- ALA dehydrase: this leads to the accumulation of ALA, which can be measured in urine.
- Coproporphyrinogen III oxidase: this leads to the accumulation of coproporphyrinogen III.
- Ferrochelatase: this leads to the accumulation of protoporphyrin IX in erythrocytes.

Overall, this results in the inhibition of haem synthesis and anaemia. Lead also binds to bone. The main clinical features and diagnostic criteria are discussed in Fig. 6.21.

Treatment

Treatment is with lead chelators such as desferrioxamine mesilate, sodium calcium edetate or penicillamine. They all bind lead, forming a complex, which can be excreted in the urine.

The porphyrias

This is a group of rare, inherited disorders in which there is a partial deficiency of one of the enzymes of haem synthesis (see Fig. 6.22). This results in the inhibition of haem synthesis and thus the formation of excessive quantities of either porphyrin precursors, for example δ-aminolevulinic acid (ALA) or porphobilinogen (PBG), or porphyrins

Fig. 6.21 Clinical features and diagnosis of lead poisoning

Clinical features	Diagnosis
Acute exposure: • severe weakness, vomiting, abdominal pain, anorexia and constipation **Chronic exposure:** • causes staining of teeth and bones, myopathy, peripheral neuropathy, renal damage and sideroblastic anaemia • eventually leads to encephalopathy and seizures • may cause mental retardation in children	Blood lead levels > 3 mg/L indicate significant exposure Urine: ↑ δ-aminolevulinic acid levels Red cell: ↑ porphyrin levels and fluorescence Blood film: anaemia with punctate basophilia; red cells may contain small, blue deposits

themselves, depending upon which enzyme is deficient (Fig. 6.22).

The inhibition of haem synthesis leads to decreased haem formation. The key, rate-limiting enzyme of haem synthesis is ALA synthase, which is normally inhibited by haem (see Fig. 6.24). In porphyrias, the absence of haem releases the inhibition (and thus the control) of ALA synthase, resulting in the increased formation of intermediates preceding the defective enzyme in each porphyria.

When porphyrin precursors are produced in excess (ALA and PBG), they cause mainly neuropsychiatric symptoms and abdominal pain (the precursors are neurotoxins). When porphyrins themselves are produced in excess, they cause skin photosensitivity (i.e., the skin burns and itches on exposure to light). This is because porphyrins absorb light, which excites them and induces the formation of oxygen free

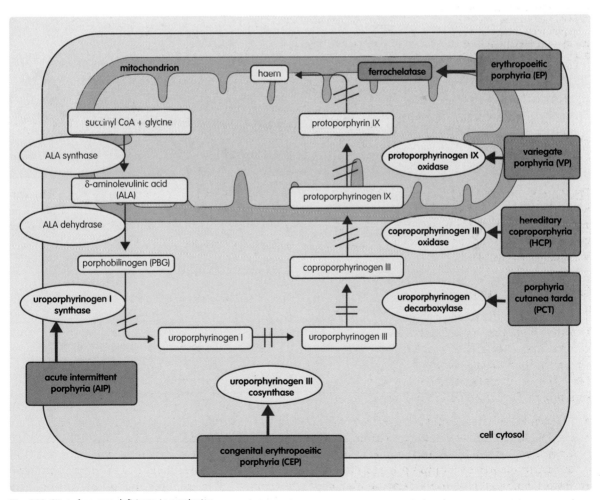

Fig. 6.22 Sites of enzyme deficiency in porphyrias.

radicals. These can attack membranes, particularly lysosomal membranes, leading to the release of enzymes which damage underlying layers of skin, rendering it susceptible to the light.

Porphyrias are diagnosed on the basis of symptoms and the pattern of porphyrins and their precursors present in the blood and urine.

Porphyrias are classified as either hepatic or erythropoeitic and also as acute or chronic (Fig. 6.23). They are all rare; the most common in the UK is acute intermittent porphyria which is discussed below. The features of other types of porphyrias are summarized in Fig 6.23.

Acute intermittent porphyria

Acute intermittent porphyria is an autosomal dominant disease with a prevalence in the UK of 1:100 000. The defect is a deficiency of uroporphyrinogen I synthase. Characteristically, acute attacks are separated by long periods of remission. The attacks are precipitated by various factors, including alcohol, barbiturates, oral contraceptives, anaesthetic agents (e.g halothane) and certain antibiotics.

Clinical features
Presentation is usually in early adult life and includes:

- Acute abdominal symptoms.
- Neuropathy.
- Neuropsychiatric symptoms (e.g depression, anxiety and psychosis).

Results of laboratory tests
Increased levels of PBG and ALA can be found in the urine of these patients. The urine darkens to a port-wine colour on exposure to air, due to the presence of PBG. The classic bedside test for excess PBG is to add Ehrlich's reagent (an aldehyde) to urine, which causes it to go pink. The colour persists when excess chloroform is added.

Management
The treatment is with fluids, pain relief and a high carbohydrate diet, which inhibits the pathway. Avoiding precipitants is important. It is important to ask about inherited disorders when pre-assessing patients for surgery.

Overall management

The effects of all porphyrias can be decreased by intravenous haemin which inhibits ALA synthase,

Porphyrias are very rare. You will seldom see or be asked about them. Figs. 6.22 and 6.23 summarize all you will ever need to know.

Fig. 6.23 The porphyrias: summary

Porphyria	Enzyme defect	Photosensitivity	Neurological symptoms	Biochemistry	
Acute intermittent (hepatic)	Uroporphyrinogen I synthase		Yes	Urine:	$\uparrow$ δ-aminolevulinic acid (ALA) and porphobilinogen (PBG)
Congenital erythropoietic	Uroporphyrinogen III cosynthase	Yes		Red cells:	$\uparrow$ UROgen I
				Urine:	$\uparrow$ UROgen I and COPROgen I
Cutaneous (hepatic)	Uroporphyrinogen decarboxylase	Yes		Urine:	$\uparrow$ UROgen I and III
				Faeces:	$\uparrow$ COPROgen
Hereditary coproporphyria (hepatic)	Coproporphyrinogen III oxidase	Yes	Yes	Urine:	$\uparrow$ ALA, PBG and COPROgen III
Variegate (hepatic)	Protoporphyrinogen IX oxidase	Yes	Yes	Urine:	$\uparrow$ PBG and ALA
				Faeces:	$\uparrow$ PROTOgen IX, COPROgen III
Erythropoietic	Ferrochelatase	Yes		Red cells:	$\uparrow$ protoporphyrin

the rate-controlling enzyme, regaining the control of haem synthesis. An increased dietary intake of antioxidant vitamins A, C and E also helps to protect against free radical damage. Intravenous haematin can be given.

Regulation of haem synthesis

The key rate-limiting enzyme of haem synthesis is ALA synthase. It is a good control point because the enzyme undergoes rapid turnover (has a half-life of 60–70 minutes). ALA synthase is inhibited by high levels of the end product haem (Fe^{2+}) and also haemin (Fe^{3+}), formed by the oxidation of haem.

In the liver, control of ALA synthase by haem is considered at three levels (numbers refer to Fig. 6.24):

1. Allosteric inhibition of the enzyme by haem. However, high concentrations of haem are necessary (10^{-5} M) and, therefore, this is not an important control mechanism.
2. Haem also inhibits the transport of newly synthesized enzyme from cytosol into mitochondria.
3. Repression of transcription of the ALA synthase gene by haem. This is probably the most effective regulation because it works at low concentrations (10^{-7} M).

In erythroid tissue, the same regulatory mechanisms apply as in the liver but additionally, under certain conditions such as chronic hypoxia or anaemia, erythropoietin production is stimulated, leading to an increase in red cell synthesis and, therefore, an increase in haem.

Induction of ALA synthase in the liver

A number of drugs, such as steroids and barbiturates, cause an increase in the amount of hepatic ALA synthase. The mechanism proceeds as follows:

Fig. 6.24 Control of haem synthesis in the hepatocyte.

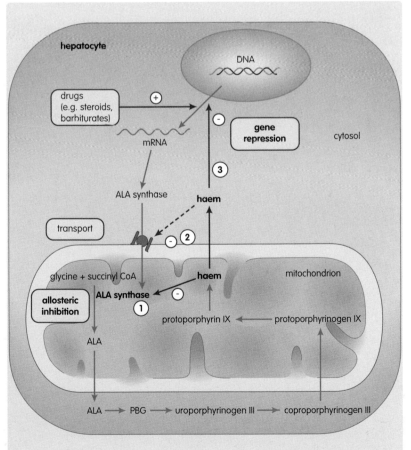

- Drugs are metabolized by microsomal cytochrome P450 enzymes, which are haem-containing proteins themselves.
- Certain drugs induce the synthesis of cytochrome P450, leading to an increase in the consumption and breakdown of haem.
- This leads to an overall decrease in the concentration of haem in the liver cells, which in turn stimulates or induces the transcription of ALA synthase and haem synthesis (see Fig. 6.24).
- Glucose blocks this induction.

Haem breakdown

About 80–85% of haem that is broken down comes from old erythrocytes; the rest comes from cytochrome turnover (Fig. 6.25).

Location/site

Kupffer cells and macrophages of the reticuloendothelial system (mainly liver, spleen and bone marrow).

Pathway

The two steps in the pathway are (steps refer to Fig. 6.25):

1. Cleavage of the porphyrin ring to form biliverdin. Haem oxygenase found in microsomes splits the porphyrin ring by breaking one of the methenyl bridges between two pyrrole rings. This produces biliverdin, Fe^{3+} and carbon monoxide (this is the only reaction *in vivo* that produces carbon monoxide).
2. Reduction of biliverdin to bilirubin in the cytosol.

Fig. 6.25 Haem breakdown.

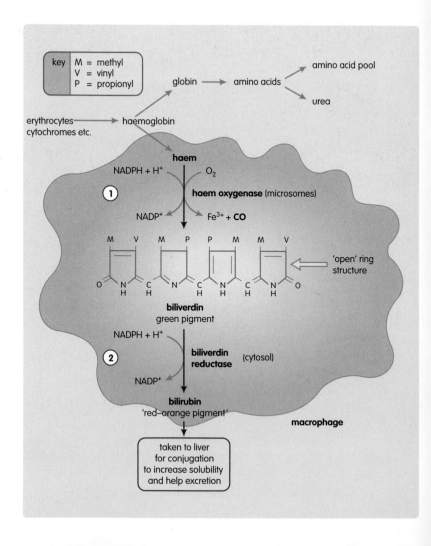

Bilirubin metabolism

Bilirubin is extremely non-polar and lipophilic and is only sparingly soluble in aqueous solutions. Within the blood, it is very tightly bound to albumin and very little remains free in solution. Bilirubin bound to albumin is taken up by the liver. Bilirubin is conjugated within the hepatic endoplasmic reticulum by a UDP glucuronyl transferase to produce bilirubin diglucuronide (Fig 6.26).

The conjugated bilirubin moves into the bile canaliculi of the liver and is then stored in the gall bladder. When stimulated by eating, bile (including the conjugated bilirubin) is secreted into the small intestine. Within the large intestine, bilirubin is further metabolized by bacteria present in the gut into urobilinogen. Some of this is absorbed from the intestine and enters the blood. Much of this in turn is taken up by the liver from the portal vein, but a small proportion enters the general circulation, is filtered at the glomerulus and enters urine (giving its characteristic yellow colour).

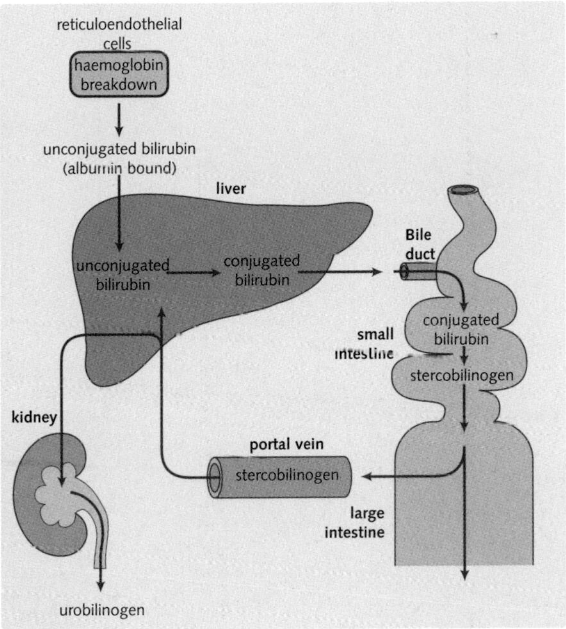

The liver has a large capacity to conjugate bilirubin and can normally cope with moderately elevated levels. However, in patients with haemolytic anaemia, such as during a sickle cell crisis, there is a very large increase in haem breakdown, resulting in high bilirubin levels, which exceed the conjugating capacity of the liver. This results in elevated plasma levels of unconjugated bilirubin, causing jaundice. In jaundice, the deposition of bilirubin leads to a yellow colouring of the skin, mucosal membranes and the whites of the eyes.

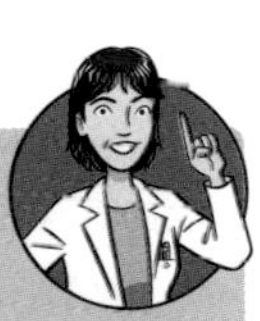

Haem breakdown occurs at sites of minor trauma underneath the skin. The changing colours of a bruise represent the different pigments produced.

Fig. 6.26 Bilirubin metabolism.

Glucose homeostasis

Objectives

You should be able to :

- Compare and contrast the fed and fasted state.
- Describe the main effects of insulin and glucagon on carbohydrate, protein and lipid metabolism.
- Compare and contrast Type 1 and Type 2 diabetes.
- Discuss the main metabolic effects of diabetes and its long-term complications.

THE STATES OF GLUCOSE HOMEOSTASIS

Glucose homeostasis can be conveniently discussed by looking at three basic states: the fed, fasted (post-absorptive) and starved state (Fig. 7.1). The starved state can be further subdivided into early and late, since different metabolic fuels are used depending on the degree of starvation (Fig. 7.2).

It is important to realize that glucose homeostasis is a dynamic process. There are no well-defined boundaries between the different states; instead, there is some degree of overlap between them.

The fed state

This is the period 0–4 hours after a meal and is summarized in Fig. 7.3. During the fed state (numbers refer to Fig. 7.3):

1. An increase in plasma glucose results in the release of insulin from the β cells in the pancreas. The availability of substrate and the increase in insulin stimulates glycogen, triacylglycerol (triglyceride), and protein synthesis by tissues; this is an anabolic state.
2. Glucose is the sole fuel for the brain; its uptake is insulin-independent.
3. Muscle and adipose tissue also use glucose; however its uptake is insulin dependent.

An increase in glucose and insulin activates glucokinase in the liver. Glucokinase, unlike hexokinase, is not inhibited by glucose-6-phosphate, enabling the liver to respond to the high blood glucose levels that occur after a meal. Glucokinase phosphorylates glucose, which can be used for synthesis of liver glycogen, therefore preventing hyperglycaemia (see Chapter 2).

Hexokinase, present in most cells, is also active when the concentration of glucose in the blood is low.

The fasted state

This is the period 4–12 hours after a meal, also called the post-absorptive state (Fig. 7.4). During the fasted state (numbers refer to Fig. 7.4):

1. The breakdown of liver glycogen stores provides glucose for oxidation by the brain. These stores are sufficient to last only between 12 and 24 hours.
2. The hydrolysis of triacylglycerols from stores releases fatty acids, which are used preferentially as a fuel by muscle and liver.
3. Muscle can also use its own glycogen as a fuel.

All these processes involved are activated by the increase in the ratio of glucagon to insulin. This activates (by phosphorylation) glycogen phosphorylase and hormone-sensitive lipase, leading, respectively to glycogen breakdown and lipolysis.

The starved state

Early starved state

Once the liver glycogen has been used up, an alternative substrate is required to provide glucose (Fig. 7.5). In short-term starvation (numbers refer to Fig. 7.5):

1. Glucagon and later cortisol activate protein breakdown in muscle, which releases amino acids (particularly alanine and glutamine).

Fig. 7.1 Three states of glucose homeostasis.

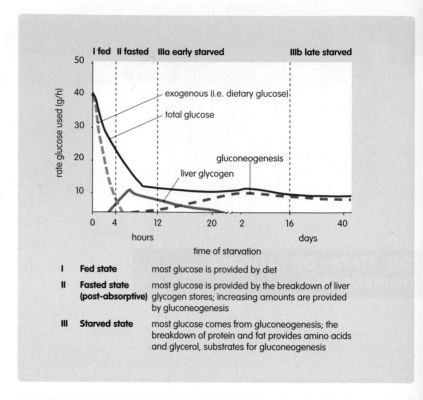

I	**Fed state**	most glucose is provided by diet
II	**Fasted state (post-absorptive)**	most glucose is provided by the breakdown of liver glycogen stores; increasing amounts are provided by gluconeogenesis
III	**Starved state**	most glucose comes from gluconeogenesis; the breakdown of protein and fat provides amino acids and glycerol, substrates for gluconeogenesis

Fig. 7.2 Three states of glucose homeostasis. (NA, noradrenaline; TG, triacylglycerol)

State	Time course	Major fuels used	Hormonal control
I Fed	0–4 h following a meal	Most tissues use glucose	↑ insulin results in: ↑ glucose uptake by peripheral tissues ↑ glycogen, TG, and protein synthesis
II Fasted (post-absorptive)	4–12 h after a meal	Brain: glucose muscle and liver: fatty acids	↑ glucagon and NA stimulate breakdown of liver glycogen and TG ↓ insulin
IIIa Early starvation	12 h → 16 days without food	Brain: glucose and some ketone bodies liver: fatty acids muscle: mainly fatty acids and some ketone bodies	↑ glucagon and NA → ↑ TG hydrolysis and ketogenesis ↑ cortisol → breakdown of muscle protein, releasing amino acids for gluconeogenesis
IIIb Prolonged starvation	> 16 days without food	Brain: uses more ketone bodies and less glucose to preserve body protein Muscle: only fatty acids	↑ glucagon and NA

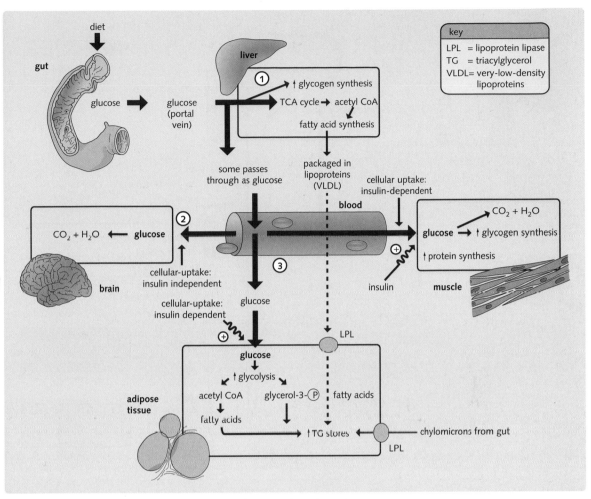

Fig. 7.3 Summary of fuel metabolism in the fed state (numbers 1–3 refer to the text).

2. Hydrolysis of triacylglycerol stores (adipose tissue) releases glycerol. Both the amino acids and glycerol are used by the liver for gluconeogenesis.

3 The glucose produced is used by the brain.

4. The fatty acids released from triacylglycerols are also used by the liver to make ketone bodies which can be used as an alternative fuel by peripheral tissues as well as the brain.

Late starved state

This is the period of starvation of longer than 16 days up until death. In prolonged starvation the breakdown of muscle protein slows down. This is because there is less need for glucose to be supplied via gluconeogenesis, because the brain adapts to using more ketone bodies. This is further helped by muscle using, almost exclusively, fatty acids as fuel.

Gluconeogenesis

Gluconeogenesis is the major source of glucose once glycogen stores are depleted. The main role of

A comparison of the fed and the fasted state is a commonly examined 'metabolic' question, because it requires overall knowledge of protein, fat and carbohydrate metabolism and its regulation. The way to answer this for each state is to think about time-course, hormonal influences, main active pathways, substrate availability and any special tissue requirements.

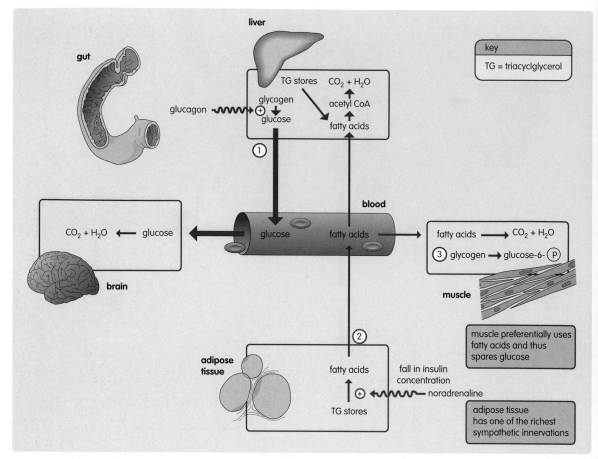

Fig. 7.4 Summary of fuel metabolism in the fasted state; that is, 4–12 h after a meal. A high glucagon to insulin ratio activates the breakdown of liver glycogen, which provides glucose for the brain. Both the fall in insulin concentration and the increase in noradrenaline promote hydrolysis of triacylglycerol stores, releasing fatty acids which can be used as a fuel by muscle and liver. Muscle uses its own glycogen as fuel (numbers refer to text on p. 131).

gluconeogenesis is the maintenance of blood glucose and the provision of glucose for the brain and erythrocytes during fasting. An increased glucagon:insulin ratio activates gluconeogenesis and causes the reciprocal inhibition of glycolysis (see Chapter 5). In muscle, cortisol activates protein breakdown, releasing, in particular, alanine and glutamine—substrates for gluconeogenesis.

Ketogenesis

Ketone body synthesis begins during the first few days of starvation and increases as the brain adapts to using ketone bodies as its major fuel, therefore reducing the need for glucose. Once significant

ketone body synthesis occurs, a decrease in the level of gluconeogenesis from amino acids is seen. This results in a reduction in the breakdown of muscle protein, thus sparing protein.

After 2–3 weeks of starvation, muscle reduces its use of ketone bodies and uses fatty acids almost exclusively; this leads to an increase in available ketone bodies for the brain.

Both ketogenesis and gluconeogenesis are balanced to ensure efficient use of metabolic fuels during starvation. Gluconeogenesis activates ketogenesis by depleting oxaloacetate, which ensures that the concentration of acetyl CoA exceeds the oxidative capacity of the TCA cycle; acetyl CoA can therefore be used for ketone body synthesis.

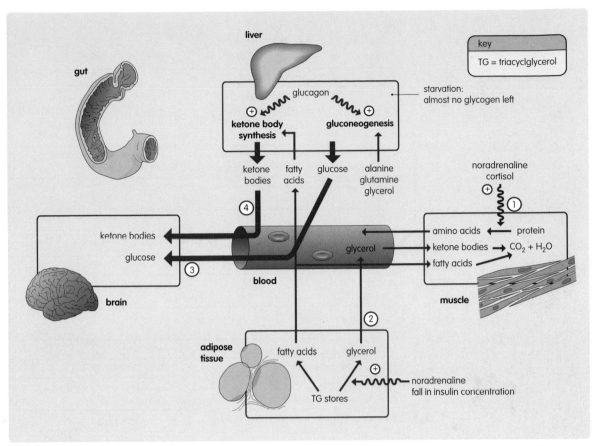

Fig. 7.5 Summary of fuel metabolism in early starvation. Noradrenaline and cortisol activate the breakdown of muscle protein to release amino acids, particularly alanine and glutamine. Noradrenaline also activates hydrolysis of triacylglycerols to release glycerol. Glycerol, alanine and glutamine are taken to the liver, where they enter gluconeogenesis and are oxidized to glucose. Glucose is used mainly by the brain. Fatty acids released from hydrolysis of triacylglycerols can be taken to the liver and used to generate ketone bodies, which can be used by brain and other tissues (numbers refer to text on p. 131).

Hormonal control of glucose homeostasis

Insulin is an anabolic hormone that increases the uptake and synthesis of glycogen, triacylglycerol and protein. Glucagon, noradrenaline, adrenaline and cortisol are catabolic hormones. The main effects of glucagon are summarized in Fig. 7.6. Noradrenaline and adrenaline (stress, or fight-and-flight hormones) have some similar effects to glucagons where they:

- Increase glycogen breakdown (in muscle only).
- Increase lipolysis in adipose tissue.
- Stimulate protein breakdown.

Glucose homeostasis in exercise

Sprinters

Sprinting is an anaerobic activity.

- In the muscle during intense activity, there is only time for anaerobic glycolysis, resulting in the build-up of lactate.
- Lactate diffuses out of muscle and is taken to the liver where it is oxidized to pyruvate, which can then be converted back to glucose via gluconeogenesis.
- The glucose formed diffuses out of the liver and returns to the muscle to be further used as fuel.

Fig. 7.6 Summary of the main effects of insulin and glucagon. (NA, noradrenaline; PPP, pentose phosphate pathway)

Pathway	Insulin: anabolic	Glucagon: catabolic
Carbohydrate metabolism		
Glycogen	Increases glycogen synthesis in muscle and liver	Increases glycogen breakdown in liver only (NA and adrenaline increase breakdown in muscle) decreases glycogen synthesis
Glycolysis/ gluconeogenesis	Increases glycolysis Inhibits gluconeogenesis	Increases gluconeogenesis inhibits glycolysis
Glucose uptake	Increases uptake by peripheral tissues, not liver	No effect
Pentose phosphate pathway	Increases PPP, producing NADPH for lipogenesis	
Lipid metabolism		
Lipolysis and β oxidation	Inhibits	Activates
Ketone body synthesis	Inhibits	Activates
Lipogenesis	Activates	Inhibits
Protein metabolism		
Uptake of amino acids by tissues	Increases uptake by most tissues	Increases uptake by the liver for gluconeogenesis
Protein synthesis	Increases rate by most tissues	Decreases
Protein breakdown	Decreases	Stimulates breakdown

This series of reactions, which 'shifts the metabolic burden from the muscle to the liver', is known as the Cori cycle (Fig. 7.7) (Compare it with the glucose–alanine cycle; see Fig. 5.33).

Long-distance running

Long-distance running is aerobic.

The body does not store enough glycogen to provide the energy necessary to run long distances. If the respiratory quotient (RQ: the ratio of the amount of O_2 consumed to the amount of CO_2 released) is measured during a run, initially it is about 1.0, indicating that mainly carbohydrate is being used. However, the RQ falls during running to a value of about 0.77 after about 1 hour, indicating that mainly fats are being oxidized.

The type and amount of substrate used varies with the intensity and duration of exercise, in a similar way to starvation. As glycogen stores are depleted,

an increase in glucagon, noradrenaline and adrenaline stimulates lipolysis, releasing fatty acids for muscle to use to conserve glucose. An increase in these hormones, along with an increase in cortisol, leads to stimulation of gluconeogenesis and protein degradation in muscle. These changes are similar to those of the fasting state; the difference is that the level of ketone bodies in the blood is low. It is not clear whether this is because they are not being synthesized or if they are being oxidized as soon as they are formed.

Mechanism of action of insulin

Insulin is an anabolic hormone. It promotes the synthesis and storage of carbohydrates, lipids and proteins and inhibits their degradation and release back into the circulation. These multiple actions of insulin are well coordinated and involve multiple signaling pathways. The full mechanism of action of

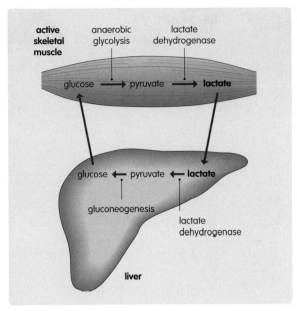

Fig. 7.7 The Cori cycle distributes the metabolic burden between the muscle and the liver. Lactate, which builds up in muscle during intense activity, is taken to the liver to be converted back to glucose via gluconeogenesis. This replenishes fuel for the muscle and prevents lactic acidosis.

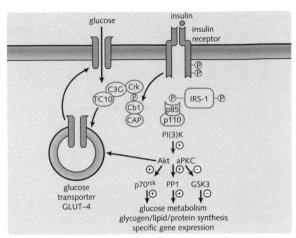

Fig 7.8 The insulin signaling pathway. Insulin binds to its receptor, resulting in autophosphorylation. This then phosphorylates the protein Cbl which is in complex with the adaptor protein CAP. Cbl/CAP complex then interacts with the adaptor protein Crk which is constitutively associated with C3G, a GTP/GDP exchange protein. C3G activates TC10, which themselves promote GLUT4 translocation to the plasma membrane. Autophosphorylation of the insulin receptor also phosphorylates insulin receptor substrate 1 (IRS-1). IRS-1 attracts p85, which binds to p110, which then activates phophatidylinositol-3 kinase (PI-3 kinase). PI 3 kinase activates protein kinase B (PKB) and Akt, which act on further pathways, resulting in glucose, lipid and protein metabolism, and specific gene expression. Akt also promotes GLUT-4 translocation to plasma membrane, resulting in increased glucose uptake.

insulin is not yet fully elucidated and is currently an active research area.

Basically, the binding of insulin to its tyrosine kinase receptor on the outside surface of the cells induces the receptor to undergo autophosphorylation at several tyrosine kinase residues located inside the cell. This autophosphorylation facilitates binding and phosphorylation of cytosolic substrate proteins, such as insulin receptor substrate-1 (IRS-1) and Cbl proteins. Upon phosphorylation, these proteins interact with other signaling molecules through their SH2 (Src-homology-2) domains, which then activates several diverse pathways.

Such pathways include activation of PI_3 kinase and TC10 (a small GTP binding protein). The net result of these diverse pathways is regulation of glucose, lipid and protein metabolism as well as cell growth and differentiation (Fig. 7.8).

DIABETES MELLITUS

Classification

Diabetes mellitus is a syndrome caused by the lack, or diminished effectiveness, of insulin. It results in a raised blood glucose known as hyperglycaemia. There are two main types:

- Type 1: formerly known as insulin-dependent diabetes mellitus (IDDM) in which there is an absolute failure of the pancreas to produce insulin.
- Type 2: formerly known as non-insulin dependent diabetes mellitus (NIDDM) in which there is a failure of the tissues to respond normally to insulin, together with a compensatory rise in plasma insulin concentration at early stages. As the disease progresses, insulin secretion deteriorates.

Type 1 diabetes mellitus

Type 1 was often referred to as juvenile-onset diabetes because it typically presents in childhood or puberty. It accounts for only 10–20% of the total number of people with diabetes and has an incidence rate of about 1 in 3000.

The aetiology of the disease is a complete deficiency of insulin that can only be corrected by life-long insulin treatment. There are three theories as to its cause:

- Auto-immune destruction of the β cells in the islets of Langerhans in the pancreas by islet cell auto-antibodies, resulting in insulin deficiency.
- Genetic factors. The evidence for a genetic cause is that, firstly, there is a 50% concordance between identical twins, which implies a mixture of both genetic and environmental factors. Secondly, there is a positive family history in approximately 10% of patients. Thirdly, more than 90% of patients with Type 1 diabetes carry HLA DR3 and DR4 antigens, compared with 40% of the general population.
- A viral cause, for example mumps or Coxsackie B, has also been considered. However, it is likely that viral infections provide the stimulus for auto-immune destruction rather than actually initiating diabetes.

Therefore, the cause is probably a mixture of all three – 'an auto-immune destruction of the β cells in genetically susceptible patients which may be precipitated by a viral infection.

The presentation of the disease is usually of rapid onset, weeks or days, with the characteristic symptoms of polyuria, polydipsia and weight loss.

Type 2 diabetes mellitus

This was also known as maturity-onset diabetes, because it typically presents after the age of 35 years. The incidence is more common, and it accounts for 80–90% of the total number of people with diabetes.

Type 2 diabetes is caused by:

- Impaired insulin secretion from the β cells; they fail to secrete enough insulin to correct the blood glucose level.
- Insulin resistance in the tissues, that is, cells failing to respond adequately to insulin.

Genetic factors are very important; there is almost 100% concordance between identical twins and about 30% of patients have a first-degree relative with Type 2 diabetes. There is no auto-immune or viral involvement.

The presentation is of an insidious onset and more than 80% of patients are obese. Sufferers are not normally prone to ketoacidosis but it can develop under stress.

In every medical examination, there will always be questions on diabetes. Know the effects of an increased glucagon/insulin ratio—the rest can be easily worked out!

Other types of diabetes

There are a number of other types of diabetes, which usually occur secondary to a predisposing factor, for example:

- Gestational diabetes that has its onset during pregnancy.
- Secondary diabetes: this may be the result of damage to the pancreas itself, for example in chronic pancreatitis or haemochromatosis, where iron may deposit in the pancreas (see Chapter 8). Diabetes may also occur secondary to the excessive secretion of catabolic hormones, resulting in hyperglycaemia and insulin resistance. For example, in acromegaly, where there is over-secretion of growth hormone, or in Cushing's syndrome, where there are high levels of glucocorticoids such as cortisol; also in poorly monitored long-term steroid therapy.

These other types of diabetes are covered in more detail in textbooks of endocrinology and clinical medicine.

Metabolic effects of diabetes mellitus

Type 1 diabetes mellitus

Insulin normally facilitates the uptake of glucose by peripheral tissues. In its absence, glucose remains in the blood, resulting in a decreased tissue availability of glucose, but a high plasma concentration of glucose. The phrase 'starvation in the midst of plenty' is frequently used to describe this. As there is a low concentration of insulin, the metabolic effects of glucagon and the other catabolic hormones are unopposed (see Fig. 7.6). This results in the predominance of catabolic processes, that is, the breakdown of carbohydrate, protein and fat (see Fig. 7.9). This aggravates hyperglycaemia, leading to keto-acidosis, hypertriglyceridaemia and importantly, dehydration (because of osmotic diuresis causing large amounts of glucose to enter urine). Keto-acidosis is life-threatening. Because cells cannot obtain glucose from the diet they have to obtain it by the breakdown of body stores or by synthesizing it from non-carbohydrate precursors (gluconeogenesis).

Thus, hyperglycaemia is caused by:

- A decreased uptake of glucose by the tissues, leading to a large increase in blood glucose.
- Glucagon-stimulated increase in the breakdown of liver glycogen and gluconeogenesis, leading to an increased hepatic output of glucose.

Ketoacidosis is caused by:

- An increase in triacylglycerol hydrolysis in adipose tissue, that releases fatty acids.
- An increase in ketone body synthesis in liver.

The release of fatty acids is much greater than in starvation; therefore, the rate of formation of ketone bodies is much greater than the rate of use, leading to ketonaemia (see Chapter 4).

Hypertriglyceridaemia is an increase in the concentration of triacylglycerols in plasma. (Note

that in clinical medicine triacylglycerols are usually referred to as triglycerides.) It is caused by:

- Some of the fatty acids released from triacylglycerols being packaged in the liver into very-low-density lipoproteins (VLDLs). Dietary triacylglycerols are assembled into chylomicrons.
- In the absence of insulin, the activity of lipoprotein lipase decreases, and the VLDLs and chylomicrons remain in the plasma, and are responsible for hypertriglyceridaemia (see Fig. 7.9).

A lot of people liken diabetes to starvation but there are some very important differences that can lead to fatal consequences for a diabetic patient (Fig. 7.10).

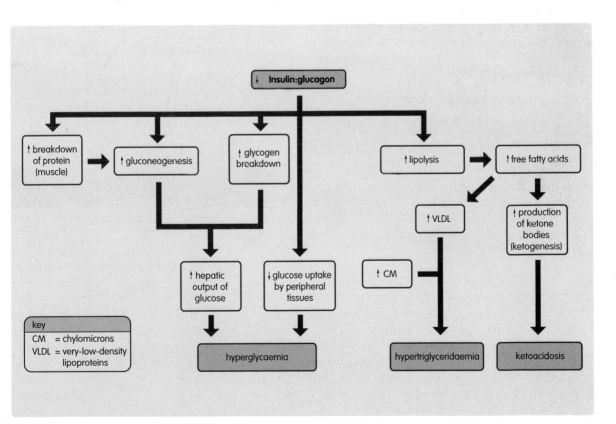

Fig. 7.9 Effect of an increased glucagon to insulin ratio in diabetes.

Type 2 diabetes mellitus

The metabolic effects are essentially the same as for Type 1 but usually they are milder because insulin is present. However:

- The amount of insulin secreted from the pancreas may be insufficient to cope with the blood glucose level.
- Target tissues or organs fail to respond correctly to insulin (they show insulin resistance).

In Type 2 diabetes, insulin resistance may be due to a number of defects, for example an abnormal insulin receptor or a defect in a glucose transporter. Insulin resistance in the liver results in uncontrolled glucose production and its decreased uptake by the peripheral tissues. Both phenomena contribute to hyperglycaemia. Hyperglycaemia in turn further stimulates insulin secretion by the pancreas. Type 2 diabetes is typically associated with older age of onset and, most importantly, with obesity.

Obesity is associated with an increase in the number and/or size of adipocytes. These cells overproduce hormones and cytokines, collectively known as adipokines, such as leptin and tumour necrosis factor-alpha, (TNF-α) which induce cellular resistance to insulin by interfering with the phosphorylation of the insulin receptor and IRS-1. Adipocytes also decrease synthesis of hormones such as adiponectin, which normally enhance insulin

During pregnancy, there is a decrease in insulin sensitivity to help provide the developing fetus with adequate glucose. However, in 3–5% of pregnant women, glucose intolerance develops. This is known as gestational diabetes mellitus (GDM), which is defined by an additional decrease in insulin sensitivity and an inability to compensate with increased insulin secretion. GDM is generally reversible after pregnancy, but about 30–50% of women with GDM go on to develop Type 2 diabetes later in life, particularly if they are obese.

responsiveness. As a result, there is insulin resistance in muscle and liver. Initially, the pancreas maintains glycaemic control by overproducing insulin but prolonged overproduction of insulin eventually results in failure of the β-cells, leading to Type 2 diabetes. However, there is still hope for improvement since insulin resistance has been shown to be reversible with weight loss and increased exercise.

Clinical features

Type 1 diabetes mellitus

The clinical features and diagnosis of Type 1 diabetes are listed in Fig. 7.11. The treatment consists of:

- Insulin. There are three main types of insulin: short acting, intermediate acting and long-acting. The duration of action of insulin is increased by

Fig. 7.10 Important differences between Type 1 diabetes mellitus and starvation

Feature	Type 1 diabetes mellitus	Starvation
Insulin	Absent or very low due to disruption of synthesis	Insulin produced but present at low level
Blood glucose	Hyperglycaemia	Normal blood glucose concentration maintained
Ketone body formation	Large increase in production of ketone bodies where rate of formation exceeds rate of use; can lead to life-threatening ketoacidosis	Increased concentration, but usually rate of formation equals rate of use

Fig. 7.11 Clinical features and diagnosis of Type 1 (insulin-dependent) diabetes mellitus

Main clinical features	Diagnostic criteria
Classically: • acute onset of symptoms (2–4 weeks) polyuria, polydipsia, accompanied by weight loss and tiredness • ketoacidosis: may present in diabetic coma	Presence of symptoms Raised random blood glucose, > 11.1 mmol/L Fasting blood glucose: venous plasma ≥7.0 mmol/L (oral glucose tolerance test is not necessary—reserved for borderline cases; glycosuria is not diagnostic due to variation in renal threshold for glucose)

forming a complex with a protamine salt and/or varying the size of the crystals.

- Diet, ensuring the correct content and timing of meals. The diet should be high in fibre and unrefined carbohydrate, low in saturated fat and refined carbohydrate.
- Education. It is crucial that patients understand their disease, and the short- and long-term benefits of treatment.

There are a number of methods for monitoring the control of diabetes and these are covered in detail in Chapter 11. They include:

- Measuring blood glucose levels, using reagent strips based on the glucose oxidase reaction, or portable glucose meters.
- Monitoring the level of glycated haemoglobin (HbA_{1c}). This provides a measure of the average blood glucose control over the past 4–6 weeks.
- The detection of ketones in urine (and blood), important for the detection of developing ketoacidosis.
- Detection and monitoring of chronic complications.

Type 2 diabetes mellitus
The diagnosis, management and treatment of Type 2 diabetes are covered in Fig. 7.12.

Complications of diabetes
These develop slowly when diabetes is poorly controlled.

Acute complications
Hypoglycaemia. The aim of treatment of Type 1 diabetes with insulin is to maintain a normal blood glucose level, which decreases the long-term effects of diabetes. However, too much insulin or too infrequent 'top ups' of blood glucose (i.e. insufficient intake of carbohydrate) lead to a low blood glucose (hypoglycaemia). Hypoglycaemia causes unpleasant autonomic symptoms, such as sweating, nausea and palpitations, and more severe neuroglycopenic symptoms as a result of a decrease in glucose supply to the brain: drowsiness, unsteadiness, confusion and coma (these patients may look drunk). This is a **very serious** condition and must be treated without delay with an intravenous 50% dextrose infusion. Mild hypoglycaemia can be treated with sugar or sweet drinks.

Fig. 7.12 Diagnosis, management and treatment of Type 2 diabetes (non-insulin dependent diabetes, NIDDM)

Clinical features	Management
• insidious onset: tiredness, polyuria, thirst, weight loss • patients usually older and typically obese • may be asymptomatic—detection of ↑ blood glucose on routine check-up **Diagnosis:** as for Type 1—symptoms usually less severe	**Diet:** often the only treatment necessary **Oral hypoglycaemic drugs:** 2 main types: • sulphonylureas, e.g. glibenclamide: ↑ insulin secretion by islet cells (inhibits ATP-sensitive K^+ channels in β cell membranes) • biguanides, e.g. metformin: ↑ glucose uptake by peripheral tissues and ↓ glucose production by liver • thiazolidinediones, e.g. rosiglitazone: ↑ insulin sensitivity N.B. acarbose inhibits intestinal enzyme, glucosidase and therefore delays the digestion of starch **insulin** is sometimes necessary when Type 2 diabetes poorly controlled

Diabetic ketoacidosis. In the absence of insulin, effects of glucagon are unopposed. Decreased uptake of glucose by tissues, coupled with an increased hepatic glucose production, leads to hyperglycaemia. This causes an osmotic diuresis, and the resulting loss of fluid and electrolytes results in dehydration. An increase in lipolysis leads to increased ketogenesis and a metabolic acidosis. Respiratory compensation results in hyperventilation. Failure to treat a patient in ketoacidosis would result in coma and death. Both dehydration and hyperglycaemia must be corrected (Fig. 7.13).

Chronic complications
In the long term the major cause of death in Type 1 diabetes are chronic complications, particularly diabetic nephropathy. In type 2 diabetes, heart disease, peripheral vascular disease and stroke are the major causes of death.

Good control of diabetes (i.e. when the blood glucose is maintained close to normal) decreases the frequency and progression of microangiopathy (but apparently not macroangiopathy) (Fig. 7.14).

The WHO criteria for diagnosis of diabetes are as follows: fasting venous plasma glucose equal or above 7 mmol/L. A glucose level of 6–7 mmol/L is defined as impaired fasting glucose (IFG). If the patient has no diabetic symptoms, diagnosis should not be based on a single glucose value.

'Compare Type 1 diabetes mellitus (IDDM) with Type 2 (NIDDM)' is a commonly asked exam question; Fig. 7.15 should help.

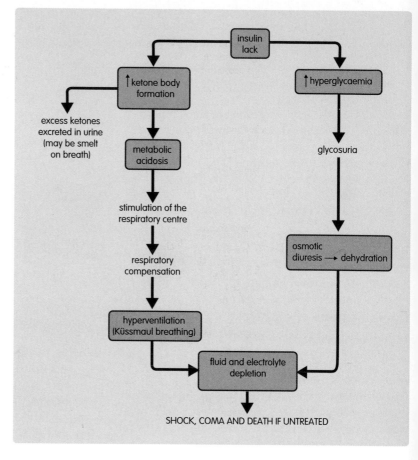

Fig. 7.13 Diabetic ketoacidosis. In the absence of insulin, hyperglycaemia causes osmotic diuresis. The loss of fluid and electrolytes results in dehydration. Increased ketogenesis causes metabolic acidosis. Respiratory compensation results in hyperventilation. Both dehydration and hyperglycaemia must be corrected in parallel with insulin treatment.

Fig. 7.14 Some long-term complications of diabetes mellitus

Complications	Proposed mechanisms
Diabetic microangiopathy affects small blood vessels: In eyes: causes retinopathy and cataracts Kidneys: causes nephropathy Peripheral and autonomic nervous system: causes neuropathy	**1. Sorbitol (polyol) pathway** (see Fig. 2.43): Glucose is converted to sorbitol by aldose reductase found particularly in lens, retina, Schwann cells of peripheral nerves and kidney In diabetes, hyperglycaemia leads to increased sorbitol formation in these tissues as they do not require insulin for glucose entry Sorbitol cannot be metabolized further or leave these cells and therefore it accumulates; it exerts a strong osmotic effect causing cells to swell, causing damage **2. Glycation of proteins** Haemoglobin is non-enzymatically glycosylated to form HbA$_{1c}$ Other proteins may also be glycated, which may mediate some of the damage as glycation may increase their oxidative potential
Diabetic macroangiopathy affects large blood vessels causing accelerated atherosclerosis	Precise mechanism is unknown The risk of cardiovascular disease in people with diabetes is 2–3 times higher than the risk of non-diabetic persons

Fig. 7.15 Comparison of Type 1 and Type 2 diabetes mellitus

	Type 1	Type 2
Usual age of onset	Young < 25 years	> 35 years
Auto-immune factors	Yes	No
Genetic factors	Risk associated with certain HLA types	Yes—polygenic inheritance
Concordance identical twins	50%	Almost 100%
Symptoms	Polyuria, polydipsia, weight loss	Similar but usually less severe presentation
Signs	Wasting, dehydration, loss of consciousness	Obesity
Ketosis	Prone	Rare; precipitated by stress
Obesity	Infrequent	Frequent

Nutrition

Objectives

You should be able to :

- Understand how energy is used by the body.
- Discuss the causes of obesity, its complications, prevention and treatment.
- Discuss protein requirements and the main causes and clinical features of protein deficiency diseases.
- Describe the main causes and clinical features of vitamin and mineral deficiency diseases, along with the diagnosis and treatment available.

BASIC PRINCIPLES OF HUMAN NUTRITION

Definitions

Nutrients

Nutrients are essential dietary factors, such as vitamins, minerals, essential amino acids and essential fatty acids, that cannot be synthesized by the body sufficiently. Sources of energy are not classed as nutrients and neither is water nor dietary fibre.

Staple foods

Staple foods are the principal sources of energy in the diet. They are specific to a particular country; for example, in parts of Africa and Asia cereals provide more than 70% of the energy in the diet. As countries become more prosperous, the percentage of energy derived from a single staple food declines. In the UK, flour and flour products provide only about 25% of food energy.

Digestion in the gastrointestinal tract (Fig. 8.1)

Digestion of carbohydrates

Digestion of carbohydrates begins in the mouth and stomach. Saliva contains an enzyme α-amylase, which hydrolyses starch into maltose and other small polymers of glucose. Digestion continues in the stomach for about an hour before the activity of salivary amylase is blocked by gastric acid.

Pancreatic secretions, like saliva, contain large quantities of α-amylase. It is identical to the α-amylase in saliva, thus virtually all the starches are digested by the time they enter the duodenum. Disaccharides and small glucose polymers are hydrolysed into monosaccharides by intestinal epithelial enzymes.

- Lactose is broken down into a molecule of galactose and a molecule of glucose.
- Sucrose is broken down into a molecule of fructose and a molecule of glucose.
- Maltose and other small glucose polymers are broken down into molecules of glucose.

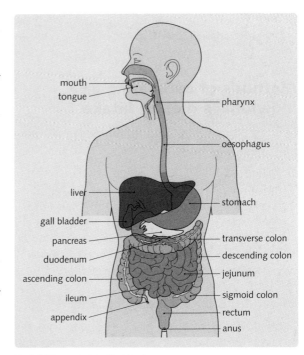

Fig 8.1 The gastrointestinal tract.

Digestion of proteins

Protein digestion begins in the stomach. The enzyme pepsin breaks down collagen to allow other enzymes to penetrate meats and digest cellular proteins. Most protein digestion occurs through the actions of pancreatic proteolytic enzymes.

- Trypsin and chymotrypsin break down protein molecules into small polypeptides.
- Carboxypolypeptidase cleaves amino acids from the carboxyl ends of the polypeptides.
- Proelastase gives rise to elastase, which then digests the elastin fibres that hold meat together.

The last stage of digestion of proteins is carried out in the intestinal lumen by enterocytes, which contain multiple peptidases that break down remaining tripeptides and dipeptides into amino acids, which then enter the blood.

Digestion of fats

Fat digestion begins with the emulsification by bile acids and lecithin, where fat globules are broken into smaller pieces to increase their surface area. Pancreatic lipase breaks down triglycerides into free fatty acids and 2-monoglycerides which are carried to the brush border of the intestinal epithelial cells by micelles. Micelles are composed of a central fat globule (containing monoglycerides and free fatty acids) with molecules of bile salt projecting outward covering the surface of the micelle.

Methods of estimating an individual's dietary intake

There are three main methods for estimating an individual's dietary intake:

- *Dietary recall.* Ask the patient what he or she has eaten. This is the least accurate because it relies on the patient's recall and willingness to cooperate.
- *Food diary.* This is slightly more accurate.
- *Complete chemical analysis.* This is the most expensive but the most accurate method.

Dietary reference values (Fig. 8.2)

The following definitions are in keeping with the dietary reference values (DRVs) for food energy and nutrients for the UK:

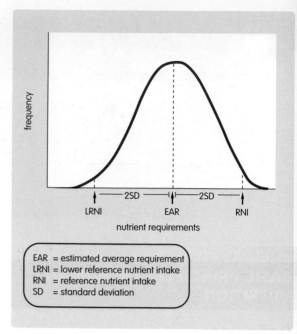

Fig. 8.2 Dietary reference values for food energy and nutrients.

EAR = estimated average requirement
LRNI = lower reference nutrient intake
RNI = reference nutrient intake
SD = standard deviation

- *Estimated average requirement* (EAR). This is the average requirement of a group of people for energy or a nutrient. About 50% of the population will need less than the EAR and 50% will need more.
- *Reference nutrient intake* (RNI). This is the amount of nutrient that is enough or more than enough for about 97% of people in the group (EAR + 2 SD).
- *Lower reference nutrient intake* (LRNI). This is the amount of nutrient that is sufficient for only a few people in a group with low needs (EAR – 2 SD).
- *Adequate intake* is the amount of nutrient enough for almost everyone, but not so much as to cause undesirable effects. This term is applied for nutrients for which there is not enough information known to estimate EAR, RNI or LRNI (e.g. vitamin E).

For instance, the DRVs for vitamin C are: LRNI, 10 mg/day; EAR, 25 mg/day; RNI, 40 mg/day. Therefore below the LRNI, symptoms of vitamin C deficiency (scurvy) are seen and above the RNI, symptoms of excess may be seen.

Fig. 8.3 Major sources of energy in the diet

Energy source	Total energy/g kcal	kJ
Fat: essential for absorption of fat-soluble vitamins (A, D, E and K)	9.2	38.6
Carbohydrate: as either starch, sugar or non-starch polysaccharide (NSP), i.e. fibre	4.0	16.8
Protein:	5.4	22.7
Alcohol: 'empty calories'	7.0	29.4

ENERGY BALANCE

Food energy

The total energy content of food is the amount of energy released when food is completely burnt in air to CO_2 and H_2O, that is, the heat of combustion (Fig. 8.3). The total energy is equal to the sum of the digestible energy and the non-digestible energy (Fig. 8.4).

- Non-digestible energy is the energy in food that we cannot break down and is lost in faeces (e.g. cellulose).
- Digestible energy is the total energy minus energy that is lost in faeces.

Metabolizable energy is the energy available to the body for use; it has three fates:

- 50% is lost as heat.
- 5–10% of energy is released during the digestion, absorption and transport of food. This is known as either the thermic effect of food, diet-induced thermogenesis (DIT), or post-prandial thermogenesis (they all mean the same thing).
- Only about 25–40% of the energy is trapped as ATP; that is, the body is only 25–40% efficient.

From Fig. 8.3, it can be seen that protein has a higher total energy content than carbohydrate. However, protein is not as efficiently oxidized (it forms urea and requires ATP for this; see Chapter 5) and only about 4 kcal/g are available as metabolizable energy. Carbohydrate is oxidized completely to CO_2 and H_2O and all the energy produced is available for use; thus the metabolizable energy is also 4 kcal/g.

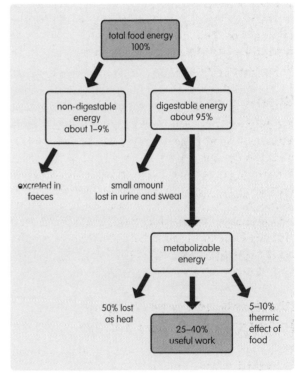

Fig. 8.4 Food energy utilization.

Body composition

An average 72 kg man is composed of:

- 15% fat.
- 85% lean body mass (LBM).

Lean body mass (LBM) is made up of (these are approximate values):

- 72% water.
- 20% protein.
- 8% bone mineral.

Generally, women have a higher fat content (about 25% fat) than men. Fat content tends to increase with age. An average 72 kg man can survive on his energy stores for about 50–60 days provided he is given water. This is mostly due to fat reserves; glycogen stores last only 12–24 hours. Fig. 8.5 summarizes the methods available to measure body composition. However, most of the methods, with the exception of anthropometry, are rarely used in clinical practice.

Energy requirements

Energy is used by the body for three main processes.

Basal metabolic rate

The basal metabolic rate (BMR) is the energy used to carry out normal body functions such as blood flow and breathing; the energy expended doing nothing. The units of BMR are kJ/hour/kg of body weight. To calculate the BMR:

Fig. 8.5 Measurement of body composition	
Measurement	**Method**
Body density	Weigh in air to give fat content (density = 0.9 mg/mL); weigh in water to give lean body mass (density = 1.1 mg/mL)
Body water	The patient is injected with a known volume of tritiated water Its concentration at equilibrium is measured This is representative of lean body mass
Total body potassium	$^{40}K^+$ is injected and its distribution assessed This is a measure of lean body mass as there is no potassium in fat
Body fat	The uptake of a fat-soluble gas, e.g. xenon or cyclopropane is measured Biopsy to measure concentration
Anthropometry	Measure: • weight and height • mid-arm circumference (biceps and triceps) • skin-fold thickness (subscapular and suprailiac) compare with normograms for weight and height

- The patient must be at rest, lying down but not asleep.
- The temperature of the environment must be moderate and constant.
- The patient must be assessed about 12 hours after the last meal or any exercise.

The BMR is usually measured first thing in the morning. It is proportional to LBM, therefore men have a higher BMR than women. Women have a greater percentage of fat which is less metabolically active. The BMR usually accounts for 50–70% of the total energy expended.

Thermic effect of food

This is the energy required for the digestion and absorption of food and accounts for 5–10% of the energy expenditure.

Physical activity

The amount of energy consumed depends on the duration and intensity of exercise. The physical activity ratio (PAR) can be measured for situations where activity is expressed as a multiple of the BMR (i.e. BMR = 1).

The PAR = metabolic rate during exercise ÷ BMR.

For example:

Lying	1.0 (equal to BMR)
Sitting	1.2
Standing	1.7
Football	7.0

The physical activity level (PAL) can also be calculated. This is equal to the total energy expenditure in 1 day divided by the BMR.

Other factors can also affect energy requirements. For example:

- Environmental temperature changes. This is a very small effect unless the temperature is either extremely high or low.
- Pregnancy and lactation. For the first 6 months of pregnancy no extra energy is necessary, but for the last 3 months, an extra 800 kJ (200 kcal) are needed each day. During lactation, an extra 2000 kJ (500 kcal) are required each day.
- Growth. The energy requirement in the first year of life is double that of adulthood.
- Age. The BMR decreases after the age of about 20 years.

How do we measure energy requirements?

Indirect calorimetry

The measurement of O_2 consumption allows indirect measurement of the metabolic rate. This is because 1 litre of O_2 consumed at rest is equal to 20 kJ of energy expenditure.

Indirect mass spectrophotometry

The incorporation of doubly labelled water ($^2H_2{}^{18}O$) into body fluids and its loss in the urine can be measured. ^2H is incorporated only into H_2O but ^{18}O is incorporated into both H_2O and CO_2. The difference between them is equal to the CO_2 produced.

Regulation of food intake

A number of systems are thought to participate in the regulation of food intake.

Overall control: the hypothalamus

There are two important areas for the control of food intake:

- The hunger or 'feeding' centre in the lateral hypothalamic area.
- The satiety centre in the ventromedial nucleus.

Lesions in the hunger centre have been shown to inhibit appetite and thus feeding, and to lead to anorexia. Lesions in the satiety centre cause overeating and obesity.

Gastric distension and gut hormones

Cholecystokinin (CCK) is known to decrease appetite. CCK slows gastric emptying, thus maintaining gastric distension, which is thought to be an important satiety signal.

Plasma concentration of glucose, insulin and glucagon

Originally it was thought that low plasma glucose levels had a direct stimulatory effect on the hunger centre. Now it is believed that it is the increased availability of glucose to tissues that produces satiety (the glucostat hypothesis). Insulin therefore promotes satiety by stimulating the uptake of glucose by peripheral tissues.

Obesity

If energy intake is equal to energy expenditure, there is no change in body mass. Obesity results from an imbalance between the input, storage and expenditure of energy; that is, it develops when energy intake is greater than energy expenditure.

Definition

Obesity can be categorized in terms of the body mass index (BMI).

$$BMI\ (kg/m^2) = weight/(height)^2$$

The categories for BMI are:

< 18.5	Underweight
18.5–24.9	Ideal weight
25.0–29.9	Overweight
>30	Obesity

Obesity is associated with an increased risk of various clinical disorders.

Currently, obesity is rising to epidemic proportions. Obesity in men, women and children is increasing rapidly in many Western and in some developing countries. This problem is beginning to replace malnutrition and infectious diseases as the most significant contributor to ill health worldwide. In developing countries, it is estimated that more than 115 million people suffer from weight-related problems.

Aetiology

Fig. 8.6 discusses some of the proposed theories for obesity. Twin studies suggest a genetic background. However, genetic factors are greatly influenced by environmental and socio-economic factors. Poor education, high alcohol intake, and less energy expenditure, increase the incidence of obesity. This may also be related to the type of food consumed, which is largely governed by financial status. The most obvious cause for obesity is an imbalance between energy input and expenditure. The reasons for overeating are usually complex and may be psychological in origin, related to stress or a life event. Only rarely are there metabolic causes.

Clinical consequences

Obesity is associated with an increased risk of:

Fig. 8.6 Causes of obesity

Cause	Evidence	Comments
Excessive intake of calories	Psychological factors, stress or social reasons	Most common cause
Genetic	Identical twins are not always the same weight Adopted children resemble their new family weightwise	Likely genetic predisposition but also modified by environmental factors (diet, social-economic status) Recent evidence suggests that there is a 'gene' for obesity
Socio-economic	In the West, low socio-economic class → obesity In the East, high socio-economic class → obesity	Survey in Finland and Scotland showed obesity is associated with: • low education • high alcohol intake • giving up smoking • getting married!
Endocrine	Adrenal hyperfunction (Cushing's syndrome), hypothyroidism, and Type 2 diabetes mellitus are all associated with obesity	But most obese people do not have endocrine problems
Energy expenditure	Diet-induced thermogenesis (DIT) is greater in lean people (N.B. basal metabolic rate is not lower in obese people!)	Maybe obese people are better atconserving energy
	80% of obese teenagers become obese adults hypothesis is that standard weight is set in infancy when fat people develop a greater number of fat cells than thin people	Not true!
	Note the recently increasing rate of child and adolescent obesity	

- Type 2 diabetes. Obesity results in persistently high insulin levels, leading to a down-regulation of insulin receptors and thus insulin resistance in the tissues.
- Coronary heart disease. There is an increase in morbidity and mortality caused by coronary heart disease in obese individuals. It may be that other risk factors are more likely to be present in obese patients.
- Hypertension.
- Respiratory problems.
- Stroke.
- Gallstones. Especially if fat, female, forty, and fertile!
- Osteoarthritis and back pain.
- Gout.

Prevention and treatment

Treatment of obesity is generally unsatisfactory. Possibilities include:

- **Reduction of energy intake.** The main treatment of an obese patient is an appropriate diet, with plenty of support and encouragement from a doctor. Lots of different weight-reducing diets have been formulated; most do not work particularly in the long term! For example, on a low-carbohydrate diet, where bread, potatoes, cakes and any starch-containing foods are cut out of the diet, initially, weight loss is fast (0.5 kg/day) but most of the loss is water. Protein is also broken down to maintain the blood glucose, but is replaced as soon as the diet is stopped. The loss of fat is the same as for a normal mixed diet. However, low carbohydrate diets improve glucose tolerance.

Other diets such as low-fat diet and low-cholesterol diet are also used to help treat obesity. Recent trials, utilizing diets low in saturated fat and supplemented with polyunsaturated fatty acids, mainly from omega-3 fatty acids (three helpings of oily fish per week, fish oil capsules and alpha-linoleic acid margarine), have shown to be beneficial in helping patients to lose weight.

Most weight-reducing diets allow an intake of 1000 kcal/day. This must be a balanced intake of protein, carbohydrate and fat (i.e. a mixed diet). Why is it that 80–100% of obese people regain lost weight? During starvation, the metabolic rate falls by 15–30%. Therefore, after dieting, to remain at a lower weight, a lower energy intake must be maintained otherwise the weight will be put straight back on. The only way to lose weight is a prolonged moderation of intake and then a permanent change in eating habits to maintain the weight loss.

- **Increase energy expenditure** in a way appropriate to age and health.
- **Drug therapy** is not generally recommended in the UK and it can only be used after dietary measures are proven to be unsuccessful. Orlistat is a pancreatic lipase inhibitor which is licensed for use together with a mildly hypocaloric diet in those with a BMI of greater than 30 kg/m^2. Part of its effect may be related to the reduction of fat intake necessary to avoid severe gastrointestinal effects such as steatorrhoea. Appetite suppressants such as phentermine (a catecholaminergic drug with minor sympathomimetic and stimulant effects) are not presently used. Currently, research is being done on unraveling the links between obesity and adipokine secretion. Adipokines are a variety of proteins with signaling properties produced in adipose tissue. An example is leptin which was discovered in 1994, and was found to signal the status of energy stores; its secretion can reduce appetite and increase energy expenditure. As a result, leptin and other adipokines are

The main cause of obesity is usually an excessive intake of calories accompanied by a decrease in energy expenditure.

Morbidity is the incidence or prevalence of disease in a population. Mortality is the number of deaths from disease in a population.

currently being investigated for use in the diagnosis and treatment of obesity.
- **Surgery.** This is extreme and performed in selected cases only. Examples include: jaw wiring, gastric plication (stapling the walls of the stomach together to form a smaller stomach), bypass of the small intestine, and gastric distension.

PROTEINS AND NUTRITION

Definitions

Reference proteins
Reference proteins contain all the amino acids in the exact proportions needed for protein synthesis. Albumin (found in egg white) and casein (milk) are closest to the ideal. Other proteins are compared with these reference proteins.

Limiting amino acids
A limiting amino acid is the essential amino acid present in a protein in the lowest amount relative to its requirement for protein synthesis. Examples of protein-containing foods and their limiting amino acids are:

- Wheat, limited by lysine.
- Meat and fish, limited by methionine and cysteine.
- Maize, limited by tryptophan.

Combining different protein-containing foods, such as meat and the pulses, ensures an adequate intake of all the amino acids, that is, protein complementation. This is particularly important in vegetarian diets.

Protein quality

The quality of any protein can be assessed using a rating system based on a number of variables.

Chemical score

The chemical score is the ratio of the amount of limiting amino acid to its requirement, expressed as percentage points. For example, if the amount of limiting amino acid in a test protein is 2% and the amount of limiting amino acid in the reference protein is 5%; the chemical score is 40%.

Biological value

The biological value is the proportion of the absorbed protein which is retained by the body for protein synthesis.

Net protein utilization

The net protein utilization (NPU) is the proportion of dietary protein which is retained by the body for protein synthesis. For example:

- For a typical mixed Western diet, NPU is 70%, meaning that 70% of the dietary protein is retained for protein synthesis.
- For a diet of mainly meat, NPU would be 75%.
- For a diet of cereals, NPU would be 50–60%.
- For a diet of eggs, NPU would be 100%.

Net dietary protein as a percentage of energy

Net dietary protein as a percentage of energy (NDPE%) is the proportion of total dietary energy provided by fully 'usable' protein. This method provides a way of comparing different diets. For example:

- Cereal-based diets provide 5–6%.
- Western diets provide 10–12%.
- In India, the diet provides 10%.

Children require an NDPE% of greater than 8%, that is, at least 8% of their diet must come from usable protein. Adults require an NDPE% of greater than 5%. In areas where the staple food is starch (e.g. yam, cassava), the diet provides only low levels of protein. It would be physically impossible to consume the amount of food necessary to satisfy the protein requirement, especially for children, and this leads to protein deficiency states. Cereal-based diets are adequate for adults but not children.

Protein requirement

Diet should provide the essential amino acids and enough amino acid nitrogen to synthesize the non-essential amino acids. These are required for:

- Maintenance of tissue proteins in adults.
- Formation of body proteins during periods of growth, pregnancy, lactation, infection, and after major trauma or illness such as cancer.

The recommended protein requirement for an adult in the UK is 0.8 g/kg/day of protein and should not be greater than 1.5 g/kg/day.

The RNI for protein is 55 g/day for men and 44 g/day for women.

Protein–energy deficiency states

Protein–energy malnutrition (PEM) arises when the body's need for protein or energy, or both, is not met by the diet. It is most commonly seen in developing countries. However, in the industrialized world, it can be present in the elderly or chronically ill patients.

Causes of PEM

These can be one or a combination of the following:

- Decreased dietary intake.
- Malabsorption.
- Increased requirement; for example, in preterm infants, infection (septic state increases catabolism), major trauma or surgery.
- Psychological; for example, depression or anorexia nervosa.

The bulk of excess protein is oxidized via gluconeogenesis to glycogen or fat and stored by the body. Therefore protein is not a slimming food. One famous diet consists of a protein-sparing modified fast (PSMF) which is hydrolysed gelatine and collagen, thus it is cheap! However, during the hydrolysis process a lot of electrolytes are lost, including potassium, which may lead to serious problems.

In developing countries, PEM manifests as two conditions in children:

- Marasmus: lack of protein and energy (i.e. starvation).
- Kwashiorkor: lack of protein only—energy supply is adequate.

Incidence

In developing countries, 20–75% of children below 5 years of age have some form of malnutrition. Five million children die every year because of malnutrition.

Aetiology and mechanisms of pathogenesis

Marasmus

Marasmus is the childhood form of starvation (Figs 8.7 and 8.8). Both protein and energy are limited, leading to a low concentration of insulin but increased levels of glucagon and cortisol, that is, a starved state (see Chapter 7). As no fuel is available for the body, muscle protein and fat are broken down to provide energy, which leads to wasting. Muscle protein is broken down to amino acids

which are used for the synthesis of albumin by the liver; therefore, this prevents oedema.

Kwashiorkor

Translated this means the 'disease the first child gets when the second child is born'. In kwashiorkor severe protein deficiency occurs but energy is maintained (Figs 8.9 and 8.10). It usually occurs when a young child is weaned from breastfeeding because of the arrival of a new baby. The first child is fed a low protein, high starch diet instead. Kwashiorkor

---

Fig. 8.8 The clinical features of marasmus

Very thin, wasted appearance
Obvious muscle wasting and loss of body fat
<60% normal body weight
Age: usually <18 months
No oedema
Wrinkled skin, hair loss and apathy
Plasma albumin is usually **normal**
Diarrhoea and infection may be present
Electrolyte disturbances: low potassium and sodium common
Anaemia

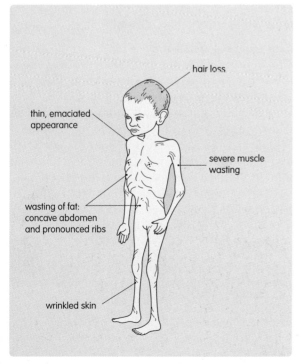

Fig. 8.7 Marasmus.

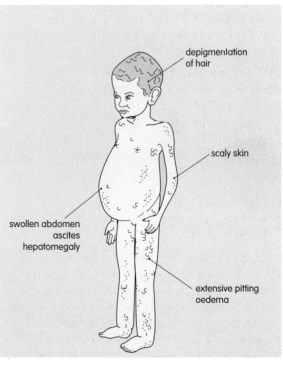

Fig. 8.9 Kwashiorkor.

Fig. 8.10 The features of kwashiorkor
Oedema: 'hides' severe wasting of underlying tissues Age: usually 2–4 years Scaly skin: 'flaky point' rash with hyperkeratosis Depigmentation of hair Distended abdomen caused by ascites and enlarged fatty liver Hypothermia and bradycardia Apathy Anaemia: due to folate, iron or copper metabolism disturbances **Low plasma albumin** Usually diarrhoea and/or infection Low potassium, sodium, glucose, and other electrolyte disturbances

Fig. 8.11 A comparison of marasmus and kwashiorkor

Feature	Marasmus	Kwashiorkor
Deficiency	Protein and energy	Protein only
Age	Usually < 18 months	Older: 1–5 years
Oedema	Absent Severe wasting of body protein and fat	Present Oedema hides wasting of body protein
Body weight	< 60% normal	60–80% normal
Cause	Severe malnutrition	Malnutrition Infection
Features	Wrinkled skin Hair loss Thin and emaciated	Scaly skin and dermatitis Sparse, depigmented hair Distended abdomen Hepatomegaly

often develops after an acute infection, such as measles or gastroenteritis, when the demand for protein is increased.

As energy is not limiting, there is a high insulin to glucagon, and insulin to cortisol ratio. Amino acids are taken up by muscle for protein synthesis. This diverts amino acids from the liver, so fewer are available for albumin synthesis: the resulting low albumin levels reduce the plasma oncotic pressure, causing oedema. The oedema causes a deceptively fat appearance and children are known as water or 'sugar' babies. It is possible there may also be some degree of energy loss in kwashiorkor and therefore other factors may contribute to, or cause, the oedema. For example:

- Excessive generation of free radicals causing membrane damage and oedema.
- Infection diverts protein synthesis from albumin to the synthesis of immunoglobulins and acute-phase proteins (e.g. C-reactive protein).

A comparison of kwashiorkor and marasmus is given in Fig. 8.11.

Management and treatment of PEM

It is important to restore fluid and electrolyte balance first. Following this:

- Any infection, hypothermia or hypoglycaemia present can be treated.
- Carefully re-feed initially, just enough to maintain a steady state to satisfy the normal daily requirement. Milk is often given with flour or maize, slowly and regularly.

- Eventually, high energy foods are given to restore weight and also any necessary vitamin and mineral supplements.

Prognosis

Mortality rates for children with severe malnutrition are about 50%. The rate is so high because adequate treatment is usually not available.

Consequences of prolonged PEM

Malnourished children are less active and more apathetic; these behavioural abnormalities are usually reversed by re-feeding. However, severe, prolonged malnutrition causes much reduced brain growth and permanent damage to both physical and mental development. Immunity is impaired, leading to delayed wound healing; protein loss from muscle may eventually include the diaphragm, leading to death. The physiological effects of severe prolonged malnutrition are listed in Fig. 8.12.

Prevention

Prevention of childhood malnutrition is a World Health Organization priority. The main targets are to provide:

- Food supplements and additional vitamins to 'at risk' groups.
- Family planning.
- Immunization programmes.

Fig. 8.12 The physiological effects of severe prolonged malnutrition

Effect	Consequence
Decreased brain development	Permanent damage to both physical and mental development
Defective immune system	Decreased cell-mediated response Immuno globulin production is maintained: this can have harmful effects as it depletes production of other proteins
Loss of protein	Firstly from muscle, then viscera → death
Electrolyte losses	May effect Na^+/K^+ pump and the maintenance of ion gradients across cells
Low haemoglobin	Anaemia
Low serum albumin (only kwashiorkor)	→ oedema
Impaired gastrointestinal function	Bacterial overgrowth and malabsorption
Fatty liver	Fat accumulates since its transport requires apolipoproteins that are deficient (not seen in marasmus)

However, drought, famine and war in affected countries often make these targets impossible to achieve.

In Western countries, a degree of PEM may be seen in hospitalized patients with the following conditions:

- Anorexia.
- Trauma, severe infection, major surgery, or burns.
- Cancer.

That is, anything that causes a negative nitrogen balance (see Chapter 5).

Malnutrition in adults in developing countries has symptoms similar to those seen in children but the results are not as devastating. This is because adults are already physically and mentally mature and are thus more resilient.

VITAMINS

Definition

A complex organic substance required in the diet in small amounts, the absence of which leads to a deficiency disease.

Vitamins can be divided into two main groups, fat-soluble and water-soluble.

Fat-soluble vitamins

Vitamins A, D, E and K. These are:

- Stored in the liver.
- Not absorbed or excreted easily.
- Can be toxic in excess (particularly A and D).

Water-soluble vitamins

The B-group vitamins and vitamin C. These are:

- Not stored extensively.
- Required regularly in the diet.
- Generally non-toxic in excess (within reason).

All B vitamins are coenzymes in metabolic pathways.

FAT-SOLUBLE VITAMINS

Vitamin A (retinol)

RNI
700 mg/day for men; 600 mg/day for women.

Sources
Animal sources are butter, whole milk, egg yolk, liver and fish liver oils; they contain retinol.

Plant sources are most green, yellow or orange vegetables; they contain β-carotene, the precursor of retinol.

Absorption and transport of vitamin A
Retinol is absorbed in the intestinal mucosa and esterified to long-chain fatty acids, forming retinyl esters. These are packaged in chylomicrons and transported to the liver for storage. When required, retinol is released and transported bound to retinol-binding protein. Retinol can be oxidized to other active forms, namely retinoic acid and retinal. β-carotene is absorbed in the intestine and converted into retinal.

Functions
There are three active forms of vitamin A:

- Retinoic acid, which acts as a typical steroid hormone. It binds to chromatin to increase the synthesis of proteins controlling cell growth and differentiation of epithelial cells. Therefore, it increases epithelial cell turnover.
- Retinal. 11-*cis* Retinal binds to opsin to form rhodopsin, the visual pigment of the rod cells in the retina involved in vision and particularly night vision (Fig. 8.13).
- β-carotene is an antioxidant. The role of antioxidants in the prevention of heart disease and lung cancer is being studied intensively, but has not yet produced any conclusive results.

Deficiency

Incidence
Vitamin A deficiency is rarely seen in developed countries because liver stores are sufficient to last 3–4 years. It is commonly found in children in developing countries such as India and parts of South-East Asia, where about 500 000 children each year are blinded as a result of vitamin A deficiency.

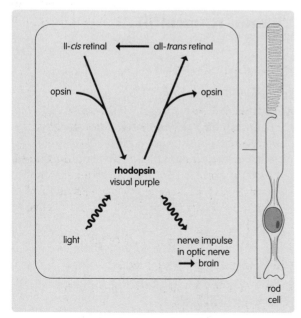

Fig. 8.13 Role of vitamin A in vision. 11-*cis* Retinal binds to opsin, converting it to rhodopsin, the visual pigment of the rod cells in the retina involved in vision and dark adaptation to light. Low light intensity (scotopic vision) activates a series of photochemical reactions that bleach rhodopsin, converting it to all-*trans* retinal, which triggers a nerve impulse in the optic nerve to the brain.

Causes
Vitamin A deficiency may be caused by a decreased dietary intake; usually only seen in very severe malnutrition. It may also occur secondary to fat malabsorption.

Clinical features
In the eye, the symptoms are progressive:

- Initially, deficiency causes impaired dark adaptation and night blindness. This is reversible.
- Severe prolonged deficiency results in xerophthalmia: a dryness of the cornea and conjunctiva due to progressive epithelial keratinization. Bitot's spots may be seen, which are white plaques of keratinized epithelial cells on the conjunctiva.
- If untreated, keratomalacia develops, causing corneal ulceration and the formation of opaque scar tissue (cataracts); this causes irreversible blindness.

In the skin, decreased epithelial cell turnover produces:

- Thickening and dryness of skin due to hyperkeratosis.
- Impaired mucosal function.

Diagnosis and treatment
Diagnosis and treatment are usually on the basis of the above clinical features. The following can also be measured:

- The plasma concentration of vitamin A and retinol binding protein.
- The response to replacement therapy.

Urgent treatment with vitamin A (as retinol palmitate) orally or intramuscularly prevents blindness. If the deficiency is severe and has already caused keratomalacia, eyesight cannot be restored. It is interesting to note that vitamin A is also used successfully to treat a number of skin problems, including acne (Fig. 8.14).

Toxicity

Hypervitaminosis A
Hypervitaminosis A is a serious toxic syndrome. Excessive intake of vitamin A causes:

- Dry, itchy skin: dermatitis.
- Mucous membrane defects and hair loss.

Fig. 8.14 Uses of vitamin A in the treatment of skin disorders

Condition	Treatment
Moderate acne	Topical retinoic acid (all *trans* retinoic acid)
Severe disfiguring acne	Isotretinoin (13-*cis* retinoic acid) orally
Psoriasis	Acitretin (Both are contraindicated in pregnancy as they are teratogenic)

- Hepatomegaly.
- Thinning and fracture of the long bones.
- Increased intracranial pressure.

Toxicity is very unlikely with normal sources but must be taken into account when prescribing high doses of retinoic acid for severe acne sufferers.

Teratogenicity

Pregnant women must not take more than 3.3 mg/day because vitamin A causes congenital defects. Therefore, they must avoid vitamin A supplements or eating liver because it contains about 13–40 mg of vitamin A per 100 g. Isotretinoin treatment for acne is absolutely contraindicated in pregnancy.

Vitamin D$_3$ (cholecalciferol)

RNI

There is no RNI for vitamin D because it is synthesized by the body.

Sources

The sources of vitamin D include:

- Diet: in fish liver oils as cholecalciferol.
- Endogenous synthesis: most vitamin D is made by the body.

Vitamin D is a derivative of cholesterol and is therefore not present in plants; vegetarians must make their own.

Synthesis

Vitamin D is manufactured in the skin by the action of sunlight of wavelength 290–310 nm. No radiation of this length is available between October and March in the UK; therefore the body relies on stores made during summer.

Cholecalciferol undergoes two hydroxylation reactions, the first in the liver and the second in the kidney to form the active form, 1,25-dihydroxy-cholecalciferol (see Fig. 8.15). Vitamin D is mostly stored as 25-hydroxycholecalciferol in the liver.

Functions

The main role of vitamin D is in calcium homeostasis, which it controls in three ways (see Fig 8.15):

- Increases uptake of calcium (and inorganic phosphate) from the intestine (main role).
- Increases the reabsorption of calcium from the kidney.
- Increases resorption of bone (when necessary) so that calcium is released.

Therefore, vitamin D increases the plasma concentration of calcium ions.

Mechanism of action

The active form, 1,25-dihydroxycholecalciferol, is a steroid hormone. In intestinal cells it binds to a cytosolic receptor. The resulting complex enters the nucleus and binds to chromatin at a specific site (enhancer region or response element) to increase the synthesis of a calcium-binding protein, calbindin, resulting in increased calcium reabsorption in the intestine.

Deficiency

Causes

- Decreased dietary intake of vitamin D.
- Inadequate exposure to sunlight of the correct wavelength.
- Renal disease leads to inadequate production of the active form 1,25-dihydroxycholecalciferol.
- Liver disease leads to decreased production of 25-hydroxycholecalciferol (precursor to active form).
- Fat malabsorption (e.g. coeliac disease).

Groups at risk of deficiency are:

- Children and women of Asian origin in sunlight-poor areas.
- Elderly and housebound individuals.
- Babies breastfed in winter because light of the correct wavelength for production of vitamin D is not available for mothers.
- Vegans (vitamin D is not present in plants).

Fig. 8.15 Synthesis, metabolism and functions of vitamin D. Active form, 1,25-dihydroxycholecalciferol has three main effects which increase the plasma calcium concentration:

1. Increases uptake of Ca^{2+} (and inorganic phosphate) from the intestine.
2. Increases reabsorption of calcium from the kidney.
3. Increases resorption of bone (when necessary) so that calcium is released.

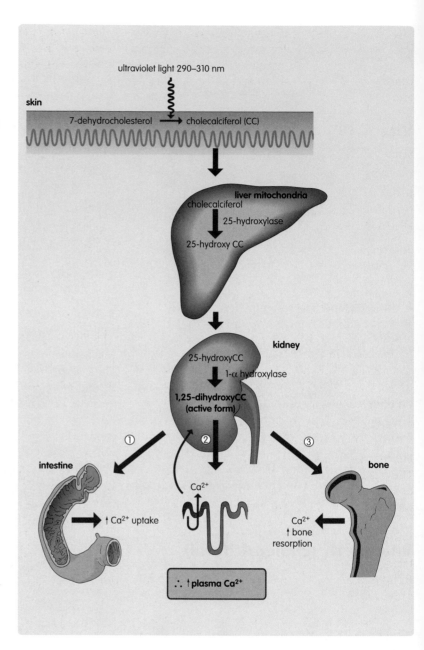

Clinical features and pathogenesis

Vitamin D deficiency disrupts bone mineralization. In children, this causes rickets; in adults, it causes osteomalacia. These disorders are covered later in this chapter with calcium deficiency.

A disruption of calcium homeostasis also causes hypocalcaemia and hypophosphataemia (low plasma calcium and phosphate). This may cause symptoms of neuromuscular irritability, numbness, parasthesiae, tetany and, possibly, seizures.

Toxicity

Vitamin D is the most toxic of all vitamins. It is fat soluble, stored in the body and slowly metabolized. Normally, it is well tolerated but in high doses over a period of time, hypervitaminosis D may occur. This condition presents with nausea, vomiting and muscle weakness. Very high levels of vitamin D result in greatly increased rates of calcium absorption and bone resorption, causing hypercalcaemia and calcium deposition in tissues, particularly the arteries, heart, liver, kidneys and pancreas. This is known as metastatic calcification and may interfere with the correct functioning of the organs, possibly causing renal stones, calcification of other arteries and heart failure.

Vitamin E (tocopherol)

Vitamin E consists of eight naturally occurring tocopherols; α-tocopherol is the most active.

RNI
None. A diet high in polyunsaturated fatty acids (PUFA) requires a high vitamin E intake.

Sources
Vegetable oils, especially wheatgerm oil, nuts and green vegetables.

Absorption and transport
Tocopherol is found 'dissolved' in dietary fat and is absorbed with it. It is transported in the blood by lipoproteins, initially in chylomicrons which deliver dietary vitamin E to the tissues. Vitamin E is transported from the liver with very-low-density lipoproteins (VLDL) and is stored in adipose tissue. Thus a defect in lipoprotein and fat metabolism may lead to a deficiency of vitamin E.

Functions and deficiency
The functions and clinical manifestations of a deficiency of vitamin E are listed in Fig. 8.16. Its mechanism of action is described in Fig. 8.17.

Deficiency

Incidence
In humans, vitamin E deficiency is very rare and is only seen in:

- Premature infants, causing haemolytic anaemia of the newborn. Vitamin E crosses the placenta in the last trimester of pregnancy; therefore,

premature infants have very small vitamin E stores. Their erythrocyte membranes are fragile and are susceptible to free radical damage, leading to lysis of erythrocytes. Vitamin E supplements are given to pregnant mothers to prevent this.
- Children and adults, secondary to severe fat malabsorption, for example, biliary atresia, cholestatic liver disease or a lipoprotein deficiency (e.g. abetalipoproteinaemia).

Clinical features
Vitamin E deficiency causes muscle weakness, peripheral neuropathy, ataxia and nystagmus. In children with abetalipoproteinaemia, vitamin E therapy can prevent the occurrence of severe spinocerebellar degeneration and gross ataxia.

Toxicity

Vitamin E is the least toxic of all the fat-soluble vitamins. The use of vitamin E supplements may help to protect against the development of heart disease by protecting low-density lipoproteins (LDL) from oxidation by free radicals.

Fig. 8.16 Vitamin E: function and effects of deficiency. PUFA, polyunsaturated fatty acid; LDL, low-density lipoprotein

Functions	Deficiency
Naturally occurring antioxidant which prevents oxidation of cell components by free radicals, e.g. PUFA present in cell membranes	Very rare except in premature infants in whom it can cause haemolytic anaemia of newborn

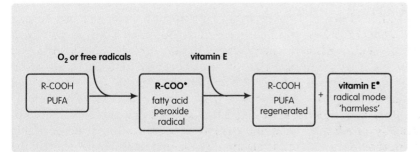

Fig. 8.17 Vitamin E as an antioxidant. Free radicals attack double bonds in polyunsaturated fatty acids to form a highly reactive fatty acid peroxide radical. This can attack other fatty acids, disrupting membrane structure and cell integrity. Vitamin E 'scavenges' fatty acid peroxide radicals to form a free radical itself. It is regenerated by other antioxidant nutrients (vitamins A and C). PUFA, polyunsaturated fatty acids.

Vitamin K

RNI
None.

Sources
The sources of vitamin K include:

- Diet: especially green vegetables, egg yolk, liver and cereals.
- It is made mostly by the normal bacterial flora of jejunum and ileum.
- Human milk contains only a small amount.

Functions and deficiency
The functions and clinical manifestations of a deficiency of vitamin K are listed in Fig. 8.18.

Deficiency

A true deficiency is rare because most of the body's vitamin K is synthesized by bacteria in the gut.

Causes
The main causes of vitamin K deficiency are:

- A decreased level of bacteria in the gut (e.g. due to long-term antibiotic therapy).
- A decrease in dietary intake.
- Newborn babies have sterile guts and cannot make vitamin K initially.
- Oral anticoagulant drugs (e.g. warfarin) are vitamin K antagonists (Fig. 8.19).

Mechanism
A deficiency of vitamin K results in low levels of the vitamin K-dependent clotting factors II, VII, IX and X and thus inhibition of the clotting cascade.

Patients will have an increased tendency to bleed and bruise.

Diagnosis and treatment
The diagnosis and treatment of vitamin K deficiency is covered in Fig. 8.20.

Deficiency in newborn babies
Newborn babies have sterile gut and have no bacteria to make vitamin K. The newborn infant has

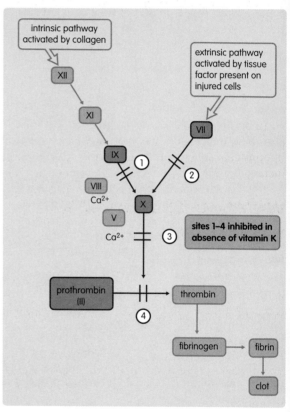

Fig. 8.19 Vitamin K deficiency: inhibition of the clotting cascade.

Fig. 8.18 Functions and deficiency of vitamin K

Functions	Deficiency
Vitamin K is a coenzyme for the carboxylation of glutamate residues of blood clotting factors II, VII, IX and X	True deficiency is rare because bacteria in the gut usually produce enough
Carboxylation activates clotting factors and thus clotting cascade	Long-term antibiotic therapy leads to ↓ bacteria and ↓ vitamin K, resulting in poor blood clotting and bleeding disorders
Anticoagulants warfarin and dicoumarol inhibit vitamin K	May result in haemorrhagic disease of the newborn

Fig. 8.20 Diagnosis and treatment of vitamin K deficiency

Diagnosis	Treatment
Clinical features: bruising and bleeding, e.g. haematuria or bleeding from the GI tract	Vitamin K supplements
Increased prothrombin time (PTT)	
Increased activated partial thromboplastin time (APTT) less marked than PTT	

HDNB is a coagulation disturbance, resulting from vitamin K deficiency and consequently impaired hepatic production of factors II, VII, IX and X. Premature infants, infants exposed to perinatal asphyxia and breastfed babies are most at risk of developing HDNB. It classically presents in the fourth day of life with gastrointestinal bleeding. Usually, the bleeding is minor but can also result in major haemorrhage and death. Therefore, every newborn baby in the UK is given prophylactic intramuscular or oral vitamin K.

Fig. 8.21 Thiamine: functions and effects of deficiency

Functions	Deficiency
Thiamine pyrophosphate is cofactor for **four key enzymes:**	
• pyruvate dehydrogenase • α-ketoglutarate dehydrogenase (TCA cycle) • branched-chain amino acid α-ketoacid dehydrogenase	Decreased activity of pyruvate dehydrogenase and α-ketoglutarate dehydrogenase causes: • accumulation of pyruvate and lactate • decreased acetyl CoA and ATP formation and thus decreased acetylcholine and central nervous system activity
• transketolase (pentose phosphate pathway)	Decreased activity of pentose phosphate pathway results in low levels of NADPH necessary for fatty acid synthesis; therefore this leads to a decrease in synthesis of myelin, which may cause peripheral neuropathy

virtually no hepatic stores of vitamin K and it is present in only low concentrations in human milk. Vitamin K deficiency causes haemorrhagic disease of the newborn (HDNB).

WATER-SOLUBLE VITAMINS

Vitamin B$_1$ (thiamine)

RNI
1.0 mg/day for men; 0.8 mg/day for women.

Sources
Wholegrain cereals, liver, pork, yeast, dairy products and legumes.

Active form
Thiamine pyrophosphate (TPP), which is formed by the transfer of a pyrophosphate group from ATP to thiamine.

Functions
The functions of thiamine are listed in Fig. 8.21, with its mechanism of action described in Fig. 8.22.

Deficiency diseases
A deficiency of thiamine causes:

- Beriberi. This occurs in two forms: wet beriberi, which results in oedema, cardiovascular symptoms and heart failure, and dry beriberi, which causes muscle wasting and peripheral neuropathy.
- Wernicke's encephalopathy, which is associated with alcoholism.
- Korsakoff's psychosis.

Beriberi

Incidence
Beriberi (Fig. 8.23) is now seen only in the poorest areas of South-East Asia where the staple food is polished rice, that is, the husk that contains most of the vitamins, including thiamine, has been removed.

Diagnosis
Diagnosis is by measurement of the transketolase activity in erythrocytes, before and after the addition of TPP. A greater than 30% increase in activity with TPP indicates a deficiency. Thiamine can now also be measured directly in plasma.

Treatment
Initially, treatment is with intramuscular injections of thiamine for approximately 3 days (varies according to severity) followed by daily, oral supplements of thiamine. For wet beriberi, treatment results in a dramatic decrease in oedema and a quick improvement of symptoms. For dry beriberi, there is a slower improvement.

Fig. 8.22 Mechanism of action of thiamine. Thiamine pyrophosphate (TPP), the active form of thiamine, acts as coenzyme for pyruvate dehydrogenase and α-ketoglutarate dehydrogenase reactions in the TCA cycle and for transketolase in the pentose phosphate pathway.

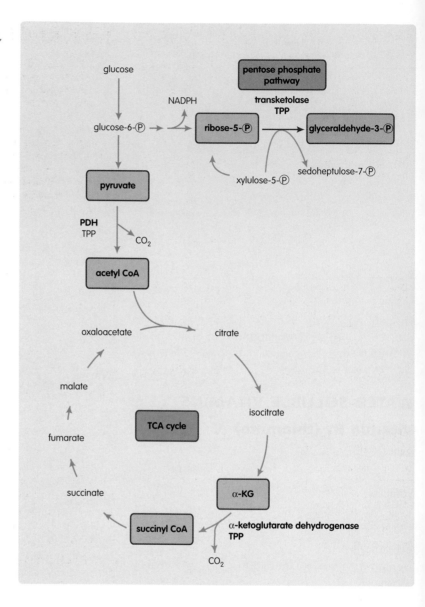

Wernicke–Korsakoff syndrome

Incidence

As thiamine is present in most foods, a dietary deficiency is rare in developed countries. The deficiency manifests itself as Wernicke's encephalopathy (Fig. 8.24). In the UK, a low thiamine intake is seen in:

- Chronic alcoholics: alcohol inhibits the uptake of thiamine.
- The elderly.
- People with diseases of the upper gastrointestinal tract (e.g. gastric cancer).

Toxicity

Toxicity is rare but an excess causes headaches, insomnia and dermatitis.

Vitamin B$_2$ (riboflavin)

RNI

1.3 mg/day for men; 1.1 mg/day for women.

Sources

Milk, eggs, liver. Riboflavin is readily destroyed by ultraviolet light.

Active forms

Riboflavin occurs in two active forms:

Fig. 8.23 Types of beriberi

	Clinical features	Signs
Wet beriberi	Oedema: spreads to involve the whole body → ascites and pleural effusions Congestive heart failure	Raised JVP Tachycardia and tachypnoea
Infantile beriberi	A form of wet beriberi that occurs in breastfed babies whose mothers are thiamine deficient	Acute onset: anorexia and oedema that can involve the larynx → aphonia Tachycardia and tachypnoea develop → death
Dry beriberi	Gradual, symmetrical, ascending peripheral neuropathy resulting in progressive paralysis	Initially, stiffness of legs → weakness, numbness, and 'pins and needles' ascends to involve trunk, arms and eventually brain

Fig. 8.24 Clinical features of Wernicke's encephalopathy and Korsakoff's psychosis

Clinical features	Causes
Wernickes' encephalopathy: • acute confusional state • ataxia; cerebellar signs • ophthalmoplegia and nystagmus • peripheral neuropathy	Alcohol Ischaemic damage to brainstem Major cause of dementia in developed countries
Diagnosis: made on clinical grounds; condition is reversible with immediate thiamine therapy	
If untreated it may develop into **Korsakoff's psychosis**: a severe irreversible syndrome characterized by loss of short-term memory	Progression from untreated Wernicke's encephalopathy

- Flavin mononucleotide (FMN).
- Flavin adenine dinucleotide (FAD).

Functions and deficiency

The functions and clinical manifestations of a deficiency of riboflavin are listed in Fig. 8.25. Riboflavin is not toxic in excess.

Fig. 8.25 Riboflavin: functions and effects of deficiency

Functions	Deficiency
FAD and FMN are coenzymes for a number of oxidases and dehydrogenases	Rare except in elderly or alcoholic individuals
They can accept two hydrogens to form $FADH_2$ and $FMNH_2$ respectively and take part in redox reactions, e.g. electron transport chain or act as antioxidants	Symptoms of deficiency: • angular stomatitis (inflammation at sides of mouth) • cheilosis (fissures at corners of the mouth) • cataracts • glossitis (inflamed tongue)

Niacin or nicotinic acid

RNI

17 mg/day for men; 13 mg/day for women.

Sources

Wholegrain cereals, meat, fish and the amino acid tryptophan.

Synthesis of niacin from tryptophan

The synthesis of niacin from trytophan is a very inefficient process: as much as 60 mg of tryptophan is needed to make 1 mg of niacin. Synthesis requires thiamine, riboflavin and pyridoxine as cofactors, and only occurs after the needs of protein synthesis are met. This means, in theory, that niacin deficiency can be treated with a high protein diet, but lots would be needed!

Active forms

NAD and NADP.

Functions and deficiency

The functions and clinical manifestations of a deficiency of niacin are listed in Fig. 8.26.

Pellagra: a disease of the skin, gastrointestinal tract and central nervous system

Incidence

Pellagra is rare and is found in areas where maize is the staple food. It is now seen only in certain parts of Africa. Maize contains niacin in a biologically unavailable form, niacytin. Niacin can only be removed from the maize by alkali treatment

Fig. 8.26 Niacin: functions and effects of deficiency

Functions	Deficiency
NAD^+ and $NADP^+$ are coenzymes for many dehydrogenases in redox reactions	Pellagra
	Symptoms, the **3Ds**: **d**ermatitis **d**iarrhoea **d**ementia leading to death
NAD is required for repair of UV light-damaged DNA in areas of exposed skin (nothing to do with redox state)	
Nicotinic acid is used for treatment of certain dyslipidaemias because it inhibits lipolysis, leading to decreased VLDL synthesis (see Chapter 4)	

Fig. 8.27 Clinical features and symptoms of pellagra

Clinical features	Symptoms
3Ds: **Dermatitis**; deficiency of NAD, inhibits DNA repair of sun-damaged skin (Fig. 8.17)	Photosensitive symmetrical skin rash occurs when skin is exposed to sunlight: • skin may crack and ulcerate • on neck, extent depends on area of skin exposed
Diarrhoea	May also see glossitis and angular stomatitis
Dementia	Dementia occurs in chronic disease and is usually irreversible; may develop tremor and encephalopathy

(Mexicans soak maize in lime juice to release the niacin). Pellagra (Fig. 8.27) can also occur in conditions in which large amounts of tryptophan are metabolized; for example, carcinoid syndrome, which is very rare.

Causes

The causes of pellagra are:

- Dietary deficiency of niacin.
- Protein deficiency (as niacin is made from tryptophan).
- Vitamin B_6 and thus pyridoxal phosphate deficiency (pyridoxal phosphate is a cofactor for niacin synthesis from tryptophan).

- Hartnup's disease: a failure to absorb tryptophan from the diet (Fig. 5.29).
- Isoniazid treatment for tuberculosis inhibits vitamin B_6, causing a decrease in tryptophan synthesis.

Diagnosis

Diagnosis is by the measurement of niacin or its metabolites (N-methylnicotinamide or 2-pyridone) in the urine.

Treatment

As niacin can be formed from tryptophan, treatment involves:

- High-dose niacin supplements.
- A high protein diet.

Mild cases are reversible, dementia usually is not, and may lead to death.

Toxicity

A high intake upsets liver function, carbohydrate tolerance and urate metabolism. More than 200 mg/day will cause vasodilatation and flushing.

Vitamin B₆

Vitamin B_6 exists in three forms: pyridoxine, pyridoxal and pyridoxamine.

RNI

1.4 mg/day for men; 1.2 mg/day for women.

Sources

Whole grains (wheat or corn), meat, fish and poultry.

Active form

All three forms can be converted to the coenzyme pyridoxal phosphate (PLP).

Functions and deficiency

The functions and clinical manifestations of a deficiency of vitamin B_6 are listed in Fig. 8.28.

Pyridoxine deficiency

Causes

Dietary deficiency is extremely rare but may be seen in:

- Newborn babies fed formula milk.
- Elderly people and alcoholics.
- Women taking oral contraceptives.
- Patients on isoniazid therapy for treatment of tuberculosis.

Fig. 8.28 Vitamin B₆: functions and effects of deficiency

Functions	Deficiency
• Pyridoxal phosphate is a coenzyme for many enzymes:	→ primary deficiency is very rare
• In amino acid metabolism: aminotransferases and serine dehydratase	→ abnormal amino acid metabolism
• In haem synthesis, ALA synthase (catalyses rate-limiting step)	→ hypochromic, microcytic anaemia
• Glycogen phosphorylase	
• Conversion of tryptophan to niacin	→ secondary pellagra
• Indirect role in serotonin and noradrenaline synthesis as they are derived from aminoacids	→ convulsions and depression

Fig. 8.29 Functions and effects of deficiency of pantothenic acid

Functions	Deficiency
As coenzyme A, it is involved in the transfer of acyl groups, e.g. acetyl CoA, succinyl CoA, fatty acyl CoA	Very rare; causes 'burning foot syndrome'
It is also a component of fatty acid synthase: acyl carrier protein (see Chapter 4)	N.B. a deficiency in rats causes depigmentation of fur, i.e. it turns grey. Not toxic in excess

The drug isoniazid binds to pyridoxal phosphate to form an inactive hydrazone derivative, which is rapidly excreted, thus causing the deficiency.

Clinical features
The main features include:

- Hypochromic, microcytic anaemia.
- Secondary pellagra.
- Convulsions and depression.

Treatment
Vitamin B₆ supplements are given to all patients on isoniazid therapy.

Toxicity

Toxicity is rare. Vitamin B₆ is actually used in the treatment of premenstrual tension (PMT). An excess is, however, associated with the development of a sensory neuropathy.

Pantothenic acid

Sources
Most foods, especially eggs, liver and yeast.

Active form
Component of coenzyme A (see Chapter 2).

Functions and deficiency
The functions and manifestations of a deficiency of pantothenic acid are listed in Fig. 8.29. Panthothenic acid is not toxic in excess.

Biotin

Sources
Most foods, especially egg yolk, offal, yeast and nuts. A significant amount is synthesized by bacteria in the intestine.

Active form
As a coenzyme for carboxylation reactions, biotin binds to a lysine residue in carboxylase enzymes (Fig. 8.30).

Functions and deficiency
The functions and clinical manifestations of a deficiency of biotin are listed in Fig. 8.31.

Vitamin B₁₂ (cobalamin)

RNI
1.5 mg/day.

Sources
Only animal sources: liver, meat, dairy foods; vegans are at risk of deficiency.

Active forms
Two active forms: deoxyadenosylcobalamin and methylcobalamin.

Absorption and transport
The absorption and transport of vitamin B₁₂ occurs in several steps (numbers refer to Fig. 8.32):

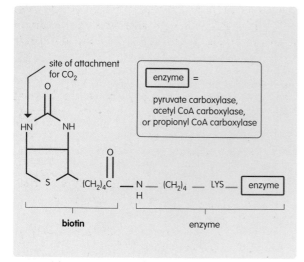

Fig. 8.30 Biotin is a coenzyme for carboxylation reactions. It binds to a lysine residue in carboxylase enzyme molecules.

Fig. 8.31 Biotin: functions and deficiency	
Functions	Deficiency
It is an activated carrier of CO_2	Very rare on a normal diet, may cause dermatitis
It is a coenzyme for: • pyruvate carboxylase in gluconeogenesis (see Chapter 5) • acetyl CoA carboxylase in fatty acid synthesis (see Chapter 4) • propionyl CoA carboxylase in β oxidation of odd-numbered fatty acids (see Fig. 8.33) • branched-chain amino acid metabolism	Can be induced by: • eating lots of raw egg whites, rich in a glycoprotein, avidin, that binds to biotin in the intestine preventing its absorption • long-term antibiotic therapy, which kills intestinal bacteria

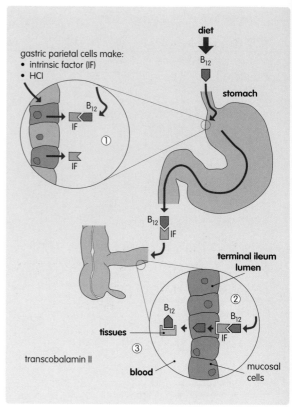

Fig. 8.32 The absorption and transport of vitamin B_{12} (numbers refer to the text).

1. Vitamin B_{12}, released from food in the stomach, becomes bound to a glycoprotein carrier, intrinsic factor (IF), produced by gastric parietal cells.
2. The complex of B_{12} and intrinsic factor binds to receptors on the mucosal cells of the terminal ileum.
3. B_{12} is absorbed and transported to tissues, attached to transcobalamin II. About 2–3 mg of B_{12} are stored by the body, mainly in the liver; this is relatively large compared with its daily requirement.

Functions

Vitamin B_{12} is a carrier of methyl groups. It is the coenzyme for two enzymes:

• Methylmalonyl CoA mutase, as deoxyadenosylcobalamin, to assist in the breakdown of odd-numbered fatty acids (Fig. 8.33).
• Homocysteine methyltransferase, as methylcobalamin, to assist in the synthesis of methionine. This reaction also reverses the methylfolate trap, regenerating tetrahydrofolate (THF) from methyl-THF (discussed below with folate).

Deficiency and toxicity

A significant amount of vitamin B_{12} is stored; it takes about 2 years for symptoms of deficiency to develop. Deficiency can cause two main problems:

• The accumulation of abnormal odd-numbered fatty acids, which may be incorporated into the

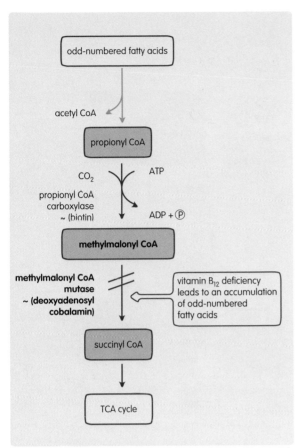

Fig. 8.33 β Oxidation of odd-numbered fatty acids. B$_{12}$ is a carrier of methyl groups. It is the coenzyme for methylmalonyl CoA mutase, assisting in the breakdown of odd-numbered fatty acids.

cell membranes of nerves, resulting in neurological symptoms, inadequate myelin synthesis and nerve degeneration.

- Secondary 'artificial' folate deficiency since folate is 'trapped' as methyl THF. This causes a decrease in nucleotide synthesis, resulting in megaloblastic anaemia (see Chapter 6).

Subacute combined degeneration of the spinal cord is the classic metabolic disorder due to vitamin B$_{12}$ deficiency. It can also be caused by folate deficiency. It is characterized by a symmetrical loss of posterior columns causing an ataxic gait, a symmetrical upper motor neurone signs in the lower limbs with absent reflexes, peripheral sensory neuropathy, optic atrophy and dementia. It is treated with intramuscular injections of hydroxycobalamin.

The most common cause of vitamin B$_{12}$ deficiency is pernicious anaemia, an auto-immune condition where antibodies are made by the body to intrinsic factor.

Causes of deficiency

Reduced intake, for example, by vegans because vitamin B$_{12}$ is only found in animal-derived foods. Reduced absorption caused by:

- A lack of intrinsic factor (e.g. pernicious anaemia).
- Diseases of the terminal ileum which is the site of B$_{12}$ absorption (e.g. Crohn's disease or tuberculosis).
- Bypass of the B$_{12}$ absorption site (e.g. fistulae or surgical resection of gut).
- Blind-loop syndrome: parasites compete for B$_{12}$.

Body stores (mainly in the liver) are large relative to the daily requirement, therefore a reduced intake alone takes about 2–3 years to cause a deficiency.

Pernicious anaemia

Pernicious anaemia is the commonest cause of vitamin B$_{12}$ deficiency.

Incidence

It is commoner in older women and is often associated with fair-haired and blue-eyed individuals, and also the presence of other auto-immune disorders (e.g. thyroid disease and Addison's disease).

Pathogenesis

Pernicious anaemia is an auto-immune disorder where antibodies are made to either:

- Gastric parietal cells, causing atrophy or wasting of the cells, thus preventing the production of intrinsic factor and stomach acid (Fig. 8.34a).
- Intrinsic factor itself (Fig. 8.34b); antibodies bind to the intrinsic factor, preventing it from either binding to vitamin B$_{12}$ (blocking antibodies) or binding to the receptors in the terminal ileum (binding antibodies). A lack of intrinsic factor leads to a decreased uptake of vitamin B$_{12}$. The clinical features of pernicious anaemia are discussed in Fig. 8.35.

Diagnosis

Diagnosis is performed by analysis of the blood film and bone marrow specimens and by the Schilling test, which measures the absorption of vitamin B$_{12}$:

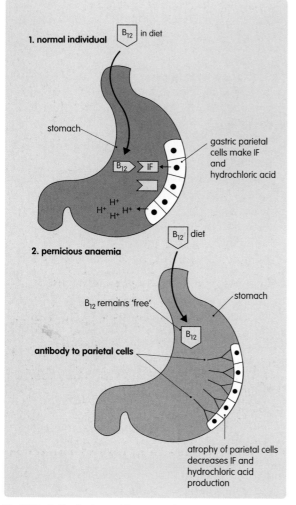

Fig. 8.34a Antibodies in pernicious anaemia.
1. In normal individuals, vitamin B_{12} released from food in the stomach becomes bound to intrinsic factor (IF) produced by gastric parietal cells.
2. In individuals with pernicious anaemia antibodies to the gastric parietal cells cause wasting of the cells and thus prevent production of intrinsic factor by them. Vitamin B_{12} is therefore not absorbed, resulting in B_{12} deficiency.

- Radioactive vitamin B_{12} is given orally.
- A 24-h urine collection is performed to measure the percentage of the dose of radioactive vitamin B_{12} excreted in the urine.
- If the subject is vitamin B_{12} deficient, less than 10% will be excreted because the vitamin B_{12} is being used to replenish depleted stores.
- If the result is abnormal, the test is repeated with the addition of intrinsic factor.
- If excretion is now normal, the diagnosis is pernicious anaemia.

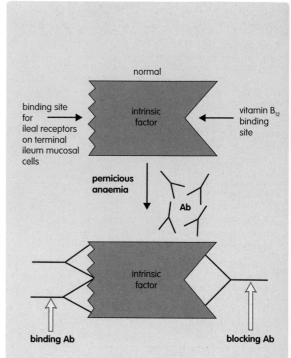

Fig. 8.34b Antibodies to intrinsic factor. Intrinsic factor contains two binding sites; one for vitamin B_{12} and a second one for ileal receptors in the terminal ileum, its site of absorption. In pernicious anaemia, antibodies produced may bind to either or both of these sites.

Treatment

The treatment of vitamin B_{12} deficiency is intramuscular injections of hydroxycobalamin for life. Initially, these are more frequent to fill the stores. Pernicious anaemia carries a slightly increased risk of carcinoma of the stomach.

The toxicity of vitamin B_{12} is low.

Folate

RNI
200 mg/day.

Sources
Green vegetables, liver and wholegrain cereals.

Active form
5,6,7,8-THF, which is involved in the transfer of one-carbon units (see Chapter 6).

Absorption and storage
Folate is absorbed in the duodenum and jejunum. About 10 mg of folate is stored, mainly in the liver.

Fig. 8.35 Clinical features and mechanism of pernicious anaemia

Clinical features	Mechanism
Megaloblastic anaemia: blood film: macrocytes (MCV > 100 fL) bone marrow: megaloblasts (developing red cells where nuclei mature more slowly than the cytoplasm)	B_{12} deficiency causes secondary folate deficiency, which leads to decreased production of DNA and defective cell division
Neurological abnormalities: peripheral neuropathy affecting sensory neurons of posterior and lateral columns of spinal cord; leads to subacute combined degeneration of spinal cord	Pathogenesis of CNS damage unknown impairment of CNS amino acid and fatty acid metabolism has been implicated
Lemon yellow colour	Combination of jaundice from red cell lysis and pallor because of anaemia
Glossitis, diarrhoea, and weight loss	
Gastric atrophy and achlorhydria (↓ hydrochloric acid production)	Antibodies to gastric parietal cells

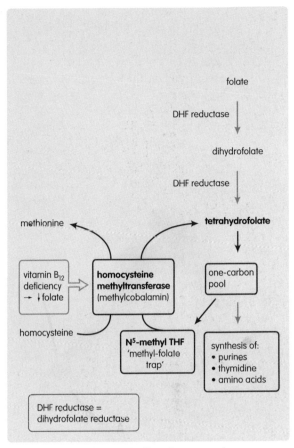

Fig. 8.36 Folate and vitamin B_{12}. The only way to re-form tetrahydrofolate is via vitamin B_{12}-dependent synthesis of methionine: the methionine salvage pathway.

The role of folate and vitamin B_{12}

All one-carbon THF units are interconvertible except N^5-methyl THF; the THF cannot be released from it and is trapped, forming the 'methyl-folate trap' (see Chapter 6).

The only way to re-form THF is via vitamin B_{12}-dependent synthesis of methionine: the methionine salvage pathway (Fig. 8.36).

Functions and deficiency

The functions and clinical manifestations of a deficiency of folate are listed in Fig. 8.37.

Folate deficiency

The stores of folate are small relative to the daily requirements, therefore a deficiency state can develop in a few months, particularly if it is associated with a period of rapid growth.

Fig. 8.37 Folate: function and deficiency

Functions	Deficiency
Synthesis of: • amino acids, e.g. glycine and methionine • purines, AMP, and GMP (see Chapter 6) • thymidine (see Chapter 6)	**Megaloblastic anaemia:** • decrease in purines and pyrimidines leads to a decrease in nucleic acid synthesis and cell division • shows up mostly in cells that are rapidly dividing, e.g. bone marrow and gut • large, immature red blood cells are present

Causes

- Decreased intake: a poor diet is the most common cause (e.g. in slimmers, elderly people and alcoholics).
- Increased requirement: during periods of rapid cell growth, such as:
- Pregnancy, infancy or adolescence.
- Cancer, inflammatory states or recovery from illness.
- Haemolytic anaemias.
- Malabsorption: in coeliac disease or after gut resection.
- Drugs:
  - Anticonvulsants impair absorption (e.g. phenytoin and phenobarbitone).
  - Dihydrofolate reductase inhibitors (e.g. methotrexate).
  - Antimalarial drugs (e.g. pyrimethamine).
- Secondary to B_{12} deficiency: vitamin B_{12} is essential to maintain an adequate supply of the active form of folate, that is 5,6,7,8-tetrahydrofolate. It regenerates THF from N^5-methyl-THF in the methionine salvage pathway (Fig. 6.3). Even if there are adequate amounts of folate in the diet, in the absence of vitamin B_{12}, folate deficiency arises.

Clinical features and diagnosis of folate deficiency

The clinical features and diagnosis of folate deficiency are covered in Fig. 8.38.

Treatment

The treatment of folate deficiency is daily oral folate supplementation.

Folate deficiency in pregnancy

The development of the neural tube in the fetus is dependent on the presence of folic acid. Pregnant women should take prophylactic folate supplements to reduce the risk of neural tube defects such as spina bifida or anencephaly. The critical time is the first few weeks after conception: women should therefore start supplements before conception to cover this period. A woman who has already had a baby with a neural tube defect has about a 1:20 risk of a second affected baby; the use of folate supplements has been shown to reduce this risk.

A comparison of folate and vitamin B_{12} deficiencies

A comparison of folate and vitamin B_{12} deficiencies is given in Fig. 8.39. A deficiency of either can cause a macrocytic, megaloblastic anaemia. Patients suspected of having either deficiency, must always be investigated for both folate and B_{12} deficiency since the administration of folic acid corrects the anaemia but masks a B_{12} deficiency. Therefore, folate should never be given alone in treatment of pernicious anaemia and other B_{12} deficiency states because it may precipitate an irreversible peripheral neuropathy.

Fig. 8.38 Clinical features and diagnosis of folate deficiency

Clinical features	Diagnosis
Megaloblastic anaemia: this is identical to vitamin B_{12} deficiency (see Fig. 8.35)	Blood film: macrocytes (MCV > 100 fL) megaloblasts in bone marrow
Growth failure	Low serum folate
N.B. peripheral neuropathy and neurological symptoms do not occur in folate deficiency	Red cell folate is a better test of folate stores normal = 135–750 mg/mL
	Must always consider and eliminate vitamin B_{12} deficiency and malignancy

Fig. 8.39 A comparison of vitamin B_{12} and folate deficiency; main differences

Characteristics	Vitamin B_{12}	Folate
Most common cause	Pernicious anaemia	↓ dietary intake
Onset	Slow, 2–3 years	Develops over weeks
Neurological symptoms	Frequent + severe	Never
Drug-related	No: vitamin B_{12} deficiency usually causes secondary folate deficiency	Yes: anticonvulsants, dihydrofolate reductase inhibitors
Folate deficiency occurs frequently on its own because of ↓ intake or ↑ demand

Vitamin C (ascorbate)

RNI
40 mg/day.

Sources
Citrus fruits, tomatoes, berries and green vegetables.

Active form
Ascorbate.

Functions and deficiency
The functions and clinical manifestations of a deficiency of ascorbate are listed in Fig. 8.40.

Vitamin C deficiency: scurvy

In the past, this used to be common among sailors who spent weeks at sea without any fresh fruit or vegetables.

Causes
Scurvy is caused by a poor dietary intake of fresh fruit and vegetables. In the UK, it is seen in elderly people, alcoholics and smokers. Smokers require twice the normal intake of vitamin C (80 mg/day). Humans have about 6 months' store of vitamin C.

Clinical features
The clinical features of scurvy are described in Fig. 8.41.

Treatment
The treatment of vitamin C deficiency is 1g daily of ascorbate and lots of fresh fruit and vegetables in the diet.

The megadose hypothesis
Some researchers believe that large doses of vitamin C cure many illnesses, such as the common cold and certain immune-mediated diseases, and even help in cancer prevention and promote fertility. The benefits of large doses are unresolved and under review. It is thought that 1–4 g/day of vitamin C can decrease the severity of symptoms of cold but not decrease the incidence. Vitamin C is an antioxidant and it is thought that, along with vitamins A and E, it might decrease the incidence of coronary heart disease and certain cancers by scavenging free radicals, thus preventing oxidative damage to cells and their components. This has not been confirmed.

Toxicity

A high intake of vitamin C may lead to the formation of kidney stones, diarrhoea and also cause

The role of ascorbate in hydroxylation reactions: Hydroxylase enzymes contain iron, which exists in two oxidation states: Fe^{3+} which is inactive, and Fe^{2+} which is reduced and active. Ascorbate is necessary to maintain iron in its reduced and active state (Fe^{2+}).

Fig. 8.40 Ascorbate: function and deficiency

Functions	Deficiency
Co-enzyme in hydroxylation reactions: • proline and lysine hydroxylases in collagen synthesis • dopamine β-hydroxylase in adrenaline and noradrenaline synthesis Powerful reducing agent: • reduces dietary Fe^{3+} to Fe^{2+} in the gut, allowing its absorption (therefore deficiency can lead to anaemia) Antioxidant and free-radical 'scavenger' • inactivates free oxygen radicals which damage lipid membranes, proteins and DNA • also protects other antioxidant vitamins A and E	**Scurvy** most symptoms are due to a decrease in collagen synthesis, leading to poor connective tissue formation and wound healing

Fig. 8.41 Clinical features of scurvy

Clinical features	Diagnosis
• Swollen, sore, spongy gums with bleeding; loose teeth • Spontaneous bruising and petechial haemorrhages • Anaemia • Poor wound healing • Swollen joints and muscle pain	Hypochromic, microcytic anaemia caused by secondary iron deficiency Low plasma ascorbate level (not very accurate) The measurement of ascorbate concentration in white blood cells provides an assessment of tissue stores

The best way to learn this sort of information is to take a large piece of paper and for each vitamin list only the main points mentioned above. Examiners love to ask about deficiency diseases.

systemic conditioning, that is, requirements increase as the body adapts to metabolizing more.

MINERALS

Classification of minerals

There are 103 known elements. Living organisms are composed mainly of 11 of these. Namely carbon, hydrogen, oxygen, nitrogen and the seven major minerals:

- Calcium, phosphorus and magnesium, which are used mainly in bone.
- Sodium, potassium and chloride, which are the main electrolytes present in the intracellular and extracellular fluid.
- Sulphur, which is used mainly in amino acids.

The RNI is greater than 100 mg/day for each of these (the exception is sulphur for which no RNI has been published).

In addition, there are at least 12 other elements that are required in the diet in smaller quantities. These are known as the essential trace elements, for which the RNI is less than 100 mg/day: iron, zinc, copper, cobalt, iodine, chromium, manganese, molybdenum, selenium, vanadium, nickel and silicon.

Calcium

Calcium is the most abundant mineral in the human body. There is about 1.2 kg of calcium in the average 70 kg adult, of which 99% is in bone.

RNI

The RNI of calcium is 700 mg/day; it is higher during periods of growth, pregnancy, lactation and after the menopause.

Sources

Milk and milk products; a lot of foods are fortified with calcium, for example, bread.

Absorption

Absorption of calcium from the diet is variable depending on the following factors:

- Lactose and basic amino acids increase absorption because they form complexes with calcium.
- Fibre decreases absorption, therefore vegans need a lot more calcium.

Active forms

The ionized form, Ca^{2+}.

Main functions

The main functions of calcium are listed in Fig. 8.42.

Regulation of calcium

Calcium levels are controlled by three hormones which also regulate plasma phosphate levels:

- Parathyroid hormone, which increases plasma calcium but decreases levels of inorganic phosphate.
- Vitamin D, which increases both plasma calcium and inorganic phosphate levels.
- Calcitonin, which decreases both plasma calcium and inorganic phosphate levels.

Calcium deficiency

In children, calcium deficiency causes rickets (derived from the old English word 'wrickken' meaning to twist). In adults, calcium deficiency causes osteomalacia. They both may occur:

- From dietary deficiency of calcium, particularly in developing countries.

Fig. 8.42 Main functions of calcium

Function	Examples
Structural role	Bone and teeth Calcium is present as calcium phosphate (hydroxyapatite) crystals
Muscle contraction	Calcium binds to troponin C
Nerve impulse transmission	Calcium is released in response to hormones and neurotransmitters
Blood clotting	Coenzyme for coagulation factors
Ion transport and cell signalling	Intracellular second messenger

- Secondary to vitamin D deficiency. Vitamin D is necessary for the intestinal absorption of calcium and phosphate (Fig. 8.15).
- From malabsorption (e.g.coeliac disease).

Pathogenesis

Both rickets and osteomalacia are the result of inadequate mineralization of bone, resulting in a reduction in its normal strength, leading to soft, easily deformed bones. The difference is that they occur at different stages of bone development. In rickets the production of undermineralized bone results in a failure of adequate growth, whereas in osteomalacia, demineralization of existing bones leads to an increased risk of fractures.

- *Rickets.* The characteristics of rickets are shown in Figs 8.43 and 8.44. Treatment is with calcium supplements and education on a balanced diet. Vitamin D supplements may also be required.
- *Osteomalacia.* This is seen particularly in elderly people and is usually secondary to vitamin D deficiency. The characteristics of osteomalacia are shown in Fig. 8.45.
- *Osteoporosis.* This is the progressive reduction of total bone mass, usually due to the effects of oestrogen deficiency post-menopause. It is prevented by the use of hormone replacement therapy, but calcium is also thought to have a role in its prevention. Adequate calcium nutrition when young helps to achieve a peak bone mass and this decreases the effects of loss and osteoporosis in later life. Calcium supplements both before and after menopause, usually with vitamin D, are recommended.

Fig. 8.44 The clinical features and diagnosis of rickets

Clinical features	Diagnosis
Bowed legs, short stature and failure to thrive	↓ serum calcium and phosphorus
Craniotabes: skull bones easily indented by finger pressure	↑ alkaline phosphatase: secreted by osteoblasts to compensate and ↑ bone formation
Rickety rosary: expansion or swelling at costochondral junctions	X-rays show defective mineralization of pelvis, long bones and ribs
Harrison sulcus: indrawing of softened ribs along attachment of diaphragm → 'hollowing'	N.B. low calcium results in ↓ neuromuscular transmission; therefore infant may present with seizures
Expansion of metaphyses especially at wrist	
Delayed dentition	

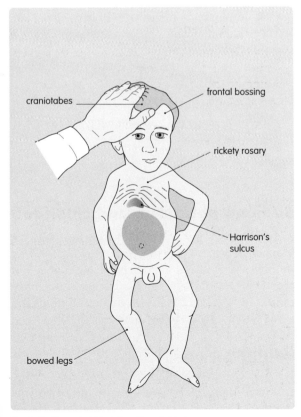

Fig. 8.43 Characteristic deformities of rickets.

Fig. 8.45 Clinical features of osteomalacia

Clinical features	Diagnosis
Spontaneous, incomplete (subclinical) fractures, often in long bones or pelvis	Low serum calcium
Bone pain	Bone biopsy shows increase in non-mineralized bone matrix
Weakness of proximal muscles causing a proximal myopathy with a characteristic waddling gait	X-rays show defective mineralization of long bones and pelvis

Calcium overload: hypercalcaemia

Causes

Major causes of hypercalcaemia are primary hyperparathyroidism and malignant disease and have nothing to do with nutrition, and are therefore beyond the scope of this book. Very rarely, hypercalcaemia is associated with the excessive ingestion of milk and antacids for the control of indigestion. This decreases the renal excretion of calcium: milk–alkali syndrome.

Clinical features

Calcium ions are normally found in cells and deposited calcium salts are present in bones and teeth. In overload, calcium salts are deposited in normal tissues, leading to tissue metastatic calcification and impaired function. This may cause renal stones, arrhythmias, heart failure and calcification of the arteries. Muscle weakness, tiredness, anorexia, constipation and a sluggish nervous response may also be seen.

Phosphorus

RNI

550 mg/day.

Sources

Most foods; a dietary deficiency has not been described.

Functions

Phosphorus works in conjunction with vitamin D and calcium:

- It has a structural role in bones and teeth.
- It is required for the production of ATP and other phosphorylated metabolic intermediates. Therefore, it is fundamental to the maintenance of function of cells in the body.

Deficiency and toxicity

The clinical manifestations of a deficiency and excess of phosphorus are listed in Fig. 8.46.

Magnesium

RNI

270 mg/day.

Sources

Most foods, especially green vegetables.

Functions

The functions of magnesium are:

Fig. 8.46 The effects of phosphorous deficiency and excess

Deficiency	Excess
If severe (< 0.3 mmol/L), will affect the function of all cells causing: • muscle weakness • in erythrocytes leads to a decrease information of 2, 3–bisphosphoglycerate and therefore reduces unloading of oxygen to tissues • rickets and osteomalacia	May combine with calcium to produce calcium phosphate and be deposited in tissues

- Structural role in bones and teeth.
- Cofactor for more than 300 enzymes in the body, that is, those enzymes that catalyse ATP-dependent reactions. Magnesium binds to ATP, forming a magnesium–ATP complex which is the substrate for enzymes such as kinases.
- Interacts with calcium to affect the permeability of excitable membranes and neuromuscular transmission.

Deficiency

Seen in alcoholics; patients with liver cirrhosis; following diuretic therapy; and in renal and intestinal disease. The symptoms are:

- Muscle weakness.
- Secondary calcium deficiency.
- Confusion, hallucinations, convulsions and other neurological symptoms.
- Can also lead to hypokalaemia.

Excess

Extremely rare.

Sodium, potassium and chloride

Sodium, potassium and chloride function together to regulate the osmolality of intracellular and extracellular fluids. Importantly, both high and low potassium concentration in plasma can cause severe cardiac problems. The characteristics of sodium and potassium are listed in Fig. 8.47.

Sulphur

The dietary intake of the sulphur-containing amino acid methionine is essential for synthesis of cysteine (see Fig. 5.5); both can then be incorporated into proteins and enzymes.

Fig. 8.47 The characteristics of sodium and potassium

	Sodium	Potassium
RNI Sources Functions	1.6g/day Salt, most foods Principal cation of ECF: plasma concentration maintained between 135 and 145 mmol/L; necessary for: • control of ECF volume • Na^+/K^+-ATPase and uptake of solutes by cell • Na^+ gradient provides driving force for secondary active transport • neuromuscular transmission	3.5g/day Most foods Principal cation of ICF: plasma concentration 3.5–5.0 mmol/L fundamental to: • Na^+/K^+-ATPase and uptake of molecules by cell • neuromuscular transmission • acid–base balance • cardiac muscle contraction
Deficiency	• disturbances common in hospitalized patients; causes of loss include: vomiting, diarrhoea, use of diuretics, Addison's disease, hyperglycaemia (causing an osmotic diuresis) or renal failure • sodium loss is usually accompanied by water loss, leading to decrease in plasma volume and signs of circulatory failure and collapse	• loss may be secondary to vomiting and the use of diuretics, diarrhoea, excess steroids, hyperaldosteronism (e.g. Conn's syndrome), Cushing's syndrome or alkalosis • high chance of cardiac arrhythmias and neuromuscular weakness • remember: intravenous insulin treatment without supplementation of potassium leads to hypokalaemia
Excess	Role in hypertension: sodium overload linked to water overload can lead to oedema and to cardiac failure	• the most common cause of potassium retention and hyperkalaemia is renal failure • both severe hypokalaemia and hyperkalaemia are dangerous and require immediate treatment

Hyperkalaemia is a medical emergency and requires immediate attention, especially when the potassium concentration is above 6 mmol/L and is accompanied by ECG changes. In such situations, it is vital to protect the cardiac membrane by giving calcium gluconate intravenously. This buys one time to treat the hyperkalaemia by giving infusion of both insulin and glucose to shift potassium ions into the cell, thus lowering the plasma potassium concentration.

Iron

RNI

The daily loss of iron from the body is 0.5–1.0 mg/day and is due to:

• Gastrointestinal tract turnover, about 0.5 mg/day.
• Desquamation of intestinal mucosal cells and biliary excretion, about 0.3 mg/day.
• Sweat and desquamation of skin cells, about 0.1 mg/day.
• Urinary losses, about 0.1 mg/day.

Small daily losses are accounted for by the absorption of dietary iron in the duodenum. The demand for iron increases during growth, pregnancy and menstruation (1 ml of blood loss is equal to 0.5 mg of iron). The daily iron requirements are:

• Adult male	1.0 mg
• Child	1.5 mg
• Menstruating woman	2.0 mg
• Pregnant woman	3.0 mg

Only 10% of dietary iron is absorbed, therefore the amount ingested daily is equal to the daily requirement $\times 10$. Therefore, the RNI = 10–20 mg/day.

Sources

Liver, meat, green vegetables and cereals. Dietary iron exists in two forms:

• Haem iron, which is derived from haemoglobin or myoglobin in meat and is rapidly absorbed.
• Non-haem iron, which is present in vegetables and cereals and is absorbed slowly.

Absorption, transport and storage

A summary of the absorption, transport, and functions of iron is given in Fig. 8.48. Total body iron is about 3–5 g. About 60% is in haemoglobin and most of the rest is stored mainly as ferritin, which is

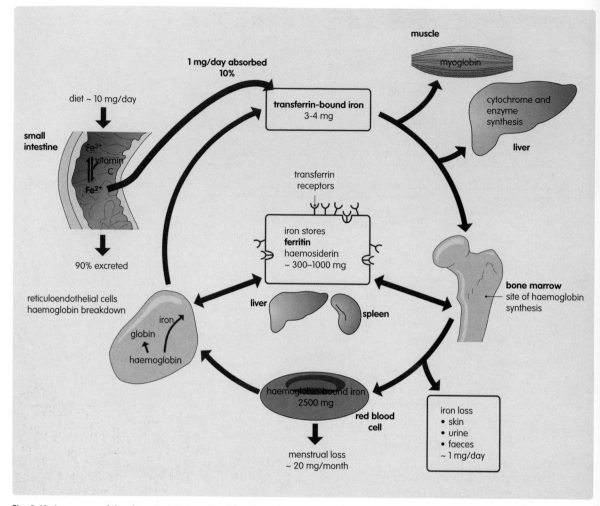

Fig. 8.48 A summary of the absorption, transport and functions of iron. Iron is transported in the blood bound to transferrin; each molecule of transferrin binds two Fe^{2+} ions. This transports iron from sites of absorption and haemoglobin breakdown to storage sites: mainly the reticuloendothelial cells (bone marrow, spleen), hepatocytes (liver) and muscle cells. These cells have transferrin receptors enabling iron to be taken up by receptor-mediated endocytosis. Iron is also transported to these sites for production of haemoglobin (bone marrow), myoglobin (muscle) or production of enzymes (liver).

a protein-iron complex. A small amount of iron is also stored as haemosiderin.

Fig. 8.49 summarizes the functions of body iron.

Iron deficiency anaemia

Bioavailability

Haem iron, present in meat, is readily absorbed. Inorganic (non-haem) iron, present in vegetables and cereals, is mostly in the oxidized (Fe^{3+}) state and must be reduced for absorption. Factors affecting bioavailability:

- Absorption is favoured in the ferrous (Fe^{2+}) as opposed to the ferric (Fe^{3+}) form.

- Stomach hydrochloric acid and ascorbic acid both favour absorption by reducing iron to the ferrous form.
- Increased erythropoietic activity (e.g. due to bleeding, haemolysis or high altitude) increases absorption.
- Alcohol increases absorption.
- Phosphates and phytates (from plants) form insoluble complexes with iron and prevent absorption.

Causes of deficiency

Inadequate intake. This is probably the most common cause of iron deficiency, particularly in a vegan diet.

Fig. 8.49 The distribution and function of total body iron

Site	Function	Amount of iron (mg)	Percentage total body iron
Total body iron		3500–5000	100
Haemoglobin	Oxygen transport	2500	60–70
Ferritin (2/3) and haemosiderin (1/3)	Iron storage: mainly liver, spleen and bone marrow	1000	27
Myoglobin	Oxygen transporter in muscle	130	3.5
Uncharacterized iron-binding molecules	Storage	80	2.2
Cytochromes and other iron-containing enzymes	Electron transport chain Cytochrome P450 (drug metabolism) Catalase (H_2O_2 breakdown) peroxidase	8	0.2
Transferrin	Transports iron from intestines to tissues	3	0.08

Increased requirement. This occurs in premature babies as iron is transferred to the fetus during the last trimester of pregnancy. It also occurs during infancy, adolescence and pregnancy, that is, during periods of increased growth.

Blood loss. 1 mL of blood contains 0.5 mg of iron. Therefore, a small blood loss of 3–4 mL/day over a period of weeks to months can cause chronic iron deficiency. Losses can be from:

- The gut (e.g. due to peptic ulcer, hiatus hernia, cancer of the stomach or caecum and ulcerative colitis)
- Menstrual loss, if periods are particularly heavy.

Always look for causes of chronic blood loss in a person with iron deficiency anaemia.

Malabsorption. Due to high levels of phytates in the diet, secondary to vitamin C deficiency or after surgery (partial or total gastrectomy).

Often, there is more than one cause, for example, a poor quality diet and heavy periods in an adolescent.

Groups in the population at risk of deficiency

Infants, toddlers, adolescents, pregnant women, menstruating women and elderly people are all at risk of iron deficiency.

Bioavailability is the efficiency (%) with which any dietary nutrient is used in the body. A number of factors can influence the absorption and use of nutrients. For example:
1. The chemical form of the nutrient.
2. Antagonistic or facilitatory ligands.
3. The breakdown of the nutrient.
4. The pH and redox state.
5. Anabolic requirements, endocrine influences, infection, and so on.

Clinical features and diagnosis of iron deficiency anaemia

The clinical features and diagnosis of iron deficiency anaemia are covered in Fig. 8.50.

Management and treatment

Finding the cause is essential. The treatment for iron deficiency anaemia is oral iron supplements (e.g. ferrous sulphate or gluconate). If malabsorption is suspected, use intramuscular or intravenous iron. Iron supplements should be given for long enough to correct the haemoglobin level; when this is

Fig. 8.50 Clinical features and diagnosis of iron deficiency anaemia

Signs and symptoms	Diagnosis
↓ **Production of haemoglobin**: less oxygen reaches the tissues especially the brain and heart muscle causing **pallor, tiredness, shortness of breath, giddines, palpitations** symptoms usually occur when haemoglobin < 8 g/dL **Epithelial abnormalities**: angular stomatitis (cracked corners of mouth) glossitis (sore tongue) koilonychia (spoon-shaped nails)	**Blood tests:** • ↓ haemoglobin, serum ferritin and iron • FBC, blood film • ↑ total iron-binding capacity (TIBC) (due to increase in 'free' transferrin) **Gold standard** for diagnosis of iron deficiency is the absence of iron stores in the bone marrow **Blood film**: microcytic, hypochromic erythrocytes, i.e. small, pale erythrocytes where: • MCV (mean cellular volume) < 80 fL • MCH (mean cell Hb) < 27 pg **N.B.** normal haemoglobin concentration is 13–18 g/dL in men, 11.5–16 g/dL in women

normal, iron must then be continued for 3–6 months to replenish stores.

Prognosis

Pathological changes are reversed by adequate replacement therapy.

Iron overload

Iron overload leads to iron deposition in the tissues, which may interfere with their function (Fig. 8.51).

Causes

There are two principal causes of iron overload. There is an inherited form, called idiopathic primary haemochromatosis, which has a homozygote prevalence in the population of 0.5%. Iron overload may also be acquired, where it occurs secondary to an increased administration of iron. This is called transfusional iron overload.

Fig. 8.51 Sites of iron deposition in iron overload

Tissue	Effect
Liver	Liver fibrosis and pigmentation resulting in cirrhosis and eventually liver failure; may progress to hepatocellular carcinoma (30%)
Pancreas	'Bronze diabetes': iron damages islet cells causing diabetes mellitus
Heart	Heart failure
Skin	Grey/bronze skin colour because of increased production of melanin
Testes	Impotence
Joints	Arthropathy

Idiopathic primary haemochromatosis

Pathogenesis. Idiopathic primary haemochromatosis is an autosomal recessive disorder characterized by the excessive absorption of iron in the small intestine. The gene defect is located on chromosome 6. Only homozygotes manifest clinical features; the accumulation of iron is gradual. It usually presents in the fifth decade when levels of iron are about 40–60 g compared with 3–5 g in a normal person. The disease is clinically manifested more commonly in men as women can compensate for the excess absorption by menstrual bleeding. The course of the disease depends on the amount of dietary iron and the presence of other dietary factors, such as vitamin C or alcohol.

Clinical consequences. Iron is deposited as insoluble haemosiderin, forming yellow granules in tissues (Fig. 8.51), which eventually interfere with tissue function. An increase in iron levels leads to an increase formation of free radicals, especially the hydroxyl radical. At normal iron levels, a reactive superoxide radical $O_2^{\bullet}$ is removed effectively by the enzyme superoxide dismutase, as shown in the reaction below:

$$2O_{2-}^{\bullet} + 2H^+ \rightarrow H_2O_2 + O_2$$

However, in iron overload, Fe^{3+} reacts with the superoxide radical to form an extremely reactive hydroxyl radical, $OH^{\bullet}$. This hydroxyl radical is capable of damaging biological molecules, particularly lipids, leading to lipid peroxidation and membrane damage (especially of lysosomal membranes).

$$O_2^{\bullet-} + Fe^{3+} \rightarrow Fe^{2+} + O_2$$
$$Fe^{2+} + H_2O_2 \rightarrow Fe^{3+} + OH^- + OH^{\bullet}$$

This results in the oxidation and destruction of cell membranes and tissues.

Treatment. The treatment for idiopathic primary haemochromatosis is regular venesection (i.e. removal of blood) to reduce the iron load. Plasma iron and ferritin levels are used to monitor the treatment. Once the excess iron is removed, the frequency of venesection is reduced.

Transfusional iron overload: transfusion siderosis

Causes. Repeated blood transfusions over a long period of time can cause iron overload. The ability of the reticuloendothelial cells (spleen, liver and bone marrow) to store iron is exceeded and iron is deposited at other sites. As with primary iron overload, iron is deposited mainly in the skin, heart, liver and pancreas. Patients with any condition requiring regular blood transfusions are regarded as high risk (e.g. thalassaemia major, aplastic anaemia).

Treatment. Chelation therapy with desferrioxamine is highly effective in chelating the iron, thus enabling its excretion.

Zinc

The daily zinc requirement is 2–3 mg/day but absorption is only about 30% effective. Therefore, the RNI is 10 mg/day. Zinc can be found in most foods. The total body zinc is 2–3 g. It is found in all tissues but high concentrations are present in the liver, kidney, bone, retina, muscle and prostate. The role of zinc in the body is described in Fig. 8.52.

Zinc deficiency

Acrodermatitis enteropathica

Acrodermatitis enteropathica is an extremely rare, autosomal recessive disorder that leads to the malabsorption of zinc in the small intestine. It presents in infancy with a severe symmetrical, eczematous rash around orifices and on the hands and feet. Frequently, the lesions become severely infected with *Candida* or bacterial infections, leading to death. Infants may also develop growth retardation, hypogonadism and poor wound healing.

Treatment

The condition is completely cured by zinc therapy. Zinc deficiency is also a very rare complication of

Fig. 8.52 The role of zinc in the body

Functions	Deficiency
Co-factor of over 100 enzymes, e.g.: • dehydrogenases, e.g. LDH • peptidases • carbonic anhydrase • enzymes of DNA and protein synthesis • superoxide dismutase	Causes: growth retardation, hypogonadism, and delayed wound healing These effects are
mainly a result of Transcription factors contain 'zinc fingers' that enable them to bind DNA	decreased activity of the enzymes of DNA synthesis

parenteral nutrition when insufficient supplementation is given.

Copper

RNI
1.2 mg/day.

Sources
Liver is a very good source.

Copper metabolism

The total body copper is about 75–150 mg. High copper concentrations are found in the liver, brain, heart and kidneys. Dietary copper is absorbed in the stomach and duodenum and transported to the liver loosely bound to albumin; the absorption is about 30% effective. It is incorporated into caeruloplasmin, a glycoprotein synthesized by the liver, which transports copper to the tissues where it can be used for the synthesis of other copper-containing enzymes. Normally, it is excreted in the bile (daily loss is approximately 2–3 mg/day). In the blood, 80–90% of the copper present is bound to caeruloplasmin.

Function

Copper is required for the synthesis of a number of copper-containing enzymes (Fig. 8.53).

Copper deficiency: Menkes' kinky hair syndrome

Menkes' kinky hair syndrome is a rare, X-linked disease with an incidence of 1 in 50 000–100 000. It is caused by the defective absorption of copper from

Fig. 8.53 The role of copper and the effects of copper deficiency

Affected enzyme	Functional role	Effect of deficiency
Caeruloplasmin	Promotes absorption of iron	Iron deficiency anaemia
Lysyl oxidase	Cross-links collagen and elastin	Weak-walled blood vessels
Tyrosinase	Melanin production	Failure of pigmentation
Dopamine β-hydroxylase	Catecholamine production	Neurological effects
Cytochrome c oxidase	Electron transport chain	Decreased ATP formation
Superoxide dismutase	Scavenges the superoxide radical and prevents lipid peroxidation and membrane damage	Tissue damage

Fig. 8.54 Clinical features of copper deficiency

Clinical features	Explanation
Depigmentation of hair 'steely hair'	↓ tyrosinase and melanin production
Arterial degeneration	↓ lysyl oxidase resulting in defective collagen and elastin
Neuronal degeneration and mental retardation	↓ catecholamine neurotransmitters
Growth failure and anaemia	↓ caeruloplasmin

Fig. 8.55 Clinical features of copper overload

Clinical effects of copper accumulation	Diagnosis
Liver: chronic hepatitis → cirrhosis

Brain: severe, progressive neurological disability including tremor, mental deterioration and loss of co-ordination

Eyes: characteristic yellow-brown Kayser-Fleischer rings around corneal limbus | Low serum concentration of caeruloplasmin

↑ urinary copper

Excess copper in liver biopsy |

the intestine, leading to a decreased synthesis of copper-containing enzymes (Fig. 8.54).

Treatment
Copper therapy has no significant effect. The life expectancy is less than 2 years.

Copper overload: Wilson's disease

Aetiology
Wilson's disease is a rare, autosomal recessive disorder (incidence of 1 in 100 000). The defect has been identified on chromosome 13 and results in failure of the liver to excrete copper in the bile. Copper incorporation into caeruloplasmin is also impaired. Copper accumulates and is deposited in the liver, basal ganglia of the brain, kidneys and the eyes, causing damage (Fig. 8.55).

Treatment
Wilson's disease is treated by daily chelation therapy with D-penicillamine. This is very effective at binding copper and eliminating it in the urine. However, the resulting liver and neurological damage is permanent.

Iodine
The human body contains about 15–20 mg of iodine, most of which is in the thyroid gland. It is essential for the synthesis of the thyroid hormones thyroxine and triiodothyronine.

Deficiency

Endemic goitre
Endemic goitre, a generalized enlargement of the thyroid gland, occurs in areas where the soil and water lack iodine such that the daily intake is less than 70 mg (usually mountainous areas). In the UK, it used to be found in people in Derbyshire, causing

the so-called Derbyshire neck. The problem has now been eliminated in most countries by the addition of iodine to table salt and its prevalence is mostly restricted to developing countries.

Pathogenesis of goitre. Normally, iodine is used to make thyroxine and triiodothyronine. Increased levels of these hormones exert a negative feedback effect on the hypothalamus and anterior pituitary, inhibiting further release of thyroid-releasing hormone and thyroid-stimulating hormone (Fig. 8.56), resulting in a decrease in their synthesis. However, low levels of iodine decrease thyroxine formation by the thyroid gland. This releases the negative feedback on the hypothalamic-pituitary axis, causing an uncontrolled increase in thyroid-stimulating hor-

mone secretion. High levels of TSH overstimulate the thyroid gland, causing hyperplasia of the thyroid epithelium and generalized enlargement (Fig. 8.57). The addition of iodine to the diet should reverse this effect.

Cretinism
Pregnant mothers who are deficient in iodine may give birth to babies who are hypothyroid. Growth and mental development in these babies are severely impaired and may be irreversible. The diagnosis is made by the neonatal screening test, the

> Hypothyroidism has an insidious onset with vague, non-specific and diverse features. It usually presents with fatigue, weight gain and cold intolerance. It may also present with bradycardia, constipation, delayed puberty, growth and mental retardation, and dry, scaly, cold and thickened skin.

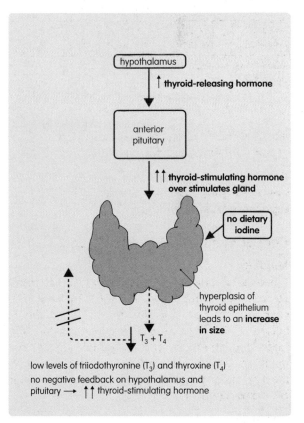

Fig. 8.56 The hypothalamic–pituitary–thyroid feedback system: normal status. In the presence of dietary iodine, thyroid hormones are produced which exert a negative feedback effect on hypothalamus and pituitary, inhibiting release of TRH and TSH.

Fig. 8.57 The hypothalamic–pituitary–thyroid feedback system: dietary iodine limiting. Decreased production of thyroid hormones releases negative feedback on hypothalamus and anterior pituitary.

Guthrie test, which is performed on all newborn babies and looks for raised thyroid-stimulating hormone levels. The same sample is used to screen for phenylketonuria. Treatment is lifelong oral replacement of thyroxine. Cretinism can be prevented by the iodination of salt in the maternal diet.

Iodine overload

Excessive dietary iodine may cause the symptoms of hyperthyroidism, that is, an overactive thyroid.

Other trace elements

The characteristics of some of the other trace elements not covered here are listed in Fig. 8.58.

Know about iron deficiency and overload, calcium deficiency, and copper overload because they are commonly asked about.

Fig. 8.58 The characteristics of some of the other trace elements

Element	Iodine	Chromium	Cobalt	Manganese	Molybdenum	Selenium	Silicon	Fluoride
Source	Supplemented salt RNI = 140 µg	Meat, liver, yeast, whole grains	Foods of animal origin			Meat, green vegetables RNI = 60 µg	Green vegetables	Drinking water
Main function	Synthesis of thyroid hormones	Possibly improves glucose tolerance	Constituent of vitamin B_{12} as cobalamin	Cofactor for enzymes: decarboxylases, transferases, superoxide dismutase	Constituent of xanthine oxidase: involved in purine breakdown	Cofactor of glutathione peroxidase	Bone calcification, glycosaminoglycan metabolism in connective tissue	Increases hardness of teeth
Deficiency	Goitre in adults Cretinism in babies	Impaired glucose tolerance (reported very rarely in patients on parenteral nutrition)	As for vitamin B_{12} deficiency	Unknown	Decreased uric acid synthesis	Endemic in parts of China → cardiomyopathy (Keshan disease)	Decrease in normal growth	Low intake leads to increased dental caries
Excess	Toxic goitre Hyperthyroidism	Non-specific: nausea, diarrhoea and irritability		Inhalation poisoning leading to psychotic symptoms and parkinsonism (rare)		Leads to hair loss, dermatitis, and irritability	Silicosis: long-term inhalation of silicon dust leads to pulmonary fibrosis	Fluorosis: where fluorine infiltrates enamel causing pitting and discoloration of teeth

CLINICAL ASSESSMENT OF METABOLIC DISEASE

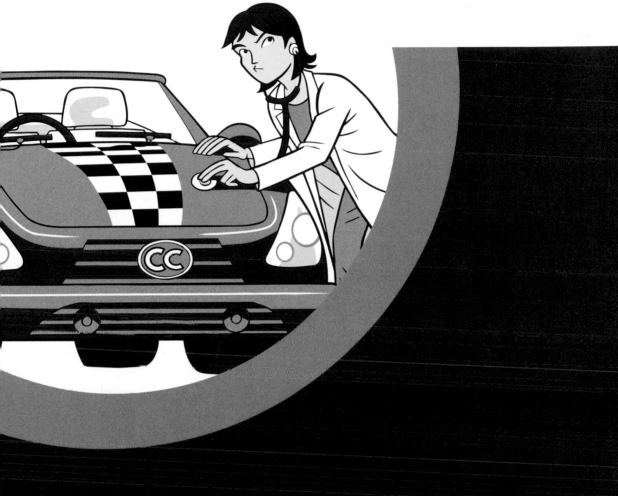

Presentation of metabolic disease

Objectives

You should be able to:

- Describe the metabolic causes of the common presenting complaints.
- Describe the symptoms of the major metabolic diseases.
- Work out a differential diagnosis for the major metabolic diseases.

COMMON PRESENTING COMPLAINTS

This section deals with some examples of common presenting complaints, and symptoms of metabolic diseases. For each complaint, the major metabolic causes are considered.

Remember, for each symptom there are also lots of non-metabolic causes, which might be more common but are beyond the scope of this book. For further discussions of these, refer to a general medicine textbook.

Fatigue

Fatigue covers a wide range of symptoms reported by patients, for example tiredness, lack of energy (one of the most common general symptoms), weakness, exhaustion, sleepiness or weariness.

Fatigue is a very common complaint and there are many causes. It is important to obtain a clear history of the complaint in terms of when it started, its progression, precipitating and relieving factors, and any associated symptoms that clearly help to eliminate other causes. Always ask whether tiredness occurs on effort. A good follow-up question is 'What slows you down when you attempt doing anything strenuous?'. The main metabolic causes of fatigue are described in Fig. 9.1.

Weight loss

Weight loss is a sign of a great many diseases. Only the main metabolic causes are considered here.

Working definition

A loss of 5% or more of the usual body weight over a period of 6 months.

It is essential to take a clear and well-documented history from the patient. It is often difficult to verify the true amount of weight lost, unless the patient is continually weighed and monitored over a period of time. Ask about:

- Changes in clothing or belt size.
- Verification from friends or relatives.

Make sure that you establish changes in diet and exercise over the period.

Involuntary weight loss is often a clue that the patient has a serious underlying disease such as

Fig. 9.1 Main metabolic causes of fatigue	
Causes	Examples and notes
Anaemia	This may be secondary to: • Iron/B_{12}/folate deficiency • haemolytic anaemia, e.g. G6PDH or pyruvate kinase deficiency (see Fig. 9.3 for other examples)
Hypothyroidism	This may be due to an iodine deficiency or an auto-immune disease, Hashimoto's thyroiditis
Malnutrition	Protein–energy malnutrition (PEM): marasmus or kwashiorkor (see Chapter 8) General vitamin deficiencies
Obesity	Tiredness, glucose intolerance, risk of hypertension
Diabetes mellitus	See types of diabetes (Fig. 9.4)
Ca^{2+} or vitamin D deficiency	Osteomalacia (weak, easily deformed bones)
Glycogen storage disorders	e.g. McArdle's syndrome (see Chapter 2)

cancer. Fig. 9.2 lists the common metabolic causes of weight loss.

Symptoms of anaemia

Anaemia occurs when the blood haemoglobin level is below the normal range for the patient's age and sex. The normal haemoglobin range in males is 13.5–18.0 g/dL and in females is 11.5–16.0 g/dL.

The symptoms depend on the severity of the anaemia; a small reduction in haemoglobin is usually asymptomatic. Most symptoms are non-specific and result from a decreased oxygen supply to the tissues:

- Fatigue.
- Headaches.
- Fainting.
- Breathlessness.
- Importantly, anaemia could unearth coronary heart disease by precipitating angina (chest pain, brought on by exercise, relieved by rest).
- Similarly, peripheral vascular disease may become symptomatic (intermittent claudication: leg pain precipitated by walking and quickly relieved by rest.
- Palpitations.

As these symptoms are relatively non-specific, to find out the cause of the anaemia, a number of laboratory tests may be performed, including:

- Full blood count, which includes the measurements of haemoglobin concentration, the red cell count, and several calculated indices, such as the mean cell volume and the mean cell haemoglobin (see Fig. 11.1).

For iron deficiency anaemia, there are unique signs and symptoms which help in clinical diagnosis. They are: painless glossitis (smooth tongue), angular stomatitis (sores at corner of the mouth), koilonychia (spoon shaped nails) and unusual dietary cravings such as pica (soil-eating).

When working out the causes of anaemia, the mean cell volume (MCV) is a very good guide to differentiating macrocytic, normocytic and microcytic anaemia (see Fig. 9.3)

- Blood film, which provides information on the morphology of cells.
- Reticulocyte count.
- Serum iron and total iron-binding capacity/transferrin.
- Serum ferritin.
- Vitamin B_{12} and folate levels.
- Schilling test. This is specific for pernicious anaemia.

These tests and their results are discussed fully in Chapter 11.

Causes of anaemia

There are many causes of anaemia, ranging from acute blood loss to hereditary haemolytic anaemias such as sickle cell anaemia. The main metabolic causes of anaemia are listed in Fig. 9.3.

Symptoms of diabetes mellitus

The presentation of the symptoms of diabetes mellitus may be acute or insidious in onset (types are listed in Fig. 9.4).

Acute

Young people often present with a brief 2–4 week history of the classical symptoms, namely polyuria, polydipsia, and weight loss, accompanied by tiredness. These patients usually have Type 1 diabetes. Remember that a patient with previously

Fig. 9.2 Common metabolic causes of weight loss	
Main cause	Differential diagnosis
Decreased calorie intake	• malnutrition: common in developing countries, and in the UK may be seen in the elderly • cancer • alcoholism • anorexia nervosa • depression
Increased loss or energy expenditure	• hyperthyroidism • poorly controlled diabetes • cancer

Fig. 9.3 Metabolic causes of anaemia

Cause	Notes
Microcytic anaemia (MCV < 75 fL)	
Iron deficiency	Decrease in haem and red blood cell production
Lead poisoning	Lead inhibits three enzymes of haem synthesis (see Chapter 6)
Vitamin C deficiency	Vitamin C is required for absorption of Fe^{2+} (see Fig 8.40)
Normocytic anaemia (MCV 76-100 fL)	
Haemolytic anaemia	Deficiency of erythrocyte enzymes such as pyruvate kinase or G6PDH (see Chapter 2)
Macrocytic anaemia (MCV > 100 fL)	
Folate/B_{12} deficiency	Folic acid and vitamin B_{12} required for DNA synthesis; results in megaloblastic anaemia (see Chapter 8)
Pernicious anaemia	Auto-immune condition in which antibodies against intrinsic factors prevent B_{12} absorption in the terminal ileum, leading to B_{12} deficiency (see Chapter 8)

Fig. 9.4 Types of diabetes mellitus

Type	Notes
Diabetes mellitus:	Overall incidence, approximately 2% in Western world
Type 1, insulin-dependent diabetes mellitus	Patients are usually younger than 25 years
Type 2, non-insulin-dependent diabetes mellitus	Patients are usually older than 25 years and often obese
Impaired glucose tolerance	Affects about 5% of population; these patients are more likely to develop diabetes when they are older
Secondary diabetes	Either due to pancreatic damage e.g. chronic pancreatitis, haemochromatosis or Wilson's disease, or due to endocrine disease, e.g. acromegaly, Cushing's disease

Note that a new category of impaired fasting glucose (>6 mmol/L) has been recently recognized

undiagnosed diabetes may present with diabetic ketoacidosis.

Subacute

The onset of symptoms is usually over months to years. Patients may still present with the classic symptoms although, quite often, tiredness is the prominent symptom, particularly Type 2 diabetes.

Asymptomatic

Glycosuria or raised blood glucose may be detected during a routine medical examination.

Diabetic ketoacidosis

If the early symptoms are not recognized, patients can present with ketoacidosis (see Fig. 7.13) where:

- Severe hyperglycaemia causes an osmotic diuresis. The consequent loss of fluid and electrolytes results in dehydration. If this is severe, the patient may be confused and be in shock. Remember to consider this diagnosis in patients presenting with abdominal pain.
- Increased production of ketone bodies results in metabolic acidosis and characteristic ketotic breath. The acidosis typically causes nausea and vomiting and further loss of fluid and electrolytes. Respiratory compensation results in hyperventilation (Kussmaul breathing). Diabetic ketoacidosis is a medical emergency: failure to treat a patient in ketoacidosis may result in coma and death.

Complications

Patients may also present with diabetic complications such as retinopathy, neuropathy or nephropathy. For example, they may present after visits to the opticians (diabetic retinopathy), or with tingling and numbness in the leg, or with leg or foot ulcers or impotence (neuropathy).

The diagnosis of diabetes is discussed fully in Chapter 7.

Symptoms of amino acid disorders

All amino acid disorders are rare. Most present in infancy as developmental delay, vomiting, failure to thrive, mental retardation and seizures. The symptoms are all non-specific, making the differential diagnosis complex. All neonates are now screened for phenylketonuria at a few days of age using the Guthrie test. The other amino acid disorders must be considered and eliminated when infants present with these symptoms without other adequate explanation; for example, in the absence of infection (Fig. 9.5). Their diagnosis depends on the measurement of metabolites in the blood and urine.

Fig. 9.5 Differential diagnosis of amino acid disorders in infants
Phenylketonuria
Inborn errors of carbohydrate metabolism, e.g. galactosaemia, glycogen storage disorders
Neurological disorders, e.g. febrile convulsions, infantile spasms
Infections (common), e.g. gastroenteritis, urinary tract infection
Coeliac disease (1 in 2000 in the UK)
Acute abdomen

Fig. 9.6 Simplified diagnostic approach to gout.

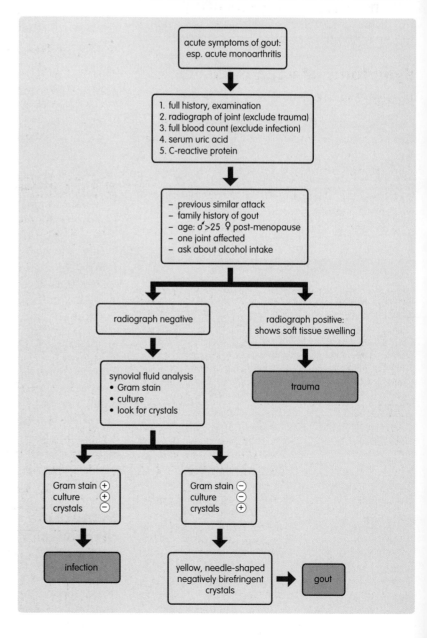

Symptoms of gout

Gout initially presents as recurrent, acute attacks of arthritis, usually affecting only one joint (monoarthropathy). The patient complains of a warm, swollen and very tender joint, usually the first metatarsophalangeal joint of the big toe. Eventually, the attacks fail to resolve completely and persistent symptoms occur because of the permanent deposition of urate crystals, leading to chronic tophaceous gout. Persistent symptoms may also be due to the presence of kidney stones (of calcium oxalate type), which can cause dysuria and renal colic. The most common differential diagnoses for the acute symptoms of gout are trauma and infection (Fig. 9.6).

Symptoms of vitamin deficiencies

Fat-soluble vitamins: A, D, E and K

The symptoms and signs of each individual vitamin deficiency are covered fully in Chapter 8 and therefore will only be covered briefly here (Fig. 9.7). General causes of deficiency are:

- Decreased intake, which may be due either to generalized malnutrition, mainly seen in developing countries; or to poor diet,

commonly seen in the elderly and in the housebound in developed countries, or it may occur in people on a vegan diet with no intake of meat.
- Fat malabsorption; for example due to liver and biliary tract disease or obstruction, meaning that no bile salts are available to facilitate absorption.

Vitamin E deficiency is very rare.

Water-soluble vitamins (B and C)

The symptoms of a deficiency of vitamins B and C are listed in Fig. 9.8.

Symptoms of mineral deficiencies

The symptoms and signs of each individual mineral deficiency are covered in detail in Chapter 8. The symptoms of the more important mineral deficiency disorders are listed in Fig. 9.9. The differential diagnosis is biased towards metabolic causes.

Fig. 9.7 Differential diagnosis of fat-soluble vitamin deficiency diseases

Vitamin deficiency	Differential diagnosis
Vitamin A: night blindness and keratomalacia	Other causes of degenerative eye changes, e.g. infection such as syphilis, gonorrhoea, chlamydia in neonates (rare)
Vitamin D: rickets or osteomalacia	- Ca^{2+} deficiency - renal disease – causing ↓ activity of 1-α hydroxylase - liver disease: causing ↓ acitivity of 25-α hydroxylase
Vitamin K: increased bleeding produces clotting problems (in newborn babies, causes haemorrhagic disease of the newborn)	- inherited coagulation disorders, e.g. haemophilia, von Willebrand's disease - anticoagulant therapy: warfarin/dicoumarol - antibiotic therapy which destroys vitamin K-producing bacteria in gut

Fig. 9.8 Symptoms of water-soluble vitamin deficiencies

Vitamin deficiency	Main symptoms
Vitamin B$_1$—thiamine: Wet beriberi	Oedema, tachycardia, shortness of breath and other signs of heart failure
Dry beriberi	Ascending peripheral neuropathy: initially weakness and numbness of legs that ascends to involve trunk, arms and eventually brain
Wernicke–Korsakoff syndrome	Confusion, ataxia, ophthalmoplegia and peripheral neuropathy
Niacin: pellagra	3 Ds: dermatitis, dementia and diarrhoea
Vitamin B$_6$: secondary pellagra	Very rare
Vitamin B$_{12}$: megaloblastic, macrocytic anaemia	See 'symptoms of anaemia' earlier
Folate: megaloblastic, macrocytic anemia	See 'symptoms of anaemia' earlier
Vitamin C: scurvy	Failure of wound healing hypochromic, microcytic anaemia Swollen, sore, spongy gums with bleeding

Fig. 9.9 Symptoms of mineral deficiencies

Symptoms	Cause
Iron deficiency: anaemia (symptoms of anaemia have been covered earlier)	May be due to: ↓ blood loss: either acute or chronic ↓ dietary intake ↓ absorption caused by: intestinal malabsorption such as ulcerative colitis, Crohn's disease and coeliac disease, ↑ phosphates and phytates in diet or vitamin C deficiency ↑ requirement: periods of growth and pregnancy
Calcium (and phosphate) **deficiency:** • in children: rickets; present with soft, easily deformed bones, short stature and failure to thrive • in adults: osteomalacia ('brittle bones')	• ↓ dietary intake • secondary to vitamin D deficiency: vitamin D is necessary for intestinal absorption of calcium and phosphate (see Chapter 8) • intestinal malabsorption • renal failure • hypothyroidism
Iodine deficiency: goitre can lead to symptoms of hypothyroidism: tiredness, weight gain, anorexia, cold intolerance, constipation	• auto-immune: Hashimoto's thyroiditis • after surgery for hyperthyroidism

History and examination

Objectives

You should be able to:

- Take a good history and perform a general examination.
- Summarise the main points of history taking and examination with an emphasis on eliciting signs and symptoms of metabolic disease.

THINGS TO REMEMBER WHEN TAKING A HISTORY

The purpose of this section is to remind you of the main points involved in taking a history from a patient.

The history is usually the most important part of the consultation.

Before you start:

- Always introduce yourself and shake hands, if appropriate. Make sure the patient is comfortable.
- Stand back and look around the bedside for clues. Is the patient being monitored, for example for blood pressure, oxygen saturation, blood glucose? Look for oxygen masks, inhalers, sputum pots, drains, walking sticks or frames; all of these provide clues to the patient's condition.
- Observe the patient. Is he or she agitated or distressed, either physically or emotionally? Are there any obvious signs, for example tremor, squint, pallor, hyperactivity?

Structure of a history

This is a basic plan designed for you to photocopy and take with you when you first start clerking patients.

Personal information:

- Name and sex.
- Age/date of birth.
- Occupation.

Presenting complaint (PC)

This should be a short statement of the symptoms the patient is complaining of, in his or her own words, for example, pain, thirst, poor appetite, tired-ness, weight loss, vomiting and so on. Remember, symptoms not diagnoses: patients do not complain of coronary heart disease, diabetes or acute intermittent porphyria!

History of presenting complaint (HPC)

Try to get the patient to tell the story in his or her own words from when he or she thought it began. For most symptoms you will need to know:

- What is the time course? When did the problem start or when did the patient first feel unwell?
- Was the onset rapid or slow?
- What is the nature of the complaint? If it is pain: what is its site, radiation and so on; if it is vomiting: how often does it happen and how much is there? What's the colour? Is there any visible blood?
- Does the symptom show a pattern? Is it continuous, intermittent or continuous with acute exacerbations?
- Are there any precipitating or relieving factors? For example, is it related to meals or the type of food eaten, or to stress? Is it helped by painkillers or any other medication?

For pain, a useful mnemonic to remember is SOCRATES.
Site
Onset
Character (e.g. sharp, dull, colicky)
Radiation
Associated symptoms (e.g. nausea, vomiting)
Timing
Exacerbation and relieving factors
Severity (e.g. on a scale of 1 to 10)

- Are there any other relevant or associated symptoms? For example, for chest pain, ask about palpitations, sweating and nausea.
- Has it happened before? Ask about any previous treatment or investigations for the complaint.

Use simple terms as much as possible and avoid medical jargon. Ask additional questions to see whether your key points were understood.

Previous medical history (PMH)

Ask the patient about previous illnesses, hospital admissions, operations and investigations, with dates. You may find the mnemonic 'MTHREADS' helpful: Myocardial infarction, Tuberculosis, Hypertension, Rheumatic fever, Epilepsy, Asthma, Diabetes, Stroke. You should always ask specifically about these conditions, as well as anaemia and jaundice.

Ask about the patient's nutritional history. A lot of metabolic and nutritional diseases present in infancy. When dealing with children, ask the parents specifically about problems during the pregnancy or birth, or when their child was a neonate; for example, problems with feeding, bowels or failure to thrive. Enquire about developmental milestones: smiling, sitting, walking, talking.

Drug history (DH)

Is the patient currently on any medication (either over the counter or prescription). Ask about the dosage. If relevant, ask about alternative therapies, herbal medicine and recreational drugs. Also remember to ask female patients if they are on the oral contraceptive pill, as many do not regard it as a drug.

Allergies

Is the patient allergic to any medicines or foods that they know of? Ask specifically about penicillin. If they say they are allergic, ask about what happened when they took the medicine or food.

Smoking

How many per day and how long ago did the patient start? If they say they have given up, you must also ask when—it might be just yesterday! A useful way of quantifying smoking is in pack years: 20 cigarettes smoked per day for 1 year equals 1 pack year.

The CAGE questionnaire is a useful screening test for alcoholism, with two or more positive answers suggesting an alcohol problem. Have you ever:
Felt you should **C**ut down on your drinking?
Been **A**nnoyed at others' concerns about your drinking?
Felt **G**uilty about drinking?
Had alcohol as an **E**ye-opener in the morning?

Alcohol

How many drinks or units each week? Remember, the limits are 21 units for males and 14 units for females per week.

Family history (FH)

Ask about any known illnesses in first-degree relatives, in particular, diabetes and heart disease. Remember to ask specifically about premature heart disease ('Has there been any talk in the family about a lot of people having heart disease at a young age?' The accepted definition of premature disease is onset below age 55 in men and 65 in women). It may help to make a quick sketch of the family tree.

A number of inborn errors of metabolism are inherited as autosomal recessive disorders and have a high incidence amongst races where marriages between first cousins are quite common, for example Ashkenazi Jews.

Be tactful when asking about a family history of malignancy.

Social history (SH)

Ask about marital status, number of children, and the type of accommodation. Ask about the patient's occupational history: current and previous jobs, exposure to chemicals or asbestos and any time off work due to illness. Ask about financial and personal worries and any risk-related behaviour, for example taking illegal drugs or any risky homosexual or heterosexual contacts.

Review of symptoms

Some of these symptoms may have already been covered in the history of the presenting complaint.

You need to use your discretion about the extent of this enquiry.

Cardiovascular system, ask specifically about:
- Chest discomfort and pain.
- Palpitations.
- Exercise tolerance (quantify by stairs climbed or distance walked before onset of breathlessness). Ask whether the patient ever felt uncomfortable or ill after an unusual effort or a hard day at work.
- Remember: Dyspnoea is shortness of breath; orthopnoea is breathlessness when lying down flat (quantify in terms of numbers of pillows the patient must sleep on to prevent dyspnoea); paroxysmal nocturnal dyspnoea is waking up at night breathless.
- Claudication (calf pain on walking). Ask how far can the patient walk without discomfort. Importantly does it happen when walking on the flat or on inclines and stairs.
- Leg pain at rest.
- Ankle oedema.

Respiratory system, ask specifically about:
- Persistent cough or wheeze.
- Sputum: amount, colour.
- Haemoptysis (coughing up blood).
- Shortness of breath.

Gastrointestinal system, ask specifically about:
- Change in appetite.
- Change in weight.
- Nausea or vomiting.
- Difficulty swallowing (dysphagia).
- Heartburn or indigestion.
- Change in bowel habit: diarrhoea, constipation, frequency, consistency, colour.

Urinary system, ask specifically about:
- Frequency.
- Urgency.
- Nocturia.
- Urine stream: hesitancy, dribbling.
- Dysuria (pain on passing water).
- Haematuria.
- Incontinence.

Skin, ask specifically about:
- Rashes or sensitive skin.
- Dermatitis.
- Eczema/psoriasis.
- Remember that the skin is frequently affected by substances encountered at work and at home.

Musculoskeletal system, ask specifically about:
- Location: generalized aches and pains or discomfort affecting a specific muscle?
- Painful joints.
- Stiffness.
- Swelling.
- Arthritis.
- Diurnal variations in symptoms (i.e. with time of the day).
- Functional deficit (i.e. can they undo buttons?).

Nervous system, ask specifically about:
- Headaches.
- Pins and needles, paresthesiae.
- Fits, faints and funny turns. Dizziness.
- Changes in vision, hearing, speech or memory.
- Anxiety, depression or suicidal thoughts.
- Changes in sleep pattern.

Menstruation and obstetric history
This should only be taken when relevant.

Make a summary

This should be a brief recall of the main points. For example: Jonathan Brown, a 4-year-old boy referred by his general practitioner, presenting with a 6-week history of increasing thirst, polyuria and weight loss. His mother has insulin-dependent diabetes mellitus. On examination …

COMMUNICATION SKILLS

Medical schools now place great emphasis on communication skills and their importance in the practice of medicine. Do not dismiss this teaching as less important than the more factual elements of the course. Newly qualified doctors often comment that this training was one of the most immediately useful things they had learnt in medical school.

Most medical school examinations now feature some form of structured clinical examination, e.g. OSCEs. You should remember some important points in relation to these:

- None of us are as good at communicating as we like to think we are.
- A lot of this material seems to be stating the obvious—but the obvious can be easy to forget under pressure, and reminding oneself of the basics is a useful exercise.

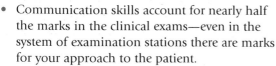

- When talking to patients, try to maintain appropriate eye contact throughout and look (be) interested.
- Take brief notes and write them up afterwards—you will be surprised at how much you can remember!

- Communication skills account for nearly half the marks in the clinical exams—even in the system of examination stations there are marks for your approach to the patient.
- Practising a few communication scenarios with friends before the exam is an easy way to pick up a lot of extra marks.
- If you get on the right side of the patient or actor in a clinical exam, they are likely to divulge their information much more easily.

The importance of communication

How you communicate is absolutely essential. Good communication makes patients more comfortable and greatly facilitates right diagnosis. On the other hand, poor communication is the most common cause of patients' complaints.

Obstacles to communication

There are many factors that can make it difficult to talk with patients and colleagues. It is important to be aware of these and address the ones you can do something about, while making allowances for those you can't. For example:

- Noisy environment and lack of privacy—try to find a quiet room or cubicle in which to see your patient if possible.
- Nervousness—both yours and the patient's. You can help yourself with practice. The patient can be put more at ease by a sensitive approach (more on this later).
- Pain—does the patient need analgesia now, rather than after the history?
- Other medical factors—breathlessness, hearing impairment and confusion (acute or chronic)

can all make communication difficult. Patience and persistence are required in these situations.
- Language and cultural barriers—if you encounter problems, try to take the history with a member of the family who can interpret. If this is not possible, it may be possible to obtain the help of an interpreter. In an acute situation, you may have to make do with smiles, drawings and gestures to establish the important points, such as the presence and site of pain.
- Hostility—some people may feel (rightly or wrongly) aggrieved by some aspect of the treatment they had already received. It is vital that you do not take this personally or be drawn into a confrontation. Try to remain calm and civil, empathize with the patient and apologise if appropriate. If all else fails, politely explain that you don't feel anything is being achieved and come back later.

Non-verbal communication skills

A large proportion of our communication 'band-width' is non-verbal. This includes body-posture, facial expression, eye movements and gestures; we are conscious of some of these things, but most are subconscious. Non-verbal cues are very important in a clinical setting, both in achieving a rapport with patients and in gaining insight into their condition.

The following points may be helpful during a consultation:

- Sit with the patient so that your eyes are on roughly the same level, preferably without a desk as a barrier between you. Maintain a comfortable distance, and try to face them while you are talking. It is also useful to make sure you have a comfortable position to write when you are taking a history—kneeling by the bedside is sometimes the best option!
- Maintain good eye contact, even if the patient doesn't. However, try not to stare: some people find it disconcerting.
- Use non-verbal cues to show you are listening, and encourage the patient: nodding, smiling and even appropriate laughter can help to put the patient at ease. Smiling is particularly important!
- It is worth having practice sessions with friends before you go into an exam, as they can point out any nervous habits that you might be unaware of.

Verbal communication skills

These are the things we say and how we say them. It is important to put the patient at ease during a consultation, although this is often easier said than done, as people are often understandably concerned in the clinical situation. The following are important skills:

- ALWAYS begin by checking the patient's identity, explaining who you are, and gaining their consent to take a history. It is a good idea to ask the patient to confirm their date of birth. Experienced doctors will tell you how many times they have seen people with the same names and surnames in one clinic session.
- Empathize with the patient: this means trying to understand their point of view and is not the same as sympathy. It is perfectly good practice to use such phrases as 'I understand' or 'That must have been very frightening', etc. when a patient is relating the details of their history.
- Use open questions at first, such as: 'What made you come to see a doctor today?' or 'Have you any other problems that have been worrying you?' Always ask the old doctor's question: 'How do you feel generally?'; you will be surprised how many things you will learn. It is a good idea to let the patient talk freely for the first minute or so, before you focus the history with closed questions such as: 'Does the pain catch you when you breathe in?'
- Avoid 'leading' questions, which direct the patient as to what to say, e.g. compare 'Does the pain go anywhere?' with 'Does the pain shoot down your left arm?'.
- Use verbal cues such as 'I see' or 'I understand' to help the flow of conversation.
- Check that you have understood what the patient has told you by repeating a summary back to him or her.
- Use plain English and avoid medical jargon. Reflect the terminology your patient uses for symptoms and diagnoses as appropriate.

Objectives in the consultation

Have a mental checklist of objectives when you go into a consultation—especially when this is part of an exam. Once again, the key to this is practice, preferably on the wards, but you can also run through mock scenarios in a study group if you are short of time. You may also need to produce this kind of list in a short-answer exam paper or viva. For example:

- Introduce yourself and establish a rapport with the patient.
- Find out why the patient has presented to you.
- Find out what the patient understands about the problem, and if they have their own theory as to what has caused it.
- What are the patient's expectations of this consultation—what do they want from you?
- Explore the problem with history and examination, and formulate a plan for further management, i.e. investigations and treatment.
- Explain your findings and plan to the patient as clearly as possible.
- Give the patient time to react to new information.
- Check the patient understands what you have said.
- Ask if there is anything else the patient is concerned about.
- Provide leaflets or write things down for the patient to take away.
- Follow-up—make sure the patient knows what the next point of contact will be: e.g. an outpatient appointment.
- The last four points can be remembered with the mnemonic 'CALF' (Check–Ask–Literature–Follow-up) and are a good way to use the last few minutes of an OSCE station to your advantage.

The following section deals with the main signs caused by an underlying metabolic disease, which may be observed on examination. It is not a comprehensive guide to clinical assessment. Some of the signs mentioned are relatively non-specific and may be related to other diseases, which may indeed be a

When interviewing the patient, remember to ask about the patient's perspective; this can gain you extra points in exams. Determine, acknowledge and appropriately explore the patient's ideas, concerns and expectations. Also ask how their problems are affecting their life and encourage the patient to express their feelings.

lot more common than the metabolic cause. Others may be specific to, and in fact be diagnostic of, a metabolic disease. Just remember, a lot of metabolic diseases are very rare and you may go through all your working life without seeing them. The section also provides some guidelines on how to examine certain parts or areas of the body and the best or simplest way to elicit signs.

> Before you examine any patient stand back and observe. Look at the patient's general appearance, level of consciousness, any obvious colour (pale or jaundiced) and whether he or she looks tired or distressed; these comments earn you extra marks.

EXAMINATION

General inspection

This section considers the main signs that are indicative of an underlying metabolic cause. These signs are often non-specific and therefore there may be other possible, non-metabolic causes that must be considered and eliminated in the differential diagnosis. In any clinical examination it is important that you are seen to generally inspect the patient. Stand at the foot of the bed and observe the patient taking a breath in and out.

The **main signs** you need to look for are detailed below.

Wasting, cachexia and obesity

The term 'wasting' is usually used to describe a mild to moderate, generalized loss of muscle and thus weight. 'Cachexia', however, is reserved for severe, generalized muscle wasting, which usually implies a serious underlying cause, for example, cancer or AIDS. An assessment of wasting and obesity in patients and the underlying metabolic causes are set out in Fig. 10.1.

Pallor and jaundice

Both pallor and jaundice are common signs, which have a number of possible causes (Fig. 10.2).

Fig. 10.1 Assessment of wasting and obesity underlying metabolic causes

Physical examination	Symptoms and signs	Possible diagnosis
Wasting: look for generalized muscle wasting	• when severe, patient has a thin emaciated appearance, almost skeletal, and it is referred to as cachexia • skin is wrinkled and there may be hair loss	• implies serious disease, principally cancer • in developing countries: probably due to malnutrition caused by marasmus • in children also consider malabsorption e.g. coeliac disease
Obesity: observe; can also: • measure weight and height and calculate body mass index (BMI) • compare with tables of ideal weight for height (mid-arm circumference and skin-fold thickness are rarely useful in practice)	• when severe it is obvious on inspection • BMI > 30 kg/m^2 is regarded as obese (see Chapter 8)	Usually energy input is greater than energy output Obesity is also seen in: • Cushing's syndrome • hypothyroidism • drug-induced, e.g. corticosteroids • consider the possibility of Type 2 diabetes mellitus

Fig. 10.2 Assessment of pallor and jaundice and underlying metabolic causes

Physical examination	Symptoms and signs	Possible diagnosis
Pallor: observe skin colour N.B. best way to assess pallor is to observe conjunctivae of eyes (see Fig. 10.8)	• normal skin colour varies according to skin thickness, circulation and pigmentation • paleness may be normal for patient or indicative of anaemia N.B. it is a poor indicator of anaemia	• iron deficiency anaemia • B_{12}/folate deficiency often secondary to pernicious anaemia causes pale-lemon skin as result of anaemia and increased haemolysis
Jaundice: observe skin colour N.B. best way to assess jaundice is to observe sclerae of eyes (see Fig. 10.8)	• yellow colour of skin is fairly insensitive indicator of mild to moderate jaundice • with severe jaundice, skin is yellow-green	Three basic causes of jaundice: • pre-hepatic: haemolytic anaemia, e.g. G6PDH deficiency • hepatocellular: viral hepatitis, paracetamol overdose • post-hepatic: obstruction of bile duct because of gallstones or carcinoma gallstones or carcinoma of head of pancreas

However, the best way to observe them is by observation of the eyes (Fig. 10.8).

Pallor is usually associated with anaemia. Jaundice refers to the yellow pigmentation of skin or sclerae of the eyes due to a raised plasma bilirubin level. Jaundice has many causes, which are classified into three main groups: pre-hepatic where there is excess unconjugated (not-liver-processed) bilirubin, for example due to increased haemolysis; intrahepatic where there is diminished liver cell function, for example due to a viral infection; and post-hepatic where there is obstruction of bile flow, for example gallstones obstructing common bile duct.

Respiratory distress

This is often best assessed by inspection (Fig. 10.3).

Tremors

The four common tremors are (Fig. 10.4):

• Essential or physiological tremor.

• Flapping tremor (CO_2 retention/chronic liver disease).
• Resting, 'pill-rolling' tremor of parkinsonism.
• Intention tremor of cerebellar disease.

Limbs

Hands

There are a number of signs on the hands and nails indicative of underlying metabolic disease. They are often subtle (Fig. 10.5). Clubbing, may be indicative of liver cirrhosis due to a number of causes, some of which are listed in Fig. 10.5. However, it is most commonly caused by suppurative lung disease or infective endocarditis and therefore these must always be highest on your list of differential diagnosis. It may also be congenital.

Limbs

Examination of the limbs for underlying metabolic disease can be conveniently divided into assessment

Fig. 10.3 Assessment of respiratory distress and its metabolic significance

Physical examination	Symptoms and signs	Possible diagnosis
Respiratory rate, rhythm, and depth of breathing are observed	• hyperventilation • 'Kussmaul respiration': deep, sighing breathing with rapid respiratory rate • smell of ketones on breath heightens suspicion	• accumulation of ketone bodies → metabolic acidosis • respiratory compensation → hyperventilation • untreated → severe diabetic ketoacidosis (see Chapter 7) • also seen in uraemia

Fig. 10.4 Assessment of tremors, and their significance in metabolic disease

Physical examination	Symptoms and signs	Possible diagnosis
Patient holds arms outstretched in front of them with hands flat Place a piece of paper on them	Look for fluttering of paper → tremor present	**Essential tremor:** normal tremor associated with anxiety, ↑ caffeine and ↑ exercise Also seen in: hypoglycaemia, alcoholism, hyperthyroid (thyrotoxic) patients, and Wilson's disease
Ask patient to hold arms outstretched with wrists hyperextended	Observe flapping motion of hands	**Flapping tremor:** CO_2 retention caused by hyperventilation may be seen in people with diabetes
Finger-nose test	Tremor arises on movement associated with cerebellar lesions	**Intention tremor:** seen in chronic alcoholics with Wernicke–Korsakoff syndrome

of vascular supply (Fig. 10.6) and skin and joint problems associated with metabolic disease (Fig. 10.7). Remember to check peripheral pulses.

Main metabolic problems to consider in examination of the limbs

Diabetic patients: Look specifically for ischaemic and neuropathic damage leading to ulceration and deformity of limbs (see Chapter 9).

Patients with peripheral vascular disease: Look for arterial ulceration and, in extreme disease, gangrene.

Examination of the limbs should include:
• Assessment of vascular supply. The quickest way to do this is to feel the pulses (Fig. 10.6). You should also observe colour, assess capillary filling time, feel for temperature and look for ankle oedema.
• Skin: look for any obvious lesions (Fig. 10.7).
• Neurological assessment. Both motor and sensory systems are particularly important in patients with diabetes.

Fig. 10.5 Main metabolic signs observed on examination of the hands

Physical examination	Symptoms and signs	Possible diagnosis
Nails:	**Clubbing:** • loss of the angle between the nail and nail-bed • underlying nail feels soft, fluctuant and 'boggy' • increased curvature in all directions **Koilonychia** spoon-shaped brittle nails, may be ridges	Liver cirrhosis caused by: • haemochromatosis ($\uparrow$ iron) • Wilson's disease ($\uparrow$ copper) • glycogen storage disorders (very rare) • alcohol Iron-deficiency anaemia
Palms:	**Palmar erythema** reddening of palms indicative of a hyperdynamic circulation	Liver cirrhosis caused by: • alcoholism or iron or copper deposition • thyrotoxicosis

Fig. 10.6 Main metabolic signs observed on examination of the limbs. Peripheral pulses provide a quick assessment of vascular supply

Physical examination	Symptoms and signs	Possible diagnosis
Arm pulses: • radial: assess rate, rhythm and volume • brachial	$\uparrow$ rate: tachycardia	• anaemia, acute blood loss/shock • thyrotoxicosis • hypoglycaemia
	$\downarrow$ rate: bradycardia	• hypothermia • hypothyroidism
	Irregular rthythm	Atrial fibrillation: hyperthyroidism
Leg pulses: • femoral • popliteal • posterior tibial • dorsalis pedis	$\downarrow$ or absent peripheral pulses (may also hear bruit over the femoral artery, indicating turbulent blood flow caused by stenosis of arteries)	Peripheral vascular disease seen in diabetes or patients with dyslipidaemias
Blood pressure (b.p.)	High	May occur secondary to endocrine or renal disease or to obesity in 95% of cases, cause of high BP is unknown; 'essential' hypertension
	Low	• severe anaemia, acute blood loss/shock • diabetic ketoacidosis • hypothyroidism

Fig. 10.7 Main metabolic signs observed on examination of the limbs: skin and joint problems associated with metabolic disease

Physical examination	Symptoms and signs	Possible diagnosis
Skin lesions: • ischaemic skin ulcers • note position, size, tenderness, edge of ulcer and note any discharge	• usually found over pressure areas: tips of toes/fingers • painful • discharge usually serum or pus, rarely blood-stained because of impaired blood supply • surrounding tissues pale and cold	Ischaemic damage seen in: • diabetes • atherosclerosis
Neuropathic ulcers	• usually found over pressure areas • painless (lack of sensation) • surrounding tissues are healthy because of good blood supply	Peripheral nerve lesions: chronic complication of diabetes
Gangrene-dead tissue	• brown/black tissue usually found on extremities and pressure points • painless and senseless	Ischaemic damage
Tendon xanthomata: look especially on Achilles tendon and finger extensors on back of hand	• fatty deposits on tendons leading to thickening • may see fat deposition in palmar creases of hand called palmar xanthomata	Characteristic of dyslipidaemias (see Chapter 4)
Gouty tophi	• deposits of urate crystals around joints, tendons and cartilage of ear lobes • cause yellow discoloration of overlying skin	Gout
Joint problems: • arthropathy • observe joints for signs of inflammation, especially big toe	Painful, red, hot, inflamed joint Acute onset	Acute gout Pseudogout

Skin manifestations of hyperlipidaemias

Tendon xanthomata, which are observed usually on the Achilles tendon or extensor tendons on the back of the hand, are often diagnostic of hyperlipidaemias. Eruptive xanthomata are a consequence of severe hypertriglyceridaemia.

Gout

This can affect any joint in the body. In an acute attack, look for a red, inflamed, painful joint. In chronic gout, look for gouty tophi: deposits of urate crystals around joints, tendons and the cartilage of ear lobes, causing yellow discolouration of the overlying skin.

Head and neck

Face

A number of metabolic and nutritional diseases result in clinical signs evident on the face. For ease,

Fig. 10.8 Observation of the eyes for signs associated with metabolic disease

Physical examination	Symptoms and signs	Possible diagnosis
Jaundice: observe colour of sclerae	Yellow discoloration of sclerae is a more sensitive indicator of jaundice than skin colour (sclerae turn yellow first)	• liver disease • haemolytic anaemia (e.g. due to G6PDH or pyruvate kinase deficiency) (see Chapter 2)
Anaemia: observe colour of conjunctiva (pull down the lower eyelid)	Pale/pink colour N.B. the best way to look for anaemia is by the colour of mucous membranes, particularly conjunctiva (also buccal mucosa)	• acute blood loss/infection • iron/B_{12}/folate deficiency • pernicious anaemia • haemolytic anaemia • hypothyroidism
Xanthelasma: look for yellow fatty lumps in skin of eyelids	Yellow fatty masses confined to the skin Non-tender	• they may or may not indicate dyslipidaemia (see Chapter 4)
Corneal arcus (arcus senilis)	Observe white rim around outer edge of iris due to cholesterol deposition Sclerosis in cornea	• common in elderly people • significant in patients < 35 years old, as it may indicate hyperlipidaemia, such as FH or familial combined hyperlipidaemia (see Chapter 4)
Kayser-Fleischer rings: examine corneal-sclera junction for ring	Green-brown ring due to copper deposition in periphery of cornea	Wilson's disease: copper overload (see Chapter 8)
Observe cornea and conjunctiva for dryness and ulceration	• dryness and ulceration: xerophthalmia • white plaques on conjunctiva: Bitot's spots • opaque scar tissue: keratomalacia and cataracts	All due to vitamin A deficiency
Progressive deterioration of vision	Loss of visual acuity	Diabetes mellitus

the signs observed are divided into those affecting either the eyes (Fig. 10.8) or the lips and mouth (Fig. 10.9).

Neck

With the exception of iodine deficiency and thyroid disease, there are very few metabolic or nutritional diseases that manifest as signs in the neck.

Thyroid disease

Look at the patient's neck and ask the patient to swallow. You will often observe a prominent goitre (a diffuse enlargement of the thyroid gland). Goitre, however, can also be seen in thyroid diseases such as Graves' disease and Hashimoto's thyroiditis. All thyroid lumps ascend on swallowing because they are attached to the trachea.

Fig. 10.9 Observation of the mouth and tongue for signs associated with metabolic disease

Physical examination	Symptoms and signs	Possible diagnosis
Colour of lips and tongue	Central cyanosis: purple-blue colour because of excess methaemoglobin in the tissues	• inadequate perfusion of tissues, methaemoglobinaemia • since methaemoglobin cannot carry oxygen, this leads to poor perfusion of tissues and cyanosis (see Chapter 3)
Colour of tongue and atrophic changes	Glossitis (red, smooth, sore tongue), loss of filiform papillae	• iron/folate/B_{12} deficiency • other B vitamin deficiencies: niacin, B_6 (pyridoxine)
Angular stomatitis: observe corners of mouth for cuts and infection	Angular stomatitis: inflamed, cracked corners of mouth; cracks may infected become with *Candida albicans*	Common in elderly due to iron deficiency or deficiency of B-group vitamins

When examining lumps and bumps, it helps to define the site, size, shape, surface, colour, temperature, tenderness, edge, composition, reducibility and state of overlying and adjacent tissues to help differentiate the diagnosis, which can range from benign hernias to malignant cancer.

Thorax

The signs associated with thorax can be divided into those related to respiratory and cardiovascular systems.

Respiratory system

Very few metabolic diseases result in obvious respiratory signs. Therefore, only a brief discussion is included here for completion.

Check list for examination of the respiratory system (Figs 10.10 and 10.11)
This is only a brief list to help you get started:

- Introduce yourself and gain consent.
- The patient should be undressed to the waist so that the appropriate part of the body is exposed.
- Position the patient so that he or she is comfortable and at the correct angle for examination (45° for respiratory and cardiovascular examination).
- Observe any respiratory distress, the level of consciousness, chest expansion (is it equal on both sides?), tachypnoea, and so on.

Begin any examination by observing the hands of the patient and work your way up the arms to the head, to the neck, and then down the chest. Remember for examination of any system follow the sequence: observation, palpation, percussion and auscultation.

Cardiovascular system

As with the respiratory system, few metabolic diseases present with cardiovascular signs. However, anaemia of any cause can precipitate angina and eventually cause heart failure and, in extreme cases, shock.

Percussion
Percussion may help to diagnose hepatomegaly in e.g. cardiac failure.

Observation and palpation
Metabolic signs that can be observed during a cardiovascular examination are listed in Fig. 10.12.

Fig. 10.10 Examination of the respiratory system in metabolic disease

Physical examination	Symptoms and signs	Possible diagnosis
Signs of respiratory distress	E.g. tachypnoea, use of accessory muscles of respiration, nasal flare and sternal recession	In starvation, severe muscle wasting can eventually cause wasting of the diaphragm, leading to respiratory distress and death
Shape of chest wall	• pigeon chest, *pectus carinatum*: prominent sternum often accompanied by indrawing of softened ribs along attachment of diaphragm, Harrison's sulcus • rickety rosary: expansion or swelling of ribs at costochondral junctions	Rickets in children
Cyanosis	• central cyanosis: observe purple-blue colour of lips • peripheral cyanosis: observe purple-blue colour of extremities (fingers and toes) caused by increased level of deoxygenated blood	Methaemoglobinaemia (see Fig. 10.9) Inadequate perfusion of tissues caused by peripheral vascular disease may be seen in diabetics patients
Respiratory rate: count for a minute; is it fast or laboured? normal is 15–20/min	• hyperventilation • deep Kussmaul respiration • breath smells of acetone • severe dehydration	• metabolic acidosis leading to diabetic ketoacidosis • respiratory compensation of metabolic acidosis results in hyperventilation

Auscultation

Anaemia of any cause can lead to an innocent ejection systolic murmur. For heart failure, you may hear a third heart sound. Checklist for auscultation:

- Always begin at the apex.
- Are there two heart sounds present? The first heart sound is due to the closure of the mitral and tricuspid valves. The second heart sound is due to the closure of the aortic and pulmonary valves. Listen over all four areas (mitral, triscupid, aortic and pulmonary).
- Listen for extra third and fourth heart sounds.
- Listen for murmurs. Murmurs are caused by turbulent blood flow. They are classified into systolic, diastolic or continuous, depending on their timing with the cardiac cycle.
- Listen over the carotid, renal and femoral arteries for bruits. These indicate turbulent

When listening for murmurs, consider the character, timing, loudness, area where loudest, radiation and accentuating manoeuvres to help determine the cause of the murmurs.

Fig. 10.11 Auscultation of the respiratory system: metabolic signs

Physical examination	Symptoms and signs	Possible diagnosis
Breath sounds	↓ breath sounds	In obese people these may be difficult to hear
Crepitations/crackles	Pulmonary oedema, often due to heart failure	Heart failure may be secondary to: • anaemia from iron/folate/B_{12}/vitamin C deficiency • kwashiorkor

Fig. 10.12 Clinical signs that may be observed during cardiovascular examination

Physical examination	Symptoms and signs	Possible diagnosis
Signs of shock and heart failure	Pallor, tachycardia, heart murmur, and cardiac enlargement Untreated progresses to heart failure	Severe anaemia (haemoglobin < 8 g/dL) causes: • blood loss • iron/folate/B_{12} deficiency • acute haemolytic crisis • hypothyroidism
Apex beat	Visible on inspection	Thin, wasted individuals
Impalpable apex beat	Normally felt at the left fifth intercostal space, mid-clavicular line	Obesity
Displaced apex beat	Heart failure → cardiomegaly	Anaemia of any cause Kwashiorkor Hypercalcaemia

blood flow caused by stenosis of arteries; they are heard in patients with disseminated atherosclerosis.

Abdomen

Most metabolic diseases that produce abdominal signs do so as a result of excessive deposition of a metabolite or nutrient in organs such as the liver, or in arteries or the skin. This interferes with the correct functioning of the organ. For example:

- In glycogen storage diseases, the deposition of glycogen in the liver causes hepatomegaly.
- In atherosclerotic disease, the deposition of fat in the walls of arteries leads to atherosclerotic plaque formation, resulting in turbulent blood

flow which may be heard as bruits over carotid or renal arteries. Aortic aneurysm may cause a palpable pulsation in the abdomen (be very careful when examining this!). Think of an abdominal aortic aneurysm in elderly male patients presenting with an abdominal or back pain. This is a medical emergency.

Useful points for the examination of the abdomen

When examining the abdomen:

- The patient should be lying as flat as possible, with arms by his or her sides.
- The patient should be exposed from the nipples to the knees; however, in the interest of privacy,

Fig. 10.13 Clinical signs that can be observed during an abdominal examination, and their underlying metabolic causes

Physical examination	Symptoms and signs	Possible diagnosis
Abdominal distension: note shape, symmetry, size of any bulge or mass	General/localized swelling	Obesity; pregnancy Ascites; kwashiorkor
	Asymmetrical enlargement	e.g. liver enlargement due to glycogen storage disorders, dyslipidaemias, kwashiorkor
Striae (stretch marks)	Purple abdominal striae	Cushing's syndrome Obesity
Spider naevi	Single, central arteriole feeding a number of small branches in a radial manner, with blanching (turning white) on pressure	Chronic liver failure and cirrhosis in: • alcoholism • haemochromatosis • Wilson's disease (copper overload) • vitamin A toxicity (see Chapter 8)
Pigmentation	Slate-grey colour	Iron overload

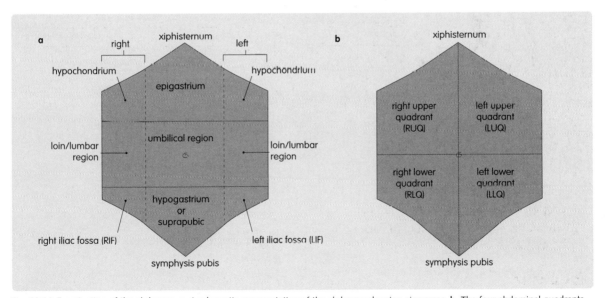

Fig. 10.14 Examination of the abdomen. **a.** A schematic representation of the abdomen showing nine areas. **b.** The four abdominal quadrants simplified.

it is best to expose in stages, beginning with xiphisternum to pubis.

- Kneel beside the bed so that you are at the same level as the patient.
- As with any system of the body, go through the sequence of observation, palpation, percussion and auscultation.

Observation

Observe the general symmetry and shape of the abdomen. The clinical signs that can be observed during an abdominal examination, and their underlying metabolic causes, are listed in Fig. 10.13.

Palpation

Points to remember when palpating the abdomen:

Fig. 10.15 Clinical signs that can be detected on palpation of the abdomen, with their underlying metabolic causes

Physical examination	Symptoms and signs	Possible diagnosis
Abdominal pain: determine site, position, radiation onset, timing, etc.	Acute, severe upper abdominal pain ± guarding and rebound tenderness	• acute pancreatitis seen in type I familial lipoprotein lipase deficiency or apoC-II hyperlipidaemia (see Chapter 4) • acute prophyria (see Chapter 6)
Liver enlargement (hepatomegaly)	• liver edge is not normally palpable below costal margin • gross hepatomegaly can fill whole abdomen	Causes: • heart failure • alcohol-induced liver disease • haemolytic anaemia, e.g. G6PDH deficiency • porphyria • iron overload: haemochromatosis • glycogen storage disorders (see Fig. 2.36) • galactosaemia (see Chapter 2)
Spleen enlargement (splenomegaly)	Spleen supposedly has a palpable notch on its medial side but it is very difficult to feel	Causes: • pernicious anaemia • galactosaemia • haemolytic anaemia
Kidneys	They are usually impalpable	• lower pole of right kidney can be felt in very thin or wasted people • renal disease and stones are associated with gout

- Before you start, ask the patient 'Have you any pain anywhere in your abdomen?'. If the answer is 'yes', begin your palpation furthest from the pain.
- The abdomen is divided either into nine areas or simply into quadrants (Fig. 10.14).

The clinical signs with their underlying metabolic causes that can be detected on palpation of the abdomen are listed in Fig. 10.15.

Percussion
Abdominal percussion has two main roles:

- To outline the liver. The liver is 'dull' to percussion and therefore it is useful in determining the degree of hepatomegaly.

- In the presence of abdominal distension, to determine whether it is due to solid, gas or free fluid (ascites) in the abdomen. The technique 'shifting dullness' can be used to distinguish the presence of ascites from solid or gas.

Ascites is seen in congestive heart failure, liver cirrhosis and secondary to wet beriberi and kwashiorkor.

Auscultation
The clinical signs that can be detected on auscultation of the abdomen, with their underlying metabolic causes, are listed in Fig. 10.16.

Fig. 10.16 Clinical signs that can be detected on auscultation of the abdomen, and their underlying metabolic causes

Physical examination	Symptoms and signs	Possible diagnosis
Bowel sounds	Absent if there is mechanical obstruction	• paralytic ileus • gallstones
Bruits	Listen along course of aorta, usually over femoral and renal arteries	• aortic aneurysm • renal artery stenosis • peripheral vascular disease, e.g. patients with diabetes or dyslipidaemias

Further investigations

Objectives

You should be able to:
- Understand the basic principles behind the routine investigations and when you should use them.
- Understand how the results of routine investigations are interpreted.
- Make a thorough assessment of the patient's nutritional status.

ROUTINE INVESTIGATIONS

This chapter describes selected aspects of clinical investigation relevant to metabolic disease. It is not a comprehensive description of laboratory tests used in clinical practice. The main tests used every day to assess metabolic function can be divided into:

- 'First-line' tests, that is, the tests most frequently requested.
- 'Second-line' tests and specialist tests.

With all routine investigations, the results should not be interpreted separately; for example in the diagnosis of anaemia, the haematology and clinical biochemistry tests are all part of the comprehensive patient assessment.

You do not need to learn normal range values for routine investigations as they will be given in exams. However, a familiarity with the common tests is helpful in appreciating the degree of abnormality when a result is abnormally high or low.

Haematology

The simplest, first-line haematology test is the full blood count (FBC). This measures red cell count and indices, total and differential white cell count and platelets. The 'second-line' tests include clotting studies and assessment of serum iron status and bone marrow iron stores (Fig. 11.1).

Clinical chemistry

First-line tests include urea and electrolytes (U&E), blood glucose, liver function tests (LFTs) and troponin (used in the diagnosis of myocardial infarction) (Fig. 11.2). Second-line tests include thyroid function tests, glycated haemoglobin, serum magnesium, ferritin, folate, lipid profile and C-reactive protein (important in the diagnosis and monitoring of infection). Other specialized tests include the measurements of vitamin and trace element concentrations performed in patients who receive total parenteral nutrition, and the specific diagnosis of genetic metabolic defects in paediatrics. The measurement of hormone levels in blood is a substantial part of specialized biochemistry testing.

Urine

Urine is commonly tested for glucose, protein and ketones (dipstick tests). Although not as sensitive as blood tests, urinalysis provides a quick and easy method of investigation (Fig. 11.4). Note that urinary ketones are important in the diagnosis of diabetic ketoacidosis.

Histopathology

These tests are usually performed to confirm a diagnosis, usually after simpler biochemical tests have been done (Fig. 11.5), and are often performed together with medical imaging tests.

Immunopathology

An example of an immunopathological investigations is listed in Fig. 11.6.

Fig. 11.1 Haematological investigations

Test	Normal range	Low/high
Full blood count (FBC) Haemoglobin g/dL	Men 13–18 Women 11.5–16	Low: anaemia High: polycythaemia
Red cell count ($\times 10^{12}$/L)	Men 4.5–6.5 Women 3.9–5.6	Low: anaemia High: polycythaemia
Mean cell volume (MCV)	76–96 fL	Low: microcytic anaemia—iron deficiency High: macrocytic anaemia—B_{12}/folate deficiency
Mean cell haemoglobin (MCH)	27–32 pg	Low: iron deficiency High: B_{12}/folate deficiency
Reticulocyte count	0.8–2%	Low: iron/B_{12}/folate deficiency anaemia thalassaemia High: haemolytic anaemia
C-reactive protein		Increases with inflammation and infection
Bone marrow iron stores		Low: iron deficiency High: thalassaemia sideroblastic anaemia
Clotting studies: • prothrombin time • activated partial thrombo-plastin time (APTT)	10–14 s 35–45 s	Both high—vitamin K deficiency Prothrombin time is a good indicator of liver function (protein synthetic capacity)
Blood film	Normocytic, normochromic erythrocytes	Microcytic, hypochromic: iron deficiency, lead poisoning, thalassaemia
		Macrocytic, hypochromic: B_{12}/folate deficiency, alcohol abuse, liver disease
		Sickle cells: sickle cell anaemia
		Irregular 'blister' cells: G6PDH deficiency (very rare)

Medical imaging

There are many medical imaging tests used, from simple radiographs and ultrasound to magnetic resonance imaging and positron emission tomography scanning. Fig. 11.7 illustrates some examples.

Remember, any patient presenting to casualty will probably require a combination of first-line tests. For example:

- Full blood count.
- Urea and electrolytes.
- Blood glucose. Bedside blood glucose can be life saving if a patient comes in unconscious or confused: he or she may be drunk or severely hypoglycaemic.
- Liver function tests.
- If there are signs of infection, blood, urine and CSF (if appropriate) sample must be taken for culture, and the measurement of C-reactive protein is useful.
- Electrocardiogram and chest radiograph if necessary.
- Troponin measurement if myocardial infarction is suspected

Investigation of glucose homeostasis

Measurement of blood glucose

Use

The measurement of blood glucose is used to confirm or reject a diagnosis of diabetes mellitus or impaired glucose tolerance and to monitor the control of blood glucose in diabetic patients.

Reference ranges for blood glucose levels are shown in Fig. 11.8.

Test

The estimation of blood glucose uses the glucose oxidase and peroxidase reaction.

Method

The test is based on the reaction catalysed by the enzymes glucose oxidase and peroxidase, and a peroxidase substrate (a dye). Glucose oxidase oxidizes glucose present in a deproteinized blood sample to gluconolactone and hydrogen peroxide. The hydrogen peroxide reacts with a dye to form a coloured complex, absorbance of which is read in a spectrophotometer. Under standard conditions, the amount of glucose in the unknown blood sample is equal to the amount of coloured product formed.

Fig. 11.2 First-line biochemical investigations on blood or serum.

Test	Normal range	Low/high
Liver function tests		

AST
ALT
	< 35 U/L
	< 35 U/L
		High: hepatocellular damage, e.g. hepatitis
		         cirrhosis
		         fatty liver

Alkaline phosphatase (ALP)	<120 U/L (different isoenzymes present in liver, bone, placenta and intestine)	High: obstruction of biliary tract or intrahepatic cholestasis: cirrhosis

γ-glutamyl transferase (GGT)	<80 U/L	High: alcohol abuse
		         obstructive liver disease
		         carcinoma of head of the pancreas
		(fairly non-specific test of liver function)

Serum total bilirubin	<22 μmol/L	High: liver disease
		         haemolytic anaemia
		         anaemia

Urea and electrolytes (U&E)		
Sodium	135–145 mmol/L	High: dehydration Low: extracellular water excess

Potassium	3.5–5.0 mmol/L	High: diabetic ketoacidosis
		         renal failure
		         potassium-sparing
		         diuretics
		Low: renal or intestinal loss
		         surgical drainage of the bowel, vomiting
		         insulin treatment of diabetic ketoacidosis
		         hyperaldosteronism, diuretics

Bicarbonate	22–32 mmol/L	High: metabolic alkalosis Low: metabolic acidosis
Urea	2.5–6.7 mmol/L	High: renal disease catabolic state
Creatinine	70 to " 150 μmol/L	High: renal damage and failure increased muscle bulk, e.g. athletes
(U&E profile also includes chloride)		
Total protein	60–80 g/L	High: myeloma
Albumin	35–50 g/L	Low: chronic liver disease
Calcium	2.12–2.65 mmol/L	Low: vitamin D deficiency High: hyperparathyroidism, malignancy
Free T_4 (thyroxine)	9–22 pmol/L	High: hyperthyroidism
Free T_3 (triiodothyronine)	5–10.2 pmol/L	Low: hypothyroidism
Troponine	< 0.5 ng/mL	High: ↑ suspicion of myocardial infarction
Thyroid-stimulating hormone (TSH)	0.5–5.7 mU/L	Low: hyperthyroidism High: hypothyroidism

AST, aspartate aminotransferase; ALT, alanine aminotransferase

Standardized solutions of glucose are processed at the same time in order to construct a calibration curve. Therefore, the amount of glucose in the unknown blood sample can be read off from the curve.

Advantages

The test is specific for glucose. A similar enzyme reaction is found in commercially available self-monitoring reagent strips: the Dextrostix/Glucometer

Fig. 11.3 Second-line biochemical investigations on blood or serum. CC, cholecalciferol

Test	Normal range	Low/high
Serum iron	13–32 μmol/L	Low: iron deficiency High: haemochroma- tosis thalassaemia
Total iron binding capacity (TIBC)	42–80 μmol/L	Low: iron deficiency
Serum B$_{12}$	160–925 ng/L	Low: pernicious anaemia
Folate	4–18 μg/L	Low: pregnancy, cancer, drugs, e.g. methotrexate
Serum urate	< 0.48 mmol/L	High: hyperuricaemia and gout
Lipid profile: Total cholesterol Triacylglycerol (triglycerides) HDL-cholesterol	< 4.0 mmol/L < 1.7 mmol/L M: ≥ 1.0 mmol/L F: ≥ 1.2 mmol/L	High: dyslipidaemias chronic liver disease
Vitamin D: 25-hydroxyCC 1, 25-dihydroxyCC	37–200 nmol/L 60–108 pmol/L	Low: rickets or osteomalacia
Copper caeruloplasmin	12–25 μmol/L 0.20–0.45 g/L	High: Wilson's disease

Fig. 11.4 Examples of urine tests

Test	Results
Glucose	High: diabetes, pregnancy, renal tubular damage, lowered renal treshold for glucose
Ketones	High: diabetic ketoacidosis and starvation
Protein	High: renal damage urinary tract infections
Porphobilinogen (PBG) and δ-aminolevulinic acid (ALA)	High: acute porphyrias (see Chapter 6)
Bilirubin	High: hepatocellular or obstructive jaundice, haemolytic anaemia
Urobilinogen	High: haemolytic or hepatocellular jaundice Low: obstructive jaundice

Fig. 11.5 Examples of histopathology investigations

Test	Results in metabolic disease
Liver biopsy	Wilson's disease: increased copper deposition leading to liver cirrhosis Haemochromatosis: iron deposition may cause cirrhosis which may progress to hepatocellular carcinoma
Synovial joint fluid analysis	Gout: the presence of yellow, needle-shaped negatively birefringent monosodium urate crystals

system (and many other systems) is commonly used at home by patients with Type 1 diabetes.

Fasting blood glucose

Use

The fasting blood glucose sample is usually used to diagnose diabetes mellitus in an asymptomatic patient or if the random blood glucose results are borderline.

Method

The patient should be fasted overnight (at least 10 hours) and have their blood glucose tested the following morning. Interpretation of fasting glucose results is shown in Fig 11.8.

Fig. 11.6 Example of immunopathology investigations

Test	Normal result	Result
Direct Coombs' test (detection of antibodies to red blood cells)	Usually no antibodies are present and therefore there is no agglutination of erythrocytes	Positive test = agglutination of erythrocytes, e.g. in haemolytic disease of the newborn or in auto-immune haemolytic anaemia

Fig. 11.7 Examples of imaging investigations

Test	Examples of diagnostic utility
Chest X-ray (CXR)	Diagnosis of heart failure: anaemia of any cause, ischaemic heart disease, hypercalcaemia, or iron overload, can all result in heart failure; on X-ray this can show up as: • an enlarged heart (cardiomegaly) • pleural effusion • increased perihilar shadowing (bat wings) due to oedema • prominent upper lobe veins • Kerley B lines
Bone X-ray, MRI	Defective bone mineralization: in rickets and osteomalacia: defective mineralization seen in pelvis, long bones and ribs in the early stages → see soft tissue swelling late stages → well-defined 'punched out' lesions in juxta-articular bone
Electrocardiogram (ECG)	Abnormalities of ECG pattern can be related to: • ischaemic damage and myocardial infarction • conduction defects (heart blocks) • arrhythmias • some electrolyte disturbances • congenital heart defects
CT scan	Used to identify abnormalities and to exclude focal lesions due to tumours or infection; essential tool in the diagnosis of space-occupying lesions

Fig. 11.8 Diagnostic concentrations of plasma glucose

	Normal (mmol/L)	IFG (mmol/L)	Diabetes (mmol/L)
Fasting plasma glucose	< 6.0	6.0–6.9	≥7.0
	Normal (mmol/L)	IGT (mmol/L)	Diabetes (mmol/L)
2h post-load blood glucose	<7.8	7.8–11.1	≥11.1

IFG = impaired fasting glycaemia, IGT = impaired glucose tolerance

Fig. 11.9 Results of an oral glucose tolerance test (OGTT)

Result	Reference range
Normal	Returns to < 7.8 mmol/L
Impaired glucose tolerance (IGT)	Fasting plasma glucose < 7.0 mmol/L and 2h value between 7.8 and 11.1 mmol/L in an OGTT
Impaired fasting glucose	Fasting plasma glucose 6–6.9 mmol/L
Diabetic	Fasting blood glucose ≥ 7.0 mmol/L and/or 2h value > 11.1 mmol/L in an OGTT

Oral glucose tolerance test

Use
The oral glucose tolerance test (OGTT) is a reference method to diagnose disturbances in glucose homeostasis. However, fasting blood glucose provides very similar information and should be used first. The use of OGTT is restricted to the detection of borderline cases.

Method
Patients should make sure that they eat a normal diet, containing adequate carbohydrate, for the preceding 3 days. This ensures that the enzymes involved in glucose metabolism are present at normal levels. After an overnight fast, an initial basal blood sample is taken and the blood glucose concentration is determined. 75 g of glucose in 250–300 mL of water is drunk and the blood glucose is measured every 30 min for the next 2 h. The blood glucose concentration is determined by the glucose oxidase method. Patients must sit comfortably during the test because stress can lead to cortisol release, which antagonizes the action of insulin, thus increasing blood glucose concentration. Figs 11.9 and 11.10 illustrate the results of an OGTT.

Assessment of glycaemic control: glycated haemoglobin

Use
The concentration of glycated haemoglobin (HbA_{1c}) provides a measure of the average blood glucose concentration over the preceding 4–6 weeks, that is, the half-life of erythrocytes. This is useful for diabetic patients to show how well their blood glucose concentration has been controlled over a period of time and for the doctor to determine the true level of control – it is a good check on the validity of glucose values entered by patients in their

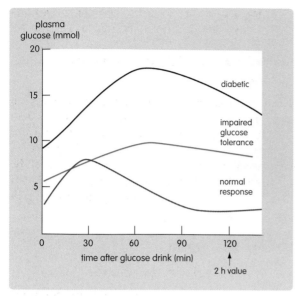

Fig. 11.10 Oral glucose tolerance test. Please note that persons with impaired glucose tolerance can have a normal fasting glucose concentration.

Fig. 11.11 Reference values for HbA$_{1c}$ expressed as a percentage of total haemoglobin

Result	Refernce values for HbA$_{1c}$
Desirable	< 6.5% (< 7.5% in patients at risk of severe hypoglycaemia)
Poorly controlled	> 10%

- Patients with dyslipidaemias and their families, and patients with a family history of premature cardiovascular disease.
- Patients with multiple risk factors; for example, patients with high blood pressure, or high cholesterol (a full list of risk factors can be found in Chapter 4).

Investigations

Screening for cholesterol levels can be done on a non-fasting sample. If a raised cholesterol is found, a full lipid profile is performed, which measures the total cholesterol, high-density lipoprotein (HDL) cholesterol, and triacylglycerols. Blood taken for lipid studies is obtained after an overnight fast. Reference values for fasting plasma lipid concentrations are shown in Fig. 11.12.

Low-density lipoprotein (LDL) cholesterol levels can also be obtained by calculation using the Friedewald equation. This is only valid if triacylglycerol levels are less than 4.5 mmol/L.

LDL mmol/L = total cholesterol − HDL − (triacylglycerol/2.2)
LDL (mg/dL) = total cholesterol − HDL − (triacylglycerol/5)

Triacylglycerol levels of greater than 10 mmol/L are associated with an increased risk of pancreatitis.

glucose result log book. The higher the value of HbA$_{1c}$, the less well-controlled the diabetes.

Method

Glucose irreversibly attaches non-enzymatically to adult haemoglobin (HbA) over the lifetime of erythrocytes. The extent to which this occurs is proportional to the blood glucose concentration. The amount of glycated haemoglobin in the blood can be measured by a number of methods including high-pressure chromatography, electrophoresis and immunoassay. It is usually expressed as a percentage of total haemoglobin (Fig. 11.11).

Investigation of lipid metabolism

Cholesterol and triacylglycerol (triglyceride) concentration

Uses

Coronary heart disease is a major cause of death in the UK. Plasma cholesterol levels are monitored routinely in 'at risk' groups and when necessary in the rest of the population. 'At risk' groups include:

- Patients with coronary heart disease (angina, post-myocardial infarction, post-angioplasty or coronary artery bypass graft), those with peripheral or cerebrovascular disease, and patients with diabetes mellitus.

Enzymes as tissue markers

Glucose-6-phosphate dehydrogenase

Use

An enzyme assay is used for the diagnosis of glucose-6-phosphate dehydrogenase deficiency, the most common erythrocyte enzyme defect (see Chapter 3). It allows patients with glucose-6-phosphate dehydrogenase deficiency to be detected in between haemolytic attacks, such that diagnosis is not just dependent on the blood picture during an attack. An enzyme activity of <2% of the normal level may be seen in very severe cases.

Fig. 11.12 Desirable values for fasting plasma lipid concentrations

Lipid	Plasma concentration (mmol/L)
Total cholesterol	< 4
LDL-cholesterol	< 2.0
HDL-cholesterol	M: ≥ 1.0
	F: ≥ 1.2
Triacylglycerol (triglyceride)	< 1.7

Pyruvate kinase assay

Use

Pyruvate kinase assay is used for the diagnosis of erythrocyte pyruvate kinase deficiency (see Chapter 2).

Test

The production of pyruvate is coupled to the reduction of a dye, with the colour change monitored spectrophotometrically. A decreased production of ATP can also be measured when radioactively labelled ^{32}P is added to erythrocytes and its incorporation into ATP is monitored.

Reference values

Patients typically need to have an enzyme level of 5–25% of the normal level to show clinical features.

Galactose and fructose

Both galactose and fructose are reducing sugars and are detected in the urine using alkaline copper (II) reagents, such as Benedict's reagent.

Galactosaemia

Galactosaemia is caused by a deficiency of the enzyme galactose-1-phosphate uridyl transferase.

Tests

Screening tests are performed in infants with suspicious symptoms:

- Test for galactosuria: Clinitest tablets or reagent strips contain copper citrate, which is reduced by galactose. The colour change observed is clear blue to green to brown to a brick red precipitate if the reduction is complete. The presence of galactose in the urine along with positive symptoms should lead to the withdrawal of galactose and lactose from the diet until a diagnostic test can be performed.

- Diagnostic test: assay erythrocytes for decreased galactose-1-phosphate uridyl transferase activity.

Fructokinase deficiency: essential fructosuria

The absence of fructokinase leads to a combination of a high fructose concentration in the blood and fructose accumulation in the urine. Both must be present to form a diagnosis. Fructose, like galactose, is a reducing sugar and its presence in urine can be detected with Clinitest tablets. Bear in mind that this is a rare diagnosis, virtually always seen in paediatric practice.

Hormone assays

Thyroid-stimulating hormone

The measurement of thyroid-stimulating hormone (TSH) levels is used as a screening test for suspected hyperthyroidism and hypothyroidism. Both hyperthyroidism and hypothyroidism influence the basal metabolic rate by over-stimulating or under-stimulating lipid and carbohydrate metabolism respectively. Elevated TSH levels signify an inadequate thyroid hormone production, while suppressed levels signify excessive unregulated production of thyroid hormone. If TSH is abnormal, decreased levels of thyroid hormones, T3 and T4, may be present; these may be measured to confirm the diagnosis.

Other investigations

Diagnosis of phenylketonuria

Every neonate is now screened for phenylketonuria as part of the neonatal screening (Guthrie test). Diagnosis is based on a high concentration of phenylalanine in the blood (see Chapter 5 for a full discussion).

The most severe and devastating form of hypothyroidism is seen in young children with congenital thyroid hormone deficiency. If the condition is not corrected by supplemental therapy through oral administration of synthetic thyroid hormone soon after birth, the child will suffer from cretinism, a form of irreversible growth and mental retardation.

It is worth knowing the different criteria for the diagnosis of diabetes and glucose intolerance as they are frequently asked in exams.

Screening test

A sample of capillary blood is taken from a heel-prick at 5–10 days after birth. The delay allows sufficient time for feeding, and therefore for protein intake to be established and for the effect of the mother's metabolism to subside. This test used to be based on a microbiological technique, using a strain of *Bacillus subtilis* which only grows if excess phenylalanine is present. However, it is now based on chromatography. Increased plasma phenylalanine levels are indicative of phenylketonuria. The neonatal screening also includes the measurement of thyroid stimulating hormone (TSH), to screen babies for hypothyroidism.

ASSESSMENT OF NUTRITIONAL STATUS

For any individual, adequate nutrition is essential to maintain growth and development and recovery from illness. It is especially important in newborn babies, infants and during pregnancy, when nutritional deficiency can lead to wasting, severe mental retardation and even death. Malnutrition must be recognized and assessed accurately, to enable decisions to be made about treatment and re-feeding methods. Assessment is divided into:

- Dietary history.
- Anthropometry.
- Physical examination.
- Laboratory tests.

Medical, social and dietary history

The main aspect of this is the dietary history, but often weight loss and poor nutrition are related to medical, psychological or financial factors (see Fig. 9.2).

Medical history

Ask specifically about:

- Loss of appetite.
- Weight loss or gain. The duration of weight change.
- Dysphagia, nausea, vomiting.
- Periods of weight loss and gain in the past; use of laxatives.
- Symptoms of hyperthyroidism: weight loss, increased appetite, irritability, preference for hot or cold temperature, and so on.
- Psychiatric history, especially if there is the possibility of depression or an eating disorder (e.g. anorexia nervosa).

Social history

In developed countries:

- Malnutrition may be related to the poor socio-economic status of a family.
- Enquire about housing, social support and income support.

In the UK, nutritional deficiency is particularly seen in:

- Elderly people ('tea and biscuit brigade') living alone who are unable to cook or shop.
- Young pregnant mothers who live off a staple diet of chips, pizzas and so on.
- Chronic alcoholics.

In developing countries, nutritional deficiency may be related to war, poor crops and the poor socio-economic status of the entire country.

Dietary history

Dietary recall
Ask specifically:

- What do you eat in a typical day?
- What do you like and dislike eating? (important in children).
- Access to food or presence of financial problems?
- Do you watch what you eat; are you on any particular diet?
- Ask specifically about alcohol intake.

Patients are often asked to keep a food diary. This is usually more accurate than simply questioning the patient, although it relies on the patient's compliance to fill the diary in, and also their willingness

The reason for weight loss or poor nutrition is often not as simple as 'not eating enough'. You must eliminate serious underlying illnesses such as cancer before you move on to diagnosis of psychiatric illness (depression or anorexia nervosa) or poor socio-economic status.

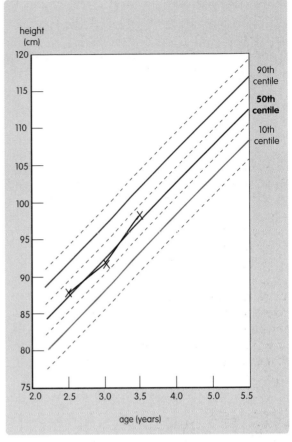

Fig. 11.13 Example of a growth chart often used to help in assessment of nutritional status in children. The line plotted here shows that the patient's height lies along the 50th centile, i.e. average height.

to provide accurate information (patients with eating disorders are not usually willing to do so).

Anthropometric measurements

The basic anthropometric measurements are:

- Height.
- Weight.
- Calculation of the body mass index (BMI): weight (kg)/height (m)^2.
- Mid-arm circumference: a measure of skeletal muscle mass (less frequently used).
- Skin-fold thickness. This helps to assess the amount of subcutaneous fat stores (needs to be done in a standardized way and is rarely used in routine assessments).

For infants, it is difficult to measure skin-fold thickness accurately and it is therefore of little value. The World Health Organization recommends that nutritional status is expressed as:

- % Weight/height: a measure of wasting as an index of acute malnutrition.
- % Height/age: a measure of growth retardation as an index of chronic malnutrition.

In infants, regular growth measurements are very valuable in assessing their nutritional status. Therefore, all infants have their height and weight plotted on a growth chart (Fig. 11.13), which allows a decrease in the rate of growth to be easily recognized and monitored as an early sign of malnutrition.

Physical clinical examination

Clinical signs

These can be a combination of any of the following:

- Wasting or cachexia.
- Pallor, which indicates anaemia, possibly caused by an iron, vitamin B_{12} or folate deficiency.
- Specific effects of vitamin deficiency; for example, deficiency of vitamin A causes Bitot's spots on the eyes, or deficiency of vitamin D and calcium causes rickets in children and osteomalacia in adults.
- Oedema.
- Bruising, for example in vitamin K deficiency.

Biochemical tests

The tests for individual nutrients, vitamins and minerals are dealt with in Chapter 8. Here, the types of tests which can be employed are considered.

Types of biochemical tests

Direct measurement

These are the measurements of the concentration of a nutrient or a metabolite in body fluid, usually in the serum or urine.

Such measurements may exploit the activation of an enzyme by a vitamin. For example, thiamine is a cofactor for erythrocyte transketolase. In thiamine deficiency, the erythrocyte enzyme activity can be measured before and after the addition of thiamine pyrophosphate (the active form of thiamine). Addition of thiamine pyrophosphate to erythrocytes should lead to an increase in enzyme activity, proving thiamine deficiency.

Measurement of stores

We measure storage forms of nutrients because:

- A decrease in the dietary intake of a nutrient leads to the mobilization of that nutrient from its stores to maintain a normal plasma concentration.
- Usually, only in severe deficiency does the plasma concentration drop significantly.
- In some cases, by measuring a decrease in the body stores we can detect a deficiency earlier.

For example, the best way to assess iron deficiency is to measure a decrease in bone marrow iron stores (serum ferritin reflects iron stores and is low in iron deficiency), and the best way to assess vitamin C deficiency is to measure a decrease in white cell vitamin C content (Fig. 11.14).

A plasma albumin of less than 30 g/L is often used as an index of malnutrition. However, albumin level is very much affected by fluid and electrolyte disorders, and in these patients, albumin is not an accurate index of nutritional status. The diagnosis of severe malnutrition is usually made on the basis of clinical assessment.

Parenteral nutrition

Nutritional support is provided for all patients who are severely malnourished or are unable to eat because of physical illness. Whenever possible, enteral nutrition is used, that is, via either a nasogastric tube, or a tube placed directly in the stomach (gastrostomy). Enteral nutrition is more natural, cheaper and far less hazardous in terms of the effects on fluid and electrolyte balance than parenteral nutrition. Enteral nutrition is always given in preference if the gastrointestinal tract is functional.

Fig. 11.14 Some biochemical tests for nutrients (FBC, full blood count; MCV, mean cell volume)

Nutrient	Tests
Protein	Serum protein, albumin, prealbumin
Fat	Total cholesterol and triglycerides
Carbohydrate	Blood glucose
Vitamin A	Plasma vitamin A, retinol binding protein
Vitamin D	↓ calcium, ↓ phosphate, ↑ alkaline phosphatase Measure vitamin D levels and parathyroid hormone
Vitamin K	↑ prothrombin time
Vitamin C	White cell vitamin C content (storage site)
B_1 (thiamine)	Erythrocyte thiamine
B_{12}	FBC, serum B_{12}, MCV
Folate	Serum and erythrocyte folate
Iron	FBC, ferritin, MCV etc., serum transferrin Best estimate is a fall in bone marrow iron stores

FBC, full blood count; MCV, mean cell volume

Indications for parenteral nutrition

Indicators for parental nutrition include:

- Intestinal failure, either as the result of surgery (gut resection) or because of a fistula or gastrointestinal tract obstruction by tumour.
- Patients with a very high energy requirement; that is, those in hypercatabolic state, for example severe trauma or burns patients and patients unable to eat.

Administration

Administration is usually via a central venous catheter into the superior vena cava, or sometimes into a peripheral vein. It involves the intravenous infusion of a mixture of high-concentration glucose, fat emulsion, amino acids, vitamins, electrolytes and trace elements.

Monitoring the patient

The most frequent complication of total parenteral nutrition (TPN) is infection of the line; therefore a meticulous aseptic technique is essential. Also, these patients require careful daily clinical monitoring to avoid complications:

- Fluid balance. The patient requires a daily fluid balance chart.
- Plasma electrolytes (sodium, potassium, chloride, bicarbonate, urea, creatinine) are monitored daily; glucose is checked even more often if required.
- Regular haematological measurements (full blood count and so on) are necessary, as is the monitoring of iron, vitamin B_{12} or folate deficiencies.
- In a patient with stable renal function, 24-h urinary urea excretion can provide an index of the body's protein status.
- Liver function tests are checked about three times a week.
- Vitamins and trace elements are periodically checked.

SELF-ASSESSMENT

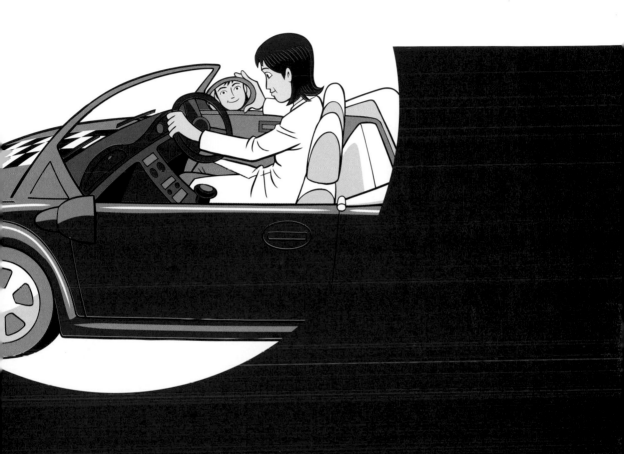

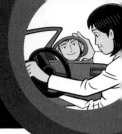

Indicate whether each answer is true or false.

Chapter 2 Carbohydrate and energy metabolism

1.   **In glycolysis:**
   a. Glucose can diffuse easily into the cells.
   b. There are three essentially irreversible reactions.
   c. The end product is lactate under anaerobic conditions.
   d. There is a net production of 12 molecules of ATP under aerobic conditions.
   e. 4 molecules of ATP are used in the production of glyceraldehyde-3-phosphate.

2.   **Pyruvate dehydrogenase:**
   a. Is inhibited by NAD^+.
   b. Is active when it is phosphorylated.
   c. Is inhibited when there is vitamin B_1 deficiency.
   d. Is regulated by PDH kinase and PDH phosphatase.
   e. Catalyses the production of acetyl CoA from glyceraldehyde-3-phosphate.

3.   **Fructose:**
   a. Requires the help of insulin to enter the cells.
   b. Is phosphorylated to fructose-6-phosphate in the liver by hexokinase.
   c. Is metabolized at the same rate as glucose.
   d. Errors in fructose metabolism are usually X-linked.
   e. Excess fructose ingestion leads to fatal lactic acidosis.

4.   **Regarding 2,3-BPG:**
   a. Concentration is decreased in patients who are long-term smokers.
   b. Blood transfusion helps increase the concentration of 2,3-BPG in patients.
   c. Fetal haemoglobin has a lower affinity for 2,3-BPG.
   d. It increases the affinity of adult haemoglobin for oxygen.
   e. Abnormality in 2,3-BPG results in haemolytic anaemia.

5.   **Regarding ethanol:**
   a. It can alter the metabolism of many drugs.
   b. Heavy drinking results in hyperglycaemia.
   c. Disulfiram is used as a treatment for alcoholics as it inhibits alcohol dehydrogenase.
   d. Metabolism of ethanol results in a high $NADH:NAD^+$ ratio.
   e. Is metabolized to acetaldehyde.

6.   **Glycogenolysis:**
   a. Occurs in the mitochondria.
   b. Glycogen phosphorylase cleaves the α-1,6 glycosidic link.
   c. Glycogen phosphorylase is inactivated when phosphorylated.
   d. Adrenaline and glucagon stimulates glycogenolysis.
   e. Calcium ions play a role in stimulating glycogenolysis.

7.   **Glycogen metabolism:**
   a. Occurs in cell cytosol.
   b. Glycogenesis does not require energy for its production.
   c. Is affected in von Gierke's disease.
   d. Adrenaline stimulates glycogen synthesis.
   e. Stores deplete over weeks.

8.   **The irreversible reactions controlling glycolysis are catalysed by:**
   a. Hexokinase.
   b. Glyceraldehyde-3-phosphate dehydrogenase.
   c. Pyruvate kinase.
   d. Phosphofructokinase-1.
   e. Phosphoglucose isomerase.

9.   **During ATP synthesis by the electron transport chain:**
   a. Protons are pumped into the mitochondrial matrix during electron transport.
   b. ATP is produced by the flow of protons through ATP synthase.
   c. Antimycin A blocks the proton channel of ATP synthase.
   d. Oxidation of NADH produces about 2.5 molecules of ATP.
   e. A low concentration of ADP stimulates ATP synthesis.

10. **The TCA cycle:**
   a. Occurs in red blood cells.
   b. The enzymes of the TCA cycle all occur in the mitochondrial matrix.
   c. Is an amphibolic pathway.
   d. Can occur in all conditions.
   e. Produces acetyl CoA as an end product.

11. **The following enzymes are inhibited by NADH:**
   a. Pyruvate dehydrogenase.
   b. Succinate dehydrogenase.
   c. Citrate synthase.

d. Isocitrate dehydrogenase.

e. α-Ketoglutarate dehydrogenase.

12. The reaction catalysed by phosphofructokinase-1 (PFK-1):

a. Is an example of an isomerization reaction.

b. Catalyses the phosphorylation of fructose-6-phoshate.

c. Is the rate-limiting reaction of the glycolytic pathway.

d. Is allosterically inhibited by fructose 2,6-bisphosphate.

e. Is allosterically inhibited by ATP and citrate.

13. Regarding glucose metabolism:

a. Under anaerobic conditions pyruvate is reduced to lactate, regenerating NAD^+.

b. The malate-aspartate shuttle has a role in the regeneration of NAD^+.

c. Net ATP yield from anaerobic glycolysis is 2 ATP.

d. Pyruvate kinase is regulated by reversible phosphorylation.

e. A deficiency of pyruvate kinase may result in haemolytic anaemia.

14. Conversion of pyruvate to acetyl CoA:

a. Is reversible.

b. Requires lipate as a cofactor.

c. Occurs in the cytosol.

d. Requires the coenzyme biotin.

e. Is inhibited in vitamin B_1 (thiamine) deficiency.

15. Acetyl CoA:

a. Serves as a donor of acetyl groups in fatty acid synthesis.

b. Cannot be formed from protein.

c. Is used to make cholesterol and ketone bodies.

d. Allosterically activates pyruvate dehydrogenase.

e. Is carboxylated by pyruvate carboxylase to form malonyl CoA.

16. α-Ketoglutarate dehydrogenase:

a. Catalyses the oxidative decarboxylation of citrate.

b. Requires thiamine pyrophosphate as a cofactor.

c. Is activated by ATP.

d. Results in the release of two molecules of CO_2.

e. Requires pyridoxal phosphate as a cofactor.

17. Oxidative phosphorylation:

a. Occurs in the inner mitochondrial space.

b. Involves the transfer of electrons from NADH or $FADH_2$ down a series of electron carriers to molecular oxygen.

c. The oxidation of NADH by the electron transport chain produces 1.5 ATP.

d. The oxidation of $FADH_2$ by the electron transport chain produces 1.5 ATP.

e. Is the process in which electron transport is coupled to the transport of protons across the inner mitochondrial membrane.

18. 2,4-Dinitrophenol:

a. Inhibits electron transport and ATP synthesis.

b. Allows electron transport to occur without ATP synthesis.

c. Inhibits electron transport without the impairment of ATP synthesis.

d. Specifically inhibits cytochrome *c*.

e. Is a competitive inhibitor of NAD^+-requiring reactions in mitochondria.

19. Gluconeogenesis:

a. Occurs exclusively in the cell cytosol.

b. Usually occurs in muscle.

c. Is important in maintaining blood glucose.

d. Is activated by fructose 2,6-bisphosphate.

e. Allows fatty acids to be converted into glucose in net amounts.

20. Glycogen:

a. Contains α-1,4 linkages that enable it to form branches.

b. Muscle glycogen is vital to the maintenance of the blood glucose concentration.

c. During fasting, liver glycogen stores last only between 12 and 24 hours.

d. Glucagon promotes glycogen breakdown in muscle.

e. Insulin promotes glycogen synthesis in both liver and muscle.

21. Glycogen storage disorders:

a. Are all inherited as autosomal dominant disorders.

b. Type I disorder is caused by a deficiency of glucose-6-phosphatase in the liver.

c. In McArdle's disease, patients tend to have an increased exercise tolerance.

d. Are only seen in boys.

e. In Pompe's disease, glycogen accumulates in lysosomes and is usually fatal before the age of 2 years.

22. Sorbitol:

a. Can be used as a sweetener in diabetic foods.

b. Is synthesized from glucose in the lens, kidney, liver and Schwann cells.

c. In the lens of the eye, sorbitol dehydrogenase oxidizes sorbitol to fructose.

d. May accumulate in diabetic patients and contribute to the formation of cataracts.

e. Is metabolized by the enzyme catalase in peroxisomes.

23. Galactosaemia:

a. Is always caused by a deficiency of galactose-1-phosphate uridyl transferase.

b. Can be caused by a deficiency of galactokinase.

c. Presents in adults.

d. Patients may become hypoglycaemic because galactose cannot be metabolized to glucose.

e. May result in cataract formation because of the high levels of glucose.

24. In the TCA cycle, the reaction catalysed by α-ketoglutarate dehydrogenase:
a. Is reversible.
b. Is inhibited by high levels of NADH.
c. Is an oxidative decarboxylation reaction.
d. Requires only NAD$^+$ as cofactor.
e. Is involved in the break-up of the oxaloacetate carrier.

25. During glycolysis, when glyceraldehyde-3-phosphate is oxidized using NAD$^+$ as a cofactor:
a. In liver, the NADH produced may be oxidized by the mitochondrial electron transport chain.
b. In erythrocytes, the NADH produced may be oxidized using pyruvate as electron acceptor.
c. Three molecules of NADH are generated per molecule of glucose oxidized.
d. One molecule of ATP will be generated in the next step of the reaction.
e. The reaction is irreversible.

26. Synthesis of glycogen in liver:
a. Is regulated primarily by substrate control.
b. Requires UTP as a key reactant.
c. Is activated by adrenaline.
d. Takes place in the cell cytosol.
e. Requires glucose as a source of monomeric units.

27. In the TCA cycle:
a. Four reactions produce NADH + H$^+$ from NAD$^+$.
b. Substrate-level phosphorylation of GDP to GTP occurs.
c. Four molecules of CO_2 are produced.
d. Four molecules of FADH$_2$ are produced.
e. Acetyl CoA can be provided by fatty acid breakdown.

28. Regarding the electron transport chain:
a. Increasing permeability of the inner mitochondrial membrane to protons increases ATP production.
b. Uncoupling occurs physiologically in brown adipose tissue.
c. Brown fat is found in abdominal fat of adults and the neck and upper back of babies.
d. Five protons need to pass through ATP synthase to make each molecule of ATP.
e. It is inhibited by a low concentration of ADP.

Chapter 3 Production of NADPH

29. The pentose phosphate pathway:
a. Is activated by a high NADPH:NADP$^+$ ratio.
b. Occurs in the cell cytosol.
c. Produces two molecules of ATP per molecule of glucose.
d. Produces one molecule of CO_2 per molecule of glucose.
e. Is regulated by the enzyme 6-phosphogluconate dehydrogenase.

30. Glucose-6-phosphate dehydrogenase deficiency:
a. Is an autosomal recessive disease.
b. Mainly affects Western European and North Americans.
c. Confers protection against malaria.
d. Results in haemolytic anaemia.
e. Can be precipitated by fava beans.

31. NADPH:
a. Is regenerated by the action of glutathione peroxidase.
b. Is used to inactivate reactive oxygen intermediates.
c. Is involved in the formation of glutathione.
d. Comes mainly from the pyruvate–malate cycle.
e. Excess NADPH causes haemolysis of RBCs.

32. Regarding the pentose phosphate pathway:
a. The net ATP yield from the pathway is 6 ATP.
b. It is located in mitochondria.
c. It generates reducing power as NADPH.
d. Glucose-6-phosphate dehydrogenase catalyses the rate-limiting step.
e. It produces five-carbon ribose sugars which can be used for nucleotide synthesis.

33. Which of the following is a function of NADPH?
a. Provides reducing power for lipid synthesis.
b. Regeneration of active glutathione.
c. Antioxidant.
d. Oxidized by the electron transport chain to make ATP.
e. May be generated during oxidative deamination of glutamate.

34. Pathways requiring NADPH include:
a. Gluconeogenesis.
b. Fatty acid synthesis.
c. Ketogenesis.
d. Cholesterol synthesis.
e. Tyrosine synthesis.

Chapter 4 Fatty acid metabolism and lipid transport

35. Lipoprotein lipase:
a. Is an intracellular enzyme.
b. Is stimulated by cAMP-mediated phosphorylation.
c. Mobilizes stored triacylglycerols from adipose tissues.
d. Produces free fatty acids and a monoacylglycerol.
e. Is stimulated by one of the apolipoproteins present in VLDL.

36. Cholesterol synthesis:
a. Occurs in erythrocytes.
b. Is regulated by its end product.

c. Takes place in the mitochondria.
d. Is limited by the rate-limiting step catalysed by the enzyme HMG-CoA synthase.
e. Requires ATP.

37. **β-Oxidation:**

a. Occurs in the cell cytosol.
b. Requires prior activation of fatty acids.
c. Requires NADH and $FADH_2$.
d. Is inhibited by malonyl CoA.
e. Is inhibited by adrenaline.

38. **Unsaturated fatty acids:**

a. Their synthesis occurs in the mitochondria.
b. Their synthesis involves an NADPH-dependent enzyme.
c. Possess double bonds of the *cis* configuration.
d. Are used to produce intracellular messengers.
e. Can produce double bonds at any position.

39. **Acetyl CoA carboxylase:**

a. Is activated by insulin.
b. Is activated by citrate.
c. Catalyses the production of malonyl-CoA for fatty acid biosynthesis.
d. Is located in the mitochondria of cells synthesizing fatty acids.
e. Catalyses a rate-controlling step in fatty acid biosynthesis.

40. **The following describes fatty acid synthesis:**

a. Oleate cannot be synthesized in the body.
b. *De novo* fatty acid synthesis occurs in mitochondria.
c. The ACP component of the fatty acid synthetase (FAS) multi-enzyme complex contains the B vitamin pantothenate.
d. Palmitate can be elongated to produce fatty acids with 18 or 20 carbons.
e. Arachidonic acid can be synthesized in the body provided we take linoleic acid in our diet.

41. **HMG-CoA reductase:**

a. Is the rate-limiting enzyme of cholesterol synthesis.
b. Is inhibited by cholesterol.
c. Is activated by reversible phosphorylation.
d. High intracellular levels of cholesterol cause repression of transcription of both HMG-CoA reductase and the LDL receptor gene.
e. Is inhibited by lovastatin.

42. **These facts about plasma lipoproteins are correct:**

a. They provide an efficient transport system for lipids.
b. Chylomicrons transport endogenously synthesized triacylglycerol and cholesterol from the liver to the tissues.
c. HDL particles are produced from LDL particles in the circulation by the action of lipoprotein lipase.

d. HDL removes 'used' cholesterol from tissues and takes it to the liver.
e. LDL formed in the circulation from VLDL binds to receptors on cells and is taken up by receptor-mediated endocytosis.

43. **Familial hypercholesterolaemia:**

a. Is inherited as an autosomal dominant disease.
b. Is caused by a deficiency of the enzyme lipoprotein lipase.
c. Homozygotes may exhibit tendon xanthomata, xanthelasma and arcus senilis.
d. Patients are able to metabolize chylomicrons normally.
e. Homozygotes are treated very effectively using fish oils.

44. **Ketone bodies are:**

a. Only produced in starvation or in poorly controlled diabetes.
b. Used by the brain in the fed state in preference to glucose.
c. Formed from acetyl CoA in mitochondria.
d. Not used as a fuel by the liver as it lacks 3-ketoacyl CoA transferase.
e. The principal fuel for erythrocytes.

45. **In the control of lipid metabolism:**

a. Fibrates inhibit HMG-CoA reductase.
b. Anion exchange resins bind bile acids in the gastrointestinal tract.
c. Increased lipoprotein lipase decreases plasma LDL levels.
d. Statins decrease plasma triacylglycerol.
e. Fish oil increases the concentration of unsaturated fatty acids.

46. **In which compartment of the liver cell are ketone bodies synthesized?**

a. Plasma membrane.
b. Cytosol.
c. Lysosome.
d. Mitochondria.
e. Endoplasmic reticulum.

47. **Regulation of fatty acid synthesis occurs at the enzymatic step catalysed by:**

a. Carnitine acyl transferase I.
b. Acetyl CoA carboxylase.
c. Pyruvate carboxylase.
d. Citrate synthase.
e. Pyruvate dehydrogenase.

48. **Ketone bodies:**

a. Are used by the liver to generate energy in the fasting state.
b. Are synthesized from proteins.
c. Produce a characteristic smell.
d. Are used in greater amounts by muscle after 2–3 weeks of starvation.
e. Are produced using the same isoenzyme of HMG-CoA used in cholesterol synthesis.

Chapter 5 Protein metabolism

49. The production of ammonia in the reaction catalysed by glutamate dehydrogenase:

a. Requires the participation of NADH.
b. May be reversed to consume ammonia if present in excess.
c. Is favoured by high levels of ATP.
d. Is inhibited when gluconeogenesis is active.
e. Produces α-ketoglutarate.

50. Aminotransferases:

a. Catalyse reactions that result in a net use or production of amino acids.
b. Catalyse irreversible reactions.
c. Require pyridoxal phosphate as a cofactor.
d. Only catalyse transamination reactions with essential amino acids.
e. Occur in the mitochondria and cytosol.

51. The following leads to a negative nitrogen balance:

a. Growth.
b. Malnutrition.
c. Pregnancy.
d. Starvation.
e. Cachexia.

52. The following are non-essential amino acids:

a. Phenylalanine.
b. Leucine.
c. Lysine.
d. Tyrosine.
e. Tryptophan.

53. Glutamate dehydrogenase:

a. Occurs in mitochondria.
b. Catalyses the removal of amino groups from most amino acids.
c. Uses either NAD^+ or $NADP^+$ as a cofactor.
d. Requires pyridoxal phosphate as a cofactor.
e. Is activated by ADP.

54. Protein degradation:

a. Can be influenced by the nature of the N-terminal amino acid.
b. Is rapid if the protein contains a [Pro-Glu-Ser-Thr] region.
c. For abnormal or cytosolic proteins, it occurs mainly in lysosomes.
d. Can be influenced by the attachment of ubiquitin to proteins.
e. Is regulated by the rate of the urea cycle.

55. The urea cycle:

a. Occurs mainly in liver hepatocytes.
b. All reactions occur in the cell cytosol.
c. Rate-limiting step is catalysed by a cytosolic enzyme, carbamoyl phosphate synthase II.
d. Net ATP consumption is 4 ATP.

e. The urea formed is insoluble and must be converted into uric acid for excretion.

56. Regarding amino acid disorders:

a. Phenylketonuria is always caused by a deficiency of the enzyme phenylalanine hydroxylase.
b. Alkaptonuria is usually caused by a deficiency of homogentisic acid oxidase.
c. Histidinaemia is usually caused by a deficiency of cystathionine synthetase.
d. In albinism, patients have low levels of pigment in the iris and retine and are prone to skin cancer.
e. The treatment of phenylketonuria involves life-long restriction of dietary phenylalanine.

57. Gluconeogenesis:

a. Occurs in muscle during exercise.
b. Occurs in the liver during exercise and fasting.
c. Occurs in adipose tissue during feeding.
d. Occurs in the kidney during periods of fasting.
e. Occurs in the brain during periods of fasting.

Chapter 6 Purines, pyrimidines and haem

58. 5,6,7,8-Tetrahydrofolate (THF):

a. Is reduced from folate by the action of dihydrofolate reductase.
b. Is a carrier of one-carbon units in purine synthesis.
c. Certain anti-cancer drugs inhibit its synthesis.
d. The methionine salvage pathway is essential for maintaining a continual supply of THF.
e. Folate deficiency can occur secondary to vitamin B_{12} deficiency.

59. Lesch–Nyhan syndrome:

a. Is caused by a deficiency of the salvage enzyme, adenine phosphoribosyl transferase (APRT).
b. Is often seen in girls.
c. Causes patients to develop severe mental retardation and to self-mutilate.
d. The salvage pathway for guanine and hypoxanthine is virtually inactive.
e. Increased levels of guanine and hypoxanthine result in hyperuricaemia and gout.

60. Gout:

a. Predominantly affects men.
b. May be caused by low levels of hypoxanthine-guanine-phosphoribosyl transferase (HGPRT).
c. Clinical features include recurrent, acute arthritic attacks, kidney stones and tophi.
d. Acute attacks are treated with xanthine oxidase inhibitors.
e. Is very effectively treated using aspirin.

61. **Concerning gout:**
    a. Gouty tophi are deposits of urate crystals in bone.
    b. Initially, gout is characterized by chronic swelling of a single joint.
    c. Gouty tophi cause yellow discoloration of overlying skin.
    d. Affected joints are tender.
    e. Renal colic is a recognized complication.

62. **Concerning porphyrias:**
    a. Neurological symptoms are rare in chronic attacks.
    b. Acute attacks commonly involve abdominal pain.
    c. Mid-stream urine sample would be useful in diagnosis.
    d. Are more common in Ashkenazi Jews.
    e. Acute attacks often come in quick succession.

63. **Haem:**
    a. Can reversibly bind O_2 for transport.
    b. Is produced mainly in erythrocytes.
    c. Synthesis is inhibited by lead.
    d. Breakdown occurs mainly in the kidneys.
    e. Phenytoin leads to a decrease in haem concentration.

64. **Gout:**
    a. Maybe caused by impaired excretion of uric acid by the kidneys.
    b. May result from a partial deficiency of hypoxanthine-guanine phosphoribosyltransferase (HGPRTase).
    c. May result from overproduction of 5-phosphoribosyl 1-pyrophosphate (PRPP).
    d. Can be treated with allopurinol.
    e. May occur in myeloproliferative disorders.

65. **The direct source of the sugar phosphate incorporated in the *de novo* synthesis of purine nucleotides is:**
    a. GMP.
    b. Ribulose-5-phosphate.
    c. UTP.
    d. Glucose-6-phosphate.
    e. 5-Phosphoribosyl 1-pyrophosphate (PRPP).

Chapter 7 Glucose homeostasis

66. **Type 1 diabetes:**
    a. Usually presents at old age.
    b. Is associated with HLA-DR4 antigens.
    c. Tends to occur in patients who are obese.
    d. Can be managed by changing the diet alone.
    e. Patients tend to develop ketoacidosis.

67. **Glucagon:**
    a. Inhibits glucose uptake in the peripheral tissues.
    b. Increases gluconeogenesis.
    c. Increases ketone body synthesis.
    d. Increases lipogenesis.
    e. Stimulates protein breakdown.

68. **The main metabolic effects found in diabetes mellitus are:**
    a. Hyperglycaemia.
    b. An increase in the rate of gluconeogenesis.
    c. A decrease in ketone body synthesis.
    d. Hypertriglyceridaemia.
    e. An increase in lipolysis.

69. **Concerning glucose homeostasis:**
    a. HBA_{1C} provides a good measure of average blood glucose concentration.
    b. The oral glucose tolerance test involves drinking 75 g of glucose in 250–300 mL of water.
    c. 7.9 mmol/L is a normal fasting glucose level according to the WHO criteria.
    d. Serum fructosamine provides a good measure of average blood glucose concentration.
    e. Impaired glucose tolerance is normally diagnosed by a random blood glucose.

70. **In the fasted state:**
    a. Uptake of glucose into muscle is insulin-dependent.
    b. The liver preferentially uses fatty acids for fuel.
    c. There is a high insulin to glucagon ratio.
    d. No food has been eaten for at least 3 hours.
    e. Noradrenaline activates hydrolysis of triacylglycerol stores.

Chapter 8 Nutrition

71. **Zinc:**
    a. Is a cofactor for the enzyme superoxide dismutase.
    b. Absorption is increased in the presence of vitamin C.
    c. Deficiency causes acrodermatitis enteropathica.
    d. Deficiency is often seen in patients on parenteral nutrition.
    e. Overload causes liver cirrhosis.

72. **Iron:**
    a. Its absorption is favoured in the ferrous state (Fe^{2+}).
    b. Is stored in the body as ferritin.
    c. Deficiency results in macrocytic anaemia.
    d. Overload can result in diabetes mellitus.
    e. Overload can be treated with penicillamine.

73. **Vitamin C:**
    a. Is a cofactor for proline and lysine hydroxylases involved in collagen synthesis.
    b. Is an antioxidant.
    c. Is a powerful oxidizing agent.
    d. Deficiency results in pellagra, characterized by swollen, sore gums and poor wound healing.
    e. Toxicity results in anaemia.

74. **Vitamin A:**
    a. Is a fat-soluble vitamin.
    b. Increases epithelial cell turnover.
    c. Deficiency results in impaired dark adaptation and night blindness.
    d. Can be used in the treatment of severe acne.
    e. Is safe to use in pregnancy, even in excess.

75. **Regarding niacin:**
    a. It can be synthesized from the amino acid tryptophan.
    b. Deficiency results in beriberi.
    c. The nutritional requirement for niacin is decreased when the diet contains large amounts of protein.
    d. The clinical features of niacin deficiency include dermatitis, diarrhoea and dementia.
    e. Nicotinic acid can be used in the treatment of hyperlipidaemia.

76. **Biotin:**
    a. Is synthesized by bacteria in the gut.
    b. Is the coenzyme for the aminotransferases.
    c. Deficiency can be induced by eating lots of raw egg whites.
    d. Deficiency results in night blindness.
    e. Deficiency may result in defective fatty acid synthesis.

77. **Vitamin B_{12}:**
    a. Is only found in food of animal origin.
    b. Is the cofactor for methylmalonyl CoA mutase, involved in the breakdown of odd-numbered fatty acids.
    c. Intrinsic factor released by gastric parietal cells is required for its absorption.
    d. The stores of vitamin B_{12} are very small.
    e. Deficiency results in both neurological symptoms and megaloblastic anaemia.

78. **Vitamin D:**
    a. Can be synthesized by the body in sufficient amounts.
    b. Active form is 25-hydroxycholecalciferol.
    c. Principal role is in calcium homeostasis.
    d. Is a recognized teratogen.
    e. Is an antioxidant.

79. **The following statements are correct:**
    a. A deficiency of vitamin A causes rickets in children.
    b. Vitamin B_{12}, C and E are all antioxidants.
    c. Vitamin A, D, E and C are all fat-soluble vitamins.
    d. A deficiency of vitamin B_{12} results in anaemia.
    e. Both vitamin K and vitamin B_{12} are synthesized by intestinal bacteria.

80. **Calcium:**
    a. Is the most abundant mineral in the human body.

    b. Deficiency can occur secondary to vitamin D deficiency.
    c. Deficiency in children causes rickets.
    d. Is inactive in its ionized form, Ca^{2+}.
    e. In overload, it is deposited in the eyes producing Kayser–Fleischer rings on the cornea.

81. **Kwashiorkor:**
    a. Is an example of protein-energy malnutrition.
    b. Is always caused by a lack of protein and energy.
    c. Is often seen in the UK.
    d. Children are usually oedematous with scaly skin.
    e. Usually occurs when a child is weaned from breastfeeding because of the arrival of a second child.

82. **Regarding the thyroid gland:**
    a. Iodine deficiency is now rare due to fortification of bread.
    b. Triiodothyronine production has a negative feedback effect on the hypothalamus and anterior pituitary.
    c. High TSH levels cause hyperplasia of thyroid epithelium.
    d. The Guthrie test is only used on babies born to hypothyroid mothers.
    e. The anterior pituitary produces thyroid-releasing hormones.

83. **Osteomalacia:**
    a. Bowed legs are a feature.
    b. Spontaneous fractures are a feature.
    c. Can be diagnosed by an increased alkaline phosphatase.
    d. Is common in childhood.
    e. Is commonly due to vitamin D deficiency.

84. **Pernicious anaemia:**
    a. Is the most common cause of vitamin B_{12} deficiency.
    b. Is an auto-immune disorder.
    c. Is diagnosed by an auto-antibody screen.
    d. Is treated by intramuscular injection of intrinsic factor.
    e. Is common in older men.

85. **Vitamin K:**
    a. Is a coenzyme for clotting factors III, V, IX and X.
    b. Needs to be taken in the diet regularly to avoid deficiency.
    c. Is given to children with intracranial haemorrhage.
    d. Deficiency will cause a decreased activated partial thromboplastin time (APTT).
    e. Is antagonized by oral anticoagulants such as warfarin.

86. **Obesity:**
    a. Can sometimes occur when energy intake is equal to energy expenditure.
    b. Is consistent with a body mass index of 20.

c. Is more common in low socio-economic class in the West.
d. Affects over 10% of women in the UK.
e. Is commonly overcome in the long term by dieting.

87. The following statements about vitamins are true:

a. Vitamin A, C and E are fat-soluble.
b. They are required in relatively small amounts.
c. Fat-soluble vitamins are stored in the liver.
d. The B-group vitamins are generally non-toxic in excess.
e. Vitamin K deficiency is relatively common.

88. Marasmus:

a. Is a protein and energy deficiency.
b. Has a high mortality rate.
c. Is characterized by a thin and emaciated appearance.
d. Often occurs in children at the age of 2 years.
e. Is treated first by correcting any infection, hypothermia or hypoglycaemia.

89. Obesity is associated with:

a. Osteoarthritis.
b. Fatty liver.
c. Gallstones.
d. Diabetes requiring treatment with insulin.
e. The development of respiratory problems.

90. Coeliac disease:

a. Can result in calcium deficiency.
b. May cause haematuria.
c. May be accompanied by normocytic anaemia.
d. Is commonly associated with weight loss.
e. Sometimes causes vitamin A deficiency.

91. Rickets:

a. Is associated with mental retardation and seizures.
b. Causes increased bone formation.
c. Results in defective mineralization of the long bones visible on X-ray.
d. Commonly develops in the elderly.
e. Is characterized by delayed dentition.

92. Regarding copper overload:

a. It is a common clinical problem in the UK.
b. A 2-month course of chelation therapy normally resolves the problem.
c. Any liver damage is irreversible.
d. It is the result of a chromosome defect.
e. The liver fails to excrete copper into the bile.

93. Wernicke-Korsakoff syndrome:

a. Is due to dietary deficiency of folic acid.
b. Causes ataxia.
c. Can lead to short-term memory loss.

d. Is seen in chronic alcholics.
e. Is irreversible.

94. In the intestine:

a. Of neonates, there are no bacteria.
b. Iron is absorbed in the ferrous (Fe^{2+}) form.
c. Fat-soluble vitamins are absorbed along with glucose.
d. Transferrin is involved in controlling iron absorption.
e. Vitamin B_{12} absorption requires ascorbic acid.

Chapter 10 History and examination

95. Tremor:

a. May be associated with hypothyroidism.
b. In Wernicke-Korsakoff syndrome will be an essential tremor.
c. Can be caused by exercise.
d. Of the flapping type is observed with outstretched arms and hands flat.
e. Can be caused by hypoglycaemia.

96. Clubbing:

a. Is caused by iron-deficiency anaemia.
b. Is defined as increased angle between the nail and nail bed.
c. Can cause underlying nail fluctuance.
d. Is a feature of cirrhosis.
e. Is commonly seen as a result of glycogen storage disorder.

97. Regarding anaemia:

a. Iron deficiency will cause a decrease in haem and erythrocyte production.
b. Macrocytic anaemia may be caused by a deficiency of erythrocyte enzymes.
c. Pernicious anaemia is an auto-immune condition causing an overload of B_{12} and folate.
d. Lead poisoning inhibits three enzymes of haem synthesis, leading to anaemia.
e. Sickle cell anaemia is a hereditary haemolytic anaemia.

Chapter 11 Further investigations

98. Regarding urea and electrolytes:

a. Creatinine is low in renal disease.
b. High serum sodium concentration indicates dehydration.
c. In renal failure, serum potassium is low.
d. Creatinine can be raised in healthy athletes.
e. Liver cirrhosis causes a high serum sodium.

99. **Regarding haematological investigations:**
   a. A haemoglobin of 12 g/dL is normal in women.
   b. A red cell count of 8×10^{12}/L is consistent with polycythaemia.
   c. A prothrombin time of 25 seconds is normal.
   d. Mean cell haemoglobin is low in folate deficiency.
   e. Microcytic, hypochromic blood film is consistent with iron deficiency.

100. **Parenteral nutrition:**
   a. Is used in preference to enteral nutrition.
   b. Is indicated when a patient is eating less than 70% of their recommended daily intake.
   c. Is often complicated by infection.
   d. Can be complicated by hyperglycaemia.
   e. Is most often given through a central venous catheter into the superior vena cave.

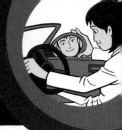

Short-answer questions (SAQs)

1. Compare and contrast fuel metabolism in skeletal muscle during:
   a. a 100 metre sprint.
   b. a marathon.

2. Describe the connection between the urea cycle and the tricarboxylic cycle.

3. NADH formed in glycolysis must be re-oxidized to NAD^+ for glycolysis to continue. Give two examples of how NAD^+ is regenerated.

4. Answer the following questions about the conversion of pyruvate to acetyl CoA.
   a. Name the enzyme that catalyses this reaction and three cofactors that it requires.
   b. What type of reaction is involved?
   c. Where in the cell does this occur?
   d. What product other than acetyl CoA is formed?
   e. What is the significance of this reaction to carbohydrate and fat metabolism?

5. What is the main difference between the action of an inhibitor and that of an uncoupler on the electron transport chain? Give a named example of each.

6. Look at the reaction shown in Fig. 1.
   a. Name substrate A and product B.
   b. Where in the cell does this reaction occur?
   c. What enzyme catalyses this reaction?
   d. Name an important cofactor of this enzyme.
   e. Name one activator and one inhibitor of this reaction.

7. Discuss the pathogenesis of familial hypercholesterolaemia.

8. What is the effect of lead on haem synthesis and what treatments are available for lead poisoning?

9. Explain how the hormone glucagon activates glycogen breakdown in the liver.

10. Briefly explain why a patient might be jaundiced, using your knowledge on bilirubin metabolism.

11. What are the main fuels that supply blood glucose during the fed state, fasted state and early and late starvation? Give an approximate time period for each state.

12. Discuss the vitamin K deficiency in newborn babies. How is it prevented?

13. What is the main function of vitamin B_1? Explain why its deficiency results in neurological disorders.

14. Give examples of the role of vitamins in:
    a. carbohydrate metabolism.
    b. amino acid metabolism.

15. A 50-year-old man is admitted to A&E with central crushing chest pain. After appropriate resuscitation, you take a full history and examination.
    a. What risk factors is it important to assess?
    b. His cholesterol level is 15 mmol/L. What action should be taken to modify this risk factor?
    c. You notice xanthelasma around his eyes. What information is it important to elicit from the history?
    d. He is prescribed simvastatin. What type of drug is this, and what is its mechanism of action?

16. A 45-year-old male New Zealander presents to your GP surgery with an acutely swollen toe. There is no previous history of trauma. He is apyrexial. He remembers his father having a similar problem but he has not been in contact with his family for several years.
    a. What is the most likely diagnosis and what is the mechanism of action of the disease?
    b. What modifiable risk factors would you enquire about?

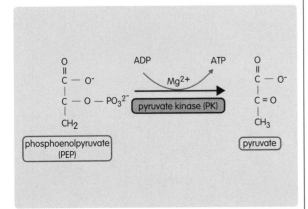

Fig. 1

233

c. What other steps would you take in addition to modifying these risk factors?

d. Three months later, he has modified some of the risk factors and has had one more attack from which he has now recovered. He is prescribed allopurinol. What is the mechanism of action of this drug?

---

17. A previously well, 17-year-old girl presents to A&E with acute onset of hyperventilation with polyuria and polydipsia. Although drowsy, she is able to give a history and you discover she has also lost a kilogram in weight in the past 3 weeks. There is no significant previous medical history. A BM test in casualty shows a blood glucose of 37 mmol/L.

a. What is the most likely diagnosis and by what mechanism does it cause these acute symptoms?

b. Under your care, she recovers from the acute illness. What long-term treatments is she likely to require?

---

18. A 17-year-old vegetarian girl presents to a GP surgery complaining of tiredness and malaise for the past 6 months. After a history and examination, you take some blood for routine tests. Haemoglobin comes back from the lab as 10 g/dL, and the blood film shows a microcytic, hypochromic anaemia.

a. What is the most likely cause of this anaemia?

b. What are the possible precipitants at this stage?

c. On further questioning it is revealed that she was diagnosed with ulcerative colitis aged 12. How will this affect management?

---

19. During your elective, you work in a clinic in Somalia. A 4-year-old boy is brought to see you in the GP clinic. His parents are concerned as he seems to be fitting. You resuscitate him and take a full history. His parents report that he does not seem to be growing as quickly as the other boys. On examination he has bowed legs, and has prominent swelling at the costochondral junctions.

a. What is the most likely diagnosis?

b. How would you confirm the diagnosis?

c. How does the presentation of this metabolic problem differ in adults?

---

20. A 37-year-old female refugee presents with a lump in her neck. She has recently given birth to a son.

a. How would you assess the lump?

b. In the part of the mountainous part of the developing world where she is from, such a lump in the neck is normal. What is the possible metabolic diagnosis?

c. Is there any risk to her baby?

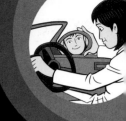

Extended-matching questions (EMQs)

For each scenario described below, choose the single most likely option from the list of options.
Each option may be used once, more than once or not at all.

1. Clinical aspects of diabetes

A. Antibiotics administration
B. Autoimmune disease with peak age of onset at 15–20 years
C. Diet and weight reduction
D. Disease caused by a single gene defect
E. Disease more common in Mediterranean than Caucasian populations
F. Disease with typical age of onset from 60 years onwards
G. Hypoglycaemia
H. Hyperglycaemia
I. Inhalation of insulin preparations
J. Injection of insulin preparations
K. Measurement of glycosylated haemoglobin
L. Random blood glucose test

For each of the following, select the SINGLE most appropriate option from the above list.

1. The onset of Type 1 diabetes.
2. The most common effective treatment of Type 1 diabetes.
3. The initial treatment of most patients with Type 2 diabetes.
4. Diabetic patient presenting with sweating, nausea, confusion and coma.
5. Method for measuring blood glucose control in the past month.

2. Metabolic transformation

A. Beta-oxidation of fatty acids
B. Cholesterol synthesis
C. Fatty acid synthesis
D. Gluconeogenesis
E. Glycogen breakdown
F. Glycogen synthesis
G. Glycolysis
H. Ketone body synthesis
I. Lipolysis
J. Lipoprotein formation
K. Transamination
L. Urea cycle

For each of the following, select ONE corresponding metabolic process from the above list.

1. The synthesis of malonyl-CoA.
2. The transfer of a carbamoyl group to ornithine.
3. The synthesis of glutamate.
4. A six-carbon sugar is broken down into two three-carbon molecules.
5. The addition of acetyl CoA to acetoacetyl CoA to form HMG-CoA.

3. Control of carbohydrate and lipid metabolism

A. Acetyl-CoA carboxylase
B. Citrate synthase
C. Fatty acid synthase
D. Fructose 1,6-bisphosphatase
E. Glucokinase
F. Glucose transporter 4 (GLUT4)
G. Glycogen phosphorylase kinase
H. Glycogen synthase
I. Hexokinase
J. Lactate dehydrogenase
K. Phosphofructokinase
L. Pyruvate kinase

For each of the following, select ONE enzyme or transporter from the above list.

1. Enzyme that is present in the liver and β cells of the pancreas, and has a low affinity for glucose.
2. Enzyme whose activity is increased during gluconeogenesis as a result of a fall in the concentration of a potent inhibitor in response to glucagon action.
3. Enzyme required for fatty acid synthesis that is activated by insulin and inhibited by glucagon.
4. Recruited to the cell membrane following insulin stimulation.
5. A multi-enzyme complex containing an acyl carrier protein.

4. Inadequate or excessive micronutrient intake

A. Calcium
B. Copper
C. Folic acid
D. Iron
E. Pyridoxal phosphate (B_6)
F. Riboflavin
G. Thiamine
H. Vitamin A
I. Vitamin C
J. Vitamin D
K. Vitamin E
L. Vitamin K

For each of the following, select the SINGLE most appropriate vitamin or mineral from the above list.

1. Lack of this substance may cause rickets.
2. Beri-beri may result from insufficient intake of this substance.
3. Deficiency in childhood causes xerophthalmia.
4. Lack of this substance causes macrocytic anaemia.
5. May contribute to osteoporosis in post-menopausal women.

5. Liver and alcohol abuse

A. Albumin
B. Alcohol
C. Bile salts
D. Bilirubin
E. Cholesterol
F. Disulfiram
G. γ-Glutamyl transferase
H. Thiamine
I. Urea
J. Vitamin A
K. Vitamin E
L. Vitamin K

For each of the following, select the SINGLE most appropriate response from the above list.

1. Jaundice arises from increased deposition of this in tissues.
2. Wernicke–Korsakoff syndrome can arise in alcoholics as a result of deficiency in this.
3. Increased risk of bruising and bleeding in alcoholics is due to deficiency in this.
4. Oedema can arise from severely depleted circulating levels of this.

5. This compound has been shown to have a beneficial effect on heart attacks and strokes when ingested in moderate amounts.

6. Locations of metabolic processes in organs and tissues

A. Adipose tissue
B. Bone marrow
C. Brain
D. Erythrocytes
E. Heart muscle
F. Intestine
G. Liver
H. Lungs
I. Lymph
J. Mitochondria
K. Pancreas
L. Skeletal muscle

For each of the following, select ONE location from the above list.

1. The release of fatty acids during fasting.
2. The synthesis of chylomicrons following ingestion of a high-fat meal.
3. The synthesis of urea.
4. Modification of glycolysis by the bisphosphoglycerate shunt.
5. The synthesis of ketone bodies from acetyl CoA.

7. Causes of anaemia

A. Anaemia of chronic disease
B. Autoimmune haemolytic anaemia
C. Coeliac disease
D. Glucose-6-phosphate dehydrogenase deficiency
E. Hypothyroidism
F. Iron deficiency
G. Multiple myeloma
H. Pernicious anaemia
I. Sickle-cell anaemia
J. Sideroblastic anaemia
K. Thalassaemia
L. Vitamin B_{12} deficiency

For each of the following, choose ONE option from the list above.

1. A 10-year-old boy presents with painful joints in the hands and feet, jaundice and anaemia. He also has splenomegaly and his blood film shows target cells.

2. A 50-year-old man presents with macrocytic anaemia. He drinks alcohol regularly.

3. A 25-year-old Greek lady presents with anaemia and jaundice following anti-malarial treatment. She is noted to have Heinz bodies.

4. A 10-month-old baby presents with anaemia and failure to thrive. His blood film shows target cells, hypochromic and microcytic cells. HbF is still present.

5. A 40-year-old woman presents with lethargy and a sore red tongue. Her blood film shows hypersegmented polymorphs, an MCV > 110 fL and a low haemoglobin.

8. Nutritional deficiencies

A. Copper
B. Folic acid
C. Nicotinic acid
D. Pyridoxine
E. Selenium
F. Thiamine
G. Vitamin A
H. Vitamin B_{12}
I. Vitamin C
J. Vitamin D
K. Vitamin K
L. Zinc

For the following, select the MOST likely cause of nutritional deficiency from the above list.

1. A 15-year-old girl complains of not being able to see very well at night.

2. A 45-year-old man with poor diet complains that his gums are bleeding easily.

3. A 30-year-old man presents with nystagmus, opthalmoplegia and ataxia. He is known to drink at least 40 units of alcohol a week.

4. A 20-year-old woman with chronic diarrhoea complains of prolonged bleeding after a small cut to her index finger. The prothrombin time is increased.

5. A 25-year-old man was recently on anti-TB treatment and now presents with dermatitis, diarrhoea and depression.

9. Clinical Investigations

A. Chest X-ray
B. CT scan
C. Direct Coombs' test
D. Fasting blood glucose
E. Glycosylated haemoglobin
F. Guthrie test
G. Lipid profile
H. Liver biopsy
I. Oral glucose tolerance test
J. Schilling test
K. Serum iron
L. Uric acid

For the following statements, choose ONE clinical investigation from the above list.

1. The doctor suspects that the patient has been misleading him regarding the control of her blood glucose levels.

2. The patient, a teetotal, has macrocytic anaemia, despite eating a healthy and sensible diet.

3. The newborn baby had a blood sample taken from a heel-prick around 7 days after birth.

4. The patient is known to have a family history of coronary heart disease.

5. The patient complains of a painful and swollen big toe, following a heavy protein meal.

10. Disorders of metabolism

A. Albinism
B. Alkaptonuria
C. Glucose-6-phosphate dehydrogenase deficiency
D. Histidinaemia
E. Homocystinuria
F. Lesch–Nyhan syndrome
G. Maple syrup urine disease
H. Menkes' kinky hair syndrome
I. Phenylketonuria
J. Porphyria
K. Sickle cell anaemia
L. Wilson's disease

For the following statements, choose ONE disorder from the above list.

1. A 6-month-old baby presents with seizures and failure to thrive. His parents are advised to follow a food restriction diet.

2. The patient presents with painful joints and complains that his urine turns black on standing.

3. The patient presents with whitish hair, grey-blue eyes and pale skin. He is advised to use high sun protection when going out.

4. A 1-month-old baby presents with metabolic acidosis, hypoglycaemia and seizures. His parents complain that his urine smells sweet.

5. A 4-month-old baby presents with self-mutilation, spasticity and kidney stones. His parents complain of an 'orange' nappy.

237

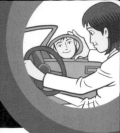

MCQ answers

Chapter 2 Carbohydrate and energy metabolism

1.
   a. False   Glucose requires the help of glucose transporters or sodium-glucose transporters to enter the cell.
   b. True   The three irreversible reactions involved are hexokinase, phosphofructokinase-1 and pyruvate kinase.
   c. True   Under anaerobic conditions, pyruvate is reduced to lactate.
   d. False   The net yield of aerobic glycolysis is 7ATP.
   e. False   Only 2 molecules of ATP are used to produce glyceraldehyde-3-phosphate.

2.
   a. False   Pyruvate dehydrogenase is inhibited by NADH (product inhibition).
   b. False   It is inactive in the phosphorylated form.
   c. True   Vitamin B$_1$ is needed for the coenzyme thiamine pyrophosphate.
   d. True   Pyruvate dehydrogenase is under the regulation of PDH kinase and PDH phosphatase.
   e. False   It catalyses the production of acetyl CoA from pyruvate.

3.
   a. False   Fructose can enter the cell without the help of insulin using GLUT-5 transporters.
   b. False   Fructose is phosphorylated to fructose-6-phosphate in the muscle.
   c. False   Is metabolized at a faster rate than glucose.
   d. False   Errors in fructose metabolism are usually autosomal recessive.
   e. True   Excess fructose ingestion depletes phosphate stores, which limits ATP production, thus activating glycolysis and production of lactic acid.

4.
   a. False   Concentration is increased to compensate for the decreased oxygen supply caused by carbon monoxide exposure.
   b. False   Transfused blood has a lower concentration of 2,3-BPG due to its storage in an acid-citrate medium.
   c. True   This helps to increase the affinity of fetal haemoglobin for oxygen to enable placental oxygen exchange from the mother's circulation.
   d. False   2,3-BPG decreases the affinity of haemoglobin for oxygen.
   e. True   Abnormal 2,3-BPG alters the ability of haemoglobin to transport oxygen, resulting in poor ATP production and haemolysis of red cells.

5.
   a. True   Ethanol induces cytochrome P450 enzyme which metabolizes many drugs.
   b. False   Heavy drinking inhibits gluconeogenesis which results in hypoglycaemia.
   c. False   Disulfiram inhibits aldehyde dehydrogenase, resulting in the side effects of nausea and flushing.
   d. True   Alcohol dehydrogenase and aldehyde dehydrogenase consumes NAD$^+$, resulting in high NADH:NAD$^+$ ratio.
   e. True   Which then enters the mitochondria for further oxidation into acetate.

6.
   a. False   It occurs in the cell cytosol.
   b. False   Glycogen phosphorylase cleaves the α-1,4 glycosidic link to release glucose-1-phosphate.
   c. False   Glycogen phosphoryalse is activated when phosphorylated by phosphorylase kinase.
   d. True   Adrenaline and glucagon activate protein kinase A which causes phosphorylation of glycogen phosphorylase.
   e. True   Calcium ions bind to calmodulin, a subunit of phosphorylase b, thus activating it.

7.
   a. True   Glycogen synthesis and degradation occurs in the cell cytosol.
   b. False   Production of glycogen requires energy from the hydrolysis of pyrophosphate.
   c. True   von Gierke's disease is caused by a deficiency of glucose-6-phosphatase, which normally hydrolyses glucose-6-phosphate.
   d. False   Adrenaline inhibits glycogen synthesis by activating protein kinase A which phosphorylates glycogen synthase, thus inactivating it.
   e. False   Occurs rapidly when the need arises to provide energy immediately.

8.
   a. True   Hexokinase irreversibly phosphorylates glucose to glucose-1-phosphate.

b. False   Glyceraldehyde-3-phosphate dehydrogenase catalyses an oxidative phosphorylation reaction.

c. True   Pyruvate kinase catalyses an irreversible substrate-level phosphorylation.

d. True   Phosphofructokinase catalyses an irreversible phosphorylation reaction.

e. False   Phosphoglucose isomerase catalyses an isomerization reaction.

9.
a. False   Electron transport is coupled to pumping of protons across the inner mitochondrial membrane into the intermembrane space.

b. True   Protons re-enter the mitochondrial matrix through the F_0 channel of ATP synthase thus producing ATP.

c. False   Antimycin A inhibits electron transfer in complex III.

d. True   Transport of NADH down the electron transport chain produces about 2.5 molecules of ATP.

e. False   ADP as a substrate is needed for ATP synthesis, thus low ADP concentration decreases ATP production.

10.
a. False   The TCA cycle occurs in the mitochondria, which red blood cells do not have.

b. False   Succinate dehydrogenase occurs on the inner face of the inner mitochondrial membrane.

c. True   It operates both catabolically and anabolically.

d. False   Only occurs in aerobic conditions.

e. False   It oxidizes acetyl CoA completely to two molecules of CO_2 releasing energy.

11.
a. True   NADH competes with NAD^+ for binding sites on pyruvate dehydrogenase.

b. False   Not inhibited by NADH.

c. True   Inhibited by NADH.

d. True   Inhibited by NADH.

e. True   Inhibited by NADH.

12.
a. False   It is a phosphorylation reaction.

b. True   It is converted to fructose 1,6-bisphosphate, a reaction unique to glycolysis.

c. True   The reaction is rate limiting in glycolysis.

d. False   Fructose 2,6-bisphosphate increases the affinity of PFK-1 for its substrate, fructose-6-phosphate, and it relieves inhibition of PFK-1 by ATP.

e. True   ATP lowers the affinity of PFK-1 for its substrate fructose-6-phosphate. Citrate enhances this effect.

13.
a. True   This is a reversible reaction determined by the ratio of NADH to NAD^+.

b. True   By transporting electrons from NADH into mitochondria for ATP regeneration by the electron transport chain.

c. True   Aerobic glycolysis yields 7 ATP.

d. True   It is also regulated by allosteric control.

e. True   Glucose-6-phosphate dehydrogenase deficiency can also cause haemolytic anaemia.

14.
a. False   The reaction is completely irreversible.

b. True   Four of the five coenzymes are vitamin B derivatives.

c. False   It occurs on the inner face of the inner mitochondrial membrane.

d. False   Biotin is a coenzyme for carboxylation reactions.

e. True   This state leads to a deficiency of the coenzyme thiamine pyrophosphate.

15.
a. True   Fatty acids and cholesterol are made from acetyl CoA in the cytosol.

b. False   Deamination and oxidation reactions can create acetyl CoA from protein.

c. True   It is also involved in steroid synthesis and is oxidized within the TCA cycle.

d. False   Acetyl CoA specifically inhibits the E2 binding site of PDH complex. This enzyme catalyses the conversion of pyruvate to acetyl CoA.

e. False   Pyruvate is carboxylated by pyruvate carboxylase to form oxaloacetate.

16.
a. False   Converts α-ketoglutarate to succinyl CoA.

b. True   It also requires FAD, lipoic acid, NAD^+ and CoA.

c. False   It is inhibited by ATP, NADH and by its products succinyl CoA and GTP.

d. False   Build up in the blood may lead to lactic acidosis.

e. False   All three regulatory enzymes in the TCA require Ca^{2+} as a cofactor.

17.
a. False   Oxidative phosphorylation occurs on the inner surface of the inner mitochondrial membrane.

b. True   This results in the formation of ATP.

c. False   Oxidation of NADH in the electron transport chain generates 2.5 ATP.

d. True $FADH_2$ oxidation bypasses the first site of proton pumping across the mitochondrial membrane.

e. True   Electron carrying groups within the four protein complexes involved include flavins, iron-sulphur proteins, haem groups and copper ions.

18. a. False Electron transport is uncoupled from ATP synthesis, so that ATP generation decreases with no effect on the electron transport chain.

b. True This is due to decreased flow of protons through ATP synthase.

c. False There is no ATP production.

d. False 2,4-DNP does not inhibit cytochrome c.

e. False NADH-requiring reactions will be inhibited.

19. a. False The first step (carboxylation of pyruvate) occurs in the mitochondria.

b. False Occurs in the liver.

c. True Ketone bodies are also produced in the liver in the early starved state.

d. False Fructose 1,6-bisphosphate is converted to fructose-6-phosphate during gluconeogenesis.

e. False Fat cannot be converted into glucose.

20. a. False α-1,6 linkages occur, enabling branch formation.

b. False Muscle cannot release glucose into blood.

c. True For this period, the stores provide oxygen for the brain.

d. False Glucagon only increases glycogen breakdown in the liver. Noradrenaline and adrenaline also increase breakdown in muscle.

e. True Insulin increases glucose uptake into muscle and activates glucokinase, which phosphorylates glucose, allowing synthesis of liver glycogen.

21. a. False They are mostly autosomal recessive disorders.

b. True Both liver and kidneys become loaded with glycogen, resulting in hypoglycaemia.

c. False They have diminished exercise tolerance.

d. False They are all autosomal recessive disorders, except VIII which is sex-linked.

e. True The accumulation of glycogen in lysosomes of all cells is usually fatal before the age of 2 years.

22. a. True It is safe as it is absorbed slowly from the intestine and also transported slowly across cell membranes.

b. True Via the enzyme aldose reductase.

c. False The lens and retina of the eye and Schwann cells can synthesize but not break down sorbitol.

d. True The strong osmotic effect causes water retention, leading to lens swelling and opacification.

e. False It is metabolized by sorbitol dehydrogenase in liver, sperm and ovaries.

23. a. False Occasionally, it is caused by deficiency in galactokinase or UDP-hexose-4-epimerase.

b. True See (a).

c. False The disease presents in neonates when lactose-containing milk feeds are introduced.

d. True Other features are poor feeding, vomiting, jaundice and hepatosplenomegaly.

e. True Also liver failure and severe mental retardation if left untreated.

24. a. False It is an irreversible rate-limiting step.

b. True NADH is produced from NAD^+ and can inhibit further production of itself allosterically.

c. True The number of carbon atoms decreases from five to four.

d. False It requires thiamine pyrophosphate (TPP), FAD, lipoic acid, NAD^+ and CoA.

e. True Between isocitrate and succinate.

25. a. True This will yield about 2.5 ATP.

b. True Under anaerobic conditions, pyruvate is reduced to lactate by lactate dehydrogenase with the simultaneous oxidation of NADH to NAD^+.

c. False Two molecules of NADH are generated per molecule.

d. True By phosphoglycerate kinase.

e. False It is a reversible reaction.

26. a. False Hormonal regulation and allosteric control are the chief mechanisms involved.

b. False Requires uridine diphosphate (UDP)-glucose pyrophosphorylase.

c. False Glucagon and adrenaline activate glycogen degradation.

d. True Synthesis does occur in the cytosol.

e. True The glucose donor UDP-glucose is essential.

27. a. False Three reactions produce $NADH + H^+$ from NAD^+.

b. True Via succinyl coenzyme A synthetase.

c. False Two molecules of CO_2 are produced at the first two steps of NADH production.

d. False Oxidation of succinate to fumarate uses FAD as an electron acceptor as the power of succinate is not sufficient to reduce NAD⁺.

e. True   Fatty acids are degraded by sequential removal of two carbon units, producing acetyl CoA.

28. a. False   Any substance with this action will allow proteins to re-enter the matrix at sites other than ATP synthase, causing uncoupling.

b. True   Brown fat contains the uncoupling protein thermogenin.

c. False   Brown fat is unique to babies and hibernating mammals.

d. False   Approximately three protons are required to make each ATP.

e. True   A reduced supply of substrate will result in decreased production of ATP.

Chapter 3 Production of NADPH

29. a. False   It is activated by a low NADPH:NADP⁺ ratio.

b. True   It occurs in the cell cytosol.

c. False   There is no net production of ATP.

d. True   One molecule of CO_2 is produced per molecule of glucose.

e. False   It is regulated by the enzyme glucose-6-phosphate dehydrogenase.

30. a. False   It is a sex-linked disease, affecting males and being carried by females.

b. False   It mainly affects South East Asia and the Mediterranean.

c. True   Heterozygotes have some protection against malaria.

d. True   Haemolytic anaemia occurs during an acute crisis.

e. True   Favism leads to haemolysis.

31. a. False   GSH is regenerated by the action of glutathione reductase.

b. True   NADPH plays an important role in detoxifying reactive oxygen intermediates.

c. True   NADPH reduces oxidized glutathione into the active reduced glutathione.

d. False   NADPH mainly comes from the pentose phosphate pathway.

e. False   NADPH helps to protect erythrocytes from excess free radicals, thus preventing haemolysis.

32. a. False   There is no net ATP generation, but there is production of NADPH to provide reducing power.

b. False   It occurs in the cell cytosol.

c. True   NADPH is a high-energy molecule which can be used for reductive synthetic reactions.

d. True   This reaction also produces one molecule of NADPH.

e. True   In erythrocytes, NADPH is used to regenerate the reduced form of the antioxidant glutathione.

33. a. True   Each cycle of lipid synthesis requires NADPH as a cofactor.

b. True   The reduced form is regenerated via glutathione reductase, which requires NADPH.

c. False   High NADPH levels ensure high activity of glutathione reductase. This provides reduced (active) glutathione which is an antioxidant.

d. False   NADPH has no role in oxidative phosphorylation.

e. True   This provides α-ketoglutarate for the TCA cycle to provide energy.

34. a. False   Gluconeogenesis does not require NADPH.

b. True   Its electrons are used for reductive biosynthesis in lipid synthesis.

c. False   Ketone body synthesis does not require NADPH.

d. True   Reduction of HMG-CoA to mevalonic acid requires NADPH as a reducing agent.

e. False   This is formed by the hydroxylation of the essential amino acid phenylalanine.

Chapter 4 Fatty acid metabolism and lipid transport

35. a. False   It is an extracellular enzyme.

b. False   It is activated by apolipoprotein C-II.

c. False   It acts on chylomicrons and VLDL to remove triacylglycerols.

d. False   It produces free fatty acids and glycerol.

e. True   It is activated by apolipoprotein C-II on the surface of VLDL.

36. a. False   It does not occur in erythrocytes.

b. True   The product cholesterol causes product inhibition.

c. False   It occurs in the cell cytosol.

d. False   The rate limiting step is catalysed by HMG-CoA reductase.

e. True   It uses ATP.

37.
a. False   It occurs in the mitochondrial matrix.
b. True   Activation of fatty acids occurs in the cytosol.
c. False   It requires NAD^+ and FAD.
d. True   Malonyl CoA inhibits carnitine acyl transferase I (CAT I), thus inhibiting acyl groups entry into the mitochondria.
e. False   Adrenaline and glucagon activate β-oxidation, while insulin inhibits it.

38.
a. False   It occurs in the smooth endoplasmic reticulum.
b. False   It is catalysed by NADH-cytochrome b_5 reductase.
c. True   Double bonds of the *cis* configuration can occur at positions Δ4, Δ5, Δ6 and Δ9.
d. True   It is required to produce prostaglandin, an intracellular messenger.
e. False   Double bonds formation can only occur at positions Δ4, Δ5, Δ6 and Δ9.

39.
a. True   Insulin promotes dephosphorylation and activation of the enzyme while glucagon causes phosphorylation.
b. True   Citrate activates acetyl CoA carboxylase.
c. True   Seven malonyl-CoA molecules are required for each palmitate synthesized.
d. False   The enzyme is in the cytosol.
e. True   The enzyme is inhibited allosterically and by hormone-dependent reversible phosphorylation.

40.
a. False   Oleate ($C_{18:1}$) is produced by the unsaturation of stearate (C_{18}) catalysed by fatty acid desaturase located in the smooth endoplasmic reticulum.
b. False   The reactions occur in the cytosol.
c. True   Pantothenate is also found in coenzyme A.
d. True   This process can occur in mitochondria where acetyl CoA is used, or in the cytosol where malonyl CoA is used.
e. True   Linoleic acid is an essential fatty acid required for the production of arachidonate, and therefore prostaglandins, leukotrienes, thromboxanes and prostacyclin.

41.
a. True   The rate-limiting enzyme HMG-CoA reductase is the primary control site.
b. True   High cholesterol causes a decrease in the rate of transcription of the gene.
c. False   Phosphorylation inhibits HMG-CoA reductase.
d. True   See b.
e. True   Statins function by inhibiting HMG-CoA reductase, decreasing cholesterol synthesis.

42.
a. True   Lipoproteins also solubilize lipids.
b. False   Chylomicrons transport dietary lipids. VLDL, IDL and LDL transport endogenously synthesized lipids from the liver to the tissues.
c. False   Lipoprotein lipase hydrolyses the triacylglycerol contained in chylomicrons to glycerol and free fatty acids.
d. True   HDL also provides apolipoproteins for other lipoproteins (CM and VLDL).
e. True   An increase in cholesterol concentration in the cell will downregulate the synthesis of LDL receptors.

43.
a. True   The cause in most patients is a defect in the LDL receptor.
b. False   It is caused by a deficiency of LDL.
c. True   Management may be with diet, drugs, plasmapheresis, liver transplant or gene therapy.
d. True   This problem is related to lipoprotein lipase or apolipoprotein CII deficiency.
e. False   Homozygotes have no receptors and die of coronary heart disease in childhood.

44.
a. False   Ketone bodies are produced at low levels all the time.
b. False   The brain only uses glucose as its only energy source in the fed state.
c. True   This is the first stage in a five-stage pathway.
d. True   Although the site of synthesis, the liver lacks 3-ketoacyl CoA transferase.
e. False   Erythrocytes cannot metabolize ketone bodies as they have no mitochondria.

45.
a. False   Fibrates activate lipoprotein lipase, thus lowering plasma triacylglycerols.
b. True   They prevent bile acid reabsorption and therefore decrease plasma LDL levels.
c. True   Increased LDL activity leads to decreased triacylglycerol.
d. False   Statins inhibit HMG-CoA reductase.
e. False   Fish oils decrease the concentration of triacylglycerols.

46.
a. False   Ketone bodies are synthesized in liver mitochondria.
b. False   Ketone bodies are synthesized in liver mitochondria.
c. False   Ketone bodies are synthesized in liver mitochondria.
d. True   Ketone bodies are synthesized in liver mitochondria.
e. False   Ketone bodies are synthesized in liver mitochondria.

47.
a. False Part of the carnitine shuttle which transports fatty acyl CoA molecules into mitochondria.
b. True This is controlled by hormone-dependent reversible phosphorylation.
c. False Enzyme involved in gluconeogenesis.
d. False Involved in the initial condensation reaction in the TCA cycle.
e. False Involved in lipid biosynthesis but not a regulatory step.

48.
a. False Despite synthesizing ketone bodies, the liver cannot use them as a fuel, as it lacks 3-ketoacyl CoA transferase.
b. False They are synthesized by the β-oxidation of fatty acids.
c. True Spontaneous decarboxylation of acetoacetate produces acetone, which produces a characteristic smell on the breath when the ketone body concentration is high.
d. False Muscle reduces its use of ketone bodies, increasing availability for the brain.
e. False Different isoenzymes of HMG-CoA reductase are used for cholesterol synthesis and ketone body formation.

Chapter 5 Protein metabolism

49.
a. False It requires NAD^+.
b. True The process is reversible which is important for reducing toxic ammonia concentration.
c. False It is inhibited by high levels of ATP.
d. False It is activated as it produces amino acid carbon skeletons for gluconeogenesis.
e. True The removal of the amino group from glutamate to form ammonia leaves behind α-ketoglutarate.

50.
a. False One amino acid is converted into another amino acid. There is no net gain or net loss.
b. False The reactions are reversible.
c. True Pyridoxal phosphate is required as a cofactor.
d. False Transamination reactions can occur with both essential and non-essential amino acids.
e. True The reaction occurs in the mitochondria and cytosol.

51.
a. False During periods of growth, there is a postive nitrogen balance.
b. True Malnutrition leads to negative nitrogen balance.
c. False Nitrogen intake will be greater than nitrogen loss during pregnancy.
d. True Starvation leads to negative nitrogen balance.
e. True Cachexia leads to negative nitrogen balance.

52.
a. False
b. False
c. False
d. True
e. False

53.
a. True Oxidative deamination occurs in the mitochondria.
b. False Glutamate dehydrogenase is specific for glutamate.
c. True Glutamate dehydrogenase is unusual in being able to use either NAD^+ or $NADP^+$ as a cofactor.
d. False See c.
e. True ATP and GTP allosterically inhibit the enzyme; GDP and ADP activate it.

54.
a. True N-terminal residues can have a stabilizing or destabilizing nature.
b. True cAMP-dependent protein kinase is an example of a protein containing the PEST region.
c. False Abnormal and short-lived cytosolic proteins are degraded by the ATP-dependent ubiquitin pathway in the cell cytosol.
d. True Rapid ubiquitin tagging increases the speed of degradation.
e. False Protein degradation is influenced by metabolic state and structural aspects of the protein.

55.
a. True Mainly in the periportal cells.
b. False Urea cycle reactions are split between the mitochondria and the cytosol.
c. False Carbamoyl phosphate synthase I catalyses the rate-limiting step in the urea cycle.
d. False Net ATP consumption is 1.5 ATP.
e. False Urea can be easily excreted by the kidneys.

56.
a. False In a small number of cases, PKU may be due to a deficiency in the enzymes that synthesize tetrahydrobiopterin, the cofactor for phenylalanine hydroxylase.
b. True This enzyme is normally involved in the breakdown of tyrosine to fumarate.

c. False   It is caused by a deficiency in histidase.

d. True   Management is with tinted contact lenses from early infancy and high sun protection.

e. True   Although too much restriction can cause poor growth and neurological symptoms.

57.   a. False   It does not occur in muscle, although lactate produced in muscle during active exercise is used in gluconeogenesis.

b. True   Gluconeogenesis occurs in the liver after starvation of longer than 12 hours and during prolonged exercise.

c. False   Fat cannot be converted to glucose, and fatty acid and glycerol synthesis is the chief response.

d. True   Gluconeogenesis can occur in the cortex of the kidney in prolonged starvation.

e. False   Gluconeogenesis does not occur in the brain.

Chapter 6 Purines, pyrimidines and haem

58.   a. True   This occurs in a two-step reaction.

b. True   They are obtained from donors such as serine, glycine or histidine and transferred to intermediates in the synthesis of other amino acids, purines or thymidines.

c. True   This is a folic acid analogue that decreases the amount available for purine and pyrimidine synthesis.

d. True   The methionine salvage pathway releases trapped THF trapped as N^5-methyl THF.

e. True   Vitamin B_{12} is essential to maintain an adequate supply of the active form of folate (5,6,7,8-tetrahydrofolate).

59.   a. False   It is caused by an absence of hypoxanthine guanine phosphoribosyl transferase (HGPRT).

b. False   It is an X-linked condition.

c. True   It also causes hyperuricaemia, leading to kidney stones, arthritis and gout.

d. True   Due to the absence of the salvage enzyme, hypoxanthine guanine phosphoribosyl transferase (HGPRT).

e. True   Guanine and hypoxanthine are broken down to form large amounts of uric acid, leading to gout.

60.   a. True   Predominantly men in middle life.

b. True   Genetic causes of gout include HPGRT deficiency.

c. True   Synovial fluid examination is used for definitive diagnosis.

d. False   Xanthine oxidase is used for long-term prophylaxis.

e. False   Aspirin causes decreased excretion of uric acid.

61.   a. False   Are deposits of urate crystals around joints, tendons and cartilage of ear lobes.

b. False   It is characterized by acute attacks of arthritis, usually affecting one joint.

c. True   Urate crystal deposition can cause discoloration of overlying skin.

d. True   Patients usually complain of warm, swollen and tender joints.

e. True   Symptoms are often due to kidney stones.

62.   a. True   Chronic exposure causes encephalopathy and seizures and may cause mental retardation in children.

b. True   Along with severe weakness, vomiting, abdominal pain and constipation.

c. True   Increased levels of porphyrin precursors PBG and ALA can be found in the urine of these patients.

d. False   Porphyrias are very rare (roughly 1 in 100 000).

e. False   Acute attacks are separated by long periods of remission.

63.   a. True   This occurs in haemoglobin and myoglobin.

b. False   Mature erythrocytes lack mitochondria and therefore cannot make haem.

c. True   Lead poisoning results in the inhibition of haem synthesis and anaemia.

d. False   Cells of the reticuloendothelial system in the liver, spleen and bone marrow are chiefly responsible for breakdown.

e. True   Some drugs, such as phenytoin and phenobarbitone, induce the activity of the cytochrome P450 enzymes which break down haem.

64.   a. True   Impaired excretion will cause hyperuricaemia since uric acid is normally eliminated via the kidneys.

b. True   That deficiency increases PRPP concentration and this turns on de novo purine synthesis, which will increase urate formation.

c. True   PRPP turns on purine nucleotide synthesis by activating PRPP-glutamine amidotransferase.

d. True   Allopurinol inhibits xanthine oxidase, thus preventing de novo purine synthesis.

e. True   There is an increase in purine turnover in myeloproliferative disorders.

65. a. False GMP is one of the products of purine synthesis.

b. False Ribulose-5-phosphate is the precursor of ribose 5-phosphate but is not directly involved in purine synthesis.

c. False UTP is a pyrimidine nucleotide important in glycogen synthesis but does not supply ribose phosphate for purine synthesis.

d. False Glucose-6-phosphate is a precursor of ribose phosphate but is not directly involved in purine synthesis.

e. True Formed in a reaction involving ribose 5-phosphate and ATP, catalysed by PRPP synthase.

Chapter 7 Glucose homeostasis

66. a. False Type 1 diabetes is also known as juvenile-onset diabetes and usually presents before the age of 25.

b. True It is associated with HLA-DR3 and HLA-DR4 antigens.

c. False Patients who are obese tend to develop Type 2 diabetes.

d. False Patients with type 1 diabetes cannot produce insulin, thus require insulin for their management.

e. True Patients with type 1 diabetes are prone to developing ketoacidosis.

67. a. False Glucagon has no effect on glucose uptake in the peripheral tissues.

b. True It stimulates gluconeogenesis to maintain blood glucose levels.

c. True It stimulates ketone body synthesis to produce ketone bodies which can be used as fuel.

d. False It inhibits lipogenesis.

e. True It stimulates protein breakdown.

68. a. True Blood glucose is raised due to lack of effectiveness of insulin.

b. True An increased glucagon:insulin ratio stimulates gluconeogenesis.

c. False Ketone body synthesis increases.

d. True Fatty acids are released from triacylglycerol, and the activity of lipoprotein lipase is decreased in the absence of insulin.

e. True An increase in free fatty acids facilitates increased production of ketone bodies.

69. a. True Glycated haemoglobin provides a measure of glucose control over the previous 6–8 weeks.

b. True Blood glucose is measured every 30 minutes for the next 2 hours.

c. False Normal fasting glucose should be less than 7.0 mmol/L, based on revised WHO criteria.

d. True Over the previous 2 weeks, so particularly useful in patients with abnormal haemoglobin and pregnancy.

e. False IGT is diagnosed with an oral glucose tolerance test.

70. a. False Hydrolysis of triacylglycerol and muscle glycogen as fuel.

b. True At the same time, glucagon activates glycogenolysis.

c. False There is a high glucagon to insulin ratio.

d. False No food has been eaten for at least 4 hours.

e. True Adipose tissue has one of the richest sympathetic innervations.

Chapter 8 Nutrition

71. a. True And for other enzymes such as LDH and carbonic anhydrase.

b. False Absorption is not affected by vitamin C.

c. True An extremely rare autosomal recessive disorder.

d. True This is a well-recognized complication.

e. False Zinc overload is not likely to cause cirrhosis.

72. a. True Dietary iron is more readily absorbed in the Fe^{2+} state.

b. True Iron is stored as ferritin and is a good measurement of iron stores in the body.

c. False Deficiency results in microcytic anaemia.

d. True Due to damage to islet cells.

e. False Overload is treated with desferrioxamine.

73. a. True Also for dopamine hydroxylase in adrenaline and noradrenaline synthesis.

b. True It inactivates free oxygen radicals which damage lipid membranes, proteins and DNA.

c. False Vitamin A,C and E are antioxidants.

d. False Deficiency causes scurvy, with spongy gums and failure of wound healing.

e. False Deficiency leads to anaemia as ascorbate is necessary to maintain iron in its reduced and active state (Fe^{2+}).

74. a. True Vitamin A, D, E and K are all fat soluble vitamins, stored in the liver and not excreted easily.

b. True   In its retinoic acid form, it binds to chromatin to increase the synthesis of proteins controlling cell growth.

c. True   Deficiency also causes increased epithelial keratinization of the cornea.

d. True   Also useful in psoriasis as acitretin.

e. False   Pregnant women must not exceed 3.3 mg/day because vitamin A causes congenital defects.

75. a. True   Although this is a very inefficient pathway.

b. False   Deficiency results in pellagra.

c. True   Although due to the inefficient nature of the process, large amounts of protein are needed for small amounts on niacin synthesis.

d. True   Mild cases of pellagra are normally reversible, although dementia is not, and may lead to death.

e. True   It inhibits lipolysis, leading to decreased VLDL and LDL.

76. a. True   Also available in most foods, especially egg yolk, offal, yeast and nuts.

b. False   It is a coenzyme in carboxylation reactions.

c. True   They contain the glycoprotein avidin that binds to biotin in the intestine, preventing its absorption.

d. False   Deficiency is rare in normal diets, but may lead to dermatitis.

e. True   It is a coenzyme for acetyl CoA carboxylase in fatty acid synthesis.

77. a. True   Therefore vegans are at risk of deficiency.

b. True   It works by carrying methyl groups.

c. True   Receptors on mucosal cells in the terminal ileum bind the complex.

c. False   It takes about 2 years for symptoms of deficiency to develop, due to the significant amounts stored.

d. True   Neurological symptoms result from inadequate myelin synthesis and nerve degeneration.

78. a. True   Manufactured in the skin by the action of sunlight of 290–310 nm wavelength.

b. False   The active form is 1,25-dihydroxycholecalciferol.

c. True   Increases uptake from intestine, reabsorption from the kidney and resorption from bone.

d. False   It is not a recognized teratogen.

e. False   Vitamin A, C and E are antioxidants.

79. a. False   Rickets is the result of inadequate bone mineralization as a result of calcium deficiency. This can be due to dietary

deficiency, malabsorption of calcium or secondary to vitamin D deficiency.

b. False   Vitamin A, C and E are antioxidants.

c. False   Vitamin A, D, E and K are fat-soluble vitamins.

d. True   Pernicious, iron deficiency, megaloblastic and macrocytic, respectively.

e. False   Vitamin K is synthesized by bacterial flora of the jejunum and ileum, but vitamin B_{12} is from animal sources only.

80. a. True   There is about 1.2 kg of calcium in the average 70 kg adult.

b. True   Also from dietary deficiency or malabsorption.

c. True   Osteomalacia occurs in adults.

d. False   It is active in the ionized form.

e. False   Copper is deposited around corneal limbus as Kayser–Fleicher rings.

81. a. True   That is, the body's need for protein or energy or both is not met by the diet.

b. False   Severe protein deficiency but energy is maintained.

c. False   Malnutrition is much more common in areas where drought, famine and war are common.

d. True   They are usually between 2 and 4 years of age.

e. True   The first child is often then fed on a low-protein, high-starch diet instead.

82. a. False   Table salt is fortified with iodine.

b. True   Both T_3 and T_4 have this negative inhibitory effect.

c. True   Uncontrolled TSH levels stimulate the thyroid, causing hyperplasia of the epithelium and generalized enlargement.

d. False   The Guthrie test is a neonatal screening test performed on all newborn babies, looking for raised TSH levels.

e. False   TRH is produced by the hypothalamus, TSH from the anterior pituitary.

83. a. False   Bow legs are a feature of rickets, which also features craniotabes, a rickety rosary, (enlargement of the ends of the ribs, where they join the costal cartilages) a Harrison sulcus and delayed dentition.

b. True   Spontaneous, incomplete fractures, often in the long bones or pelvis.

c. False   Increased alkaline phosphatase is a feature of rickets.

d. False   It is a disease of adults, particularly in the elderly.

e. True   It is commonly due to vitamin D deficiency.

84. a. True — Pernicious anaemia is the most common cause of vitamin B_{12} deficiency.

b. True — Antibodies are made to either gastric parietal cells or to intrinsic factor.

c. False — It is diagnosed by analysis of the blood film and bone marrow specimens and by the Schilling test, which measures the absorption of vitamin B_{12}.

d. False — It is treated by monthly intramuscular injections of hydroxycobalamin for life.

e. False — It is more common in older women.

85. a. False — Vitamin K is a coenzyme required for the γ-carboxylation of clotting factors II, VII, IX and X.

b. False — True deficiency is rare because most of the body's vitamin K is synthesized by bacteria in the gut.

c. False — Haemorrhagic disease of the newborn is the result of vitamin deficiency and can occur in the first week of life, and vitamin K is given to prevent this.

d. False — Deficiency will cause an increased activated partial thromboplastin time.

e. True — Oral anticoagulants are vitamin K antagonists.

86. a. False — There is no change in body mass under these circumstances.

b. False — A BMI of >30 is defined as obesity.

c. True — And high socio-economic class in the East.

d. True — 12% of women and 8% of men.

e. False — Lower energy intake must normally be maintained to avoid subsequent weight gain.

87. a. False — Vitamin A, D, E and K are fat-soluble.

b. True — Compared with protein, carbohydrate and fat, they are needed in small amounts.

c. True — They are stored in the liver.

d. True — Water-soluble vitamins are generally non-toxic in excess.

e. False — It is rare as it is synthesized in the gut by bacterial flora.

88. a. True — Kwashiorkor is a protein-only deficiency.

b. True — Treatment is often not available.

c. True — Also by wrinkled skin and hair loss.

d. False — Commonly in children under 18 months old.

e. False — The first priority is to restore fluid and electrolyte balance.

89. a. True — Osteoarthritis, and back pain as one of its symptoms, are associated with obesity.

b. False — There is no direct association with fatty liver.

c. True — Especially if fat, female, forty and fertile.

d. False — Type 2 diabetes can require treatment with insulin.

e. True — Breathlessness and respiratory problems can occur.

90. a. True — Malabsorption can result in calcium deficiency.

b. True — Decreased vitamin K absorption causes a decrease in vitamin K-dependent clotting factors and increased bleeding tendency.

c. True — Mixed B_{12}, folate and iron deficiency can often result in a normocytic anaemia.

d. True — Malabsorption will result in weight loss.

e. True — Rarely seen in the developed world as usually only seen in very severe malnutrition.

91. a. False — Seizures are the result of decreased neuromuscular transmission but calcium deficiency has no effect on the brain.

b. True — Due to increased secretion of alkaline phosphatase by osteoblasts.

c. True — X-rays show defective mineralization of pelvis, long bones and ribs.

d. False — Calcium deficiency causes rickets in children and osteomalacia in adults.

e. True — Delayed dentition is a characteristic feature.

92. a. False — Wilson's disease is a rare autosomal recessive disorder.

b. False — Wilson's disease is treated with daily chelation therapy with D-penicillamine.

c. True — Liver and neurological damage is permanent.

d. True — The defect lies on chromosome 13.

e. True — Copper incorporation into caeruloplasmin is also impaired.

93. a. False — Is due to dietary deficiency of thiamine.

b. True — Due to cerebellar effects.

c. True — Korsakoff's psychosis is a severe irreversible amnesic syndrome that develops in untreated cases.

d. True — Alcohol inhibits uptake of thiamine.

e. False — Is reversible with immediate thiamine therapy.

94. a. True — Newborn babies have sterile gut and so have no bacteria to make vitamin K.

b. True — In addition, ascorbic acid favours its absorption.

c. False — They are absorbed in phospholipid-bile salt micelles along with other fats.

d. True   Iron is transported bound to transferrin from the intestines to the tissues.

e. False   It requires intrinsic factor from the parietal cells of the stomach.

d. True   δ-ALA dehydrogenase, coproporphyrinogen III and ferrochelatase are inhibited.

e. True   High levels of haem breakdown and bilirubin levels exceeding the conjugating capacity of the liver cause jaundice.

Chapter 10 History and examination

95. a. False   Is associated with hyperthyroidism.
     b. False   Wernicke–Korsakoff syndrome will cause an intention tremor.
     c. True   A normal essential tremor can be associated with increased exercise, anxiety and caffeine.
     d. False   The hands must be hyperextended to elicit a flapping tremor.
     e. True   Essential tremor is also seen in hypoglycaemia, alcoholism, hyperthyroidism and Wilson's disease.

96. a. False   Koilonychia is caused by iron deficiency anaemia.
     b. False   Is defined as a decrease in angle between the nail and nail bed.
     c. True   Underlying nail can feel soft, fluctuant and 'boggy'.
     d. True   Caused by metabolic disturbances such as haemochromatosis, Wilson's disease, glycogen storage disorder and alcoholism.
     e. False   Glycogen storage disorders are a rare cause of clubbing.

97. a. True   This leads to microcytic, hypochromic cells.
     b. False   Deficiency of erythrocyte enzymes such as pyruvate kinase or G6PDH causes haemolytic anaemia.
     c. False   Antibodies to intrinsic factor prevent B_{12} absorption, leading to deficiency in B_{12} and folate in pernicious anaemia.

Chapter 11 Further investigations

98. a. False   Creatinine is high in renal disease.
     b. True   Dehydration causes a high serum sodium.
     c. False   Serum potassium is high in renal failure and increases during treatment with potassium-sparing diuretics.
     d. True   Due to increased muscle bulk.
     e. False   Water excess due to liver cirrhosis causes a low serum sodium.

99. a. True   Values between 12 and 13 g/dL are normal in women.
     b. True   Normal values are between 4 and 5.2×10^{12}/L in women and 4.5 and 6.8×10^{12}/L in men.
     c. False   Normal values are between 12 and 16 s.
     d. False   MCH is high in B_{12}/folate deficiency.
     e. True   A macrocytic picture is seen in B_{12}/folate deficiency.

100. a. False   Enteral nutrition is always given in preference if the gastrointestinal tract is functional.
     b. False   Is indicated in intestinal failure.
     c. True   Infection and sepsis associated with the central catheter is the most important complication.
     d. True   Glucose intolerance and hyperglycaemia are common side effects.
     e. True   Or sometimes into a peripheral vein.

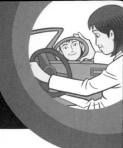

1. a. During a 100 metre sprint, anaerobic metabolism of glucose occurs in the skeletal muscle, resulting in the build-up of lactate. Lactate diffuses out of the muscle and is taken to the liver where it is oxidized to pyruvate, which can be converted back to glucose via gluconeogenesis. The formed glucose diffuses out of the liver and returns to the muscle to be further used as fuel.
    b. During a marathon, aerobic metabolism of glucose occurs in the skeletal muscle. However, the body does not have sufficient glycogen to sustain the energy required. As glycogen stores become depleted, an increase in glucagon, noradrenaline and adrenaline stiumulates lipolysis, releasing fatty acids for use by the muscle. As a result, there is fall in the respiratory quotient (RQ).

2. In the urea cycle, carbamoyl phosphate is formed from ammonia, carbon dioxide and ATP via the action of carbamoyl phosphate synthetase I. Carbamoyl phosphate then interacts with ornithine to produce citrulline. This is followed by the formation of argininosuccinate from citrulline and aspartate, via the action of argininosuccinate synthase. Following this, argininosuccinate is converted to arginine and fumarate. Arginine is hydrolysed to form urea, and ornithine is regenerated for the continued operation of the urea cycle.
    The fumarate formed is an intermediate of the TCA cycle, which is converted to malate and then oxaloacetate via the action of fumarase and malate dehydrogenase respectively. Oxaloacetate can undergo transamination to form aspartate, which is an intermediate of the urea cycle. Thus, both the urea cycle and TCA cycle are dependent on one another for continous operation.

3. a. Under anaerobic conditions, pyruvate is reduced to lactate by lactate dehydrogenase (LDH) with the simultaneous oxidation of NADH to NAD^+. The reaction occurs in the cell cytosol and is important in red blood cells (no mitochondria) because it is their only pathway for NAD^+ regeneration; it is also important in active skeletal muscle when oxygen is limiting. N.B. It is always best to illustrate your answers wherever possible with the relevant equation or a quick sketch of a pathway.
    b. Under anaerobic conditions, NADH is oxidized to NAD^+ by the electron transport chain in mitochondria, generating energy. NADH first has to enter the mitochondria. The inner mitochondrial membrane is impermeable to NADH and therefore only its two high-energy electrons are transported into the mitochondria by either the glycerol-3-phosphate shuttle or the malate–aspartate shuttle.

    In the malate–aspartate shuttle, NADH is used to reduce oxaloacetate to malate, regenerating cytosolic NAD^+. In the glycerol-3-phosphate shuttle, NADH is used to reduce dihydroxyacetone-3-phosphate to glycerol-3-phosphate, regenerating NAD^+. The answer to this part is best illustrated with a simple sketch of both shuttles, as shown in Figs 2.6 and 2.7.

4. a. Pyruvate dehydrogenase complex (PDH). The three cofactors required are thiamine pyrophosphate, FAD and lipoate.
    b. Oxidative decarboxylation.
    c. Mitochondrial matrix.
    c. CO_2.
    e. The reaction is completely irreversible, such that pyruvate cannot be formed from acetyl CoA. Therefore, carbohydrates can form fats but not vice versa, meaning there can be no net synthesis of glucose from fatty acids!

5. This answer is best illustrated with a quick sketch of the electron transport chain, showing the action of inhibitors and uncouplers.
    Inhibitors of the electron transport chain bind to specific components of the chain, blocking the transfer of electrons at that site. For example, rotenone and amytal bind to, and inhibit, electron transfer within NADH dehydrogenase (complex I), causing inhibition of the chain. Normally, electron transport is accompanied by pumping of protons across the inner mitochondrial membrane into the inner mitochondrial space. The inhibition of electron transport results in the inhibition of the proton pump and thus of ATP synthesis.
    Uncouplers (for example, 2,4-dinitrophenol) increase the permeability of the inner mitochondrial membrane to protons, so that they can re-enter the matrix at sites other than ATP synthase. This dissipates the proton gradient without ATP production. Normally, the proton gradient couples electron transport to oxidative phosphorylation (ATP synthesis). Uncouplers dissipate the proton gradient so that electron transport still occurs normally, but without ATP production.

6. a. A = acetyl CoA. B = malonyl CoA.
    b. The cell cytosol.
    c. Acetyl CoA carboxylase.
    d. Biotin.
    e. Activators are either citrate (allosteric activator) or insulin (causes reversible dephosphorylation). Inhibitors are either palmitoyl CoA or glucagon (causes reversible phosphorylation).

7. Familial hypercholesterolaemia (FH) is an autosomal dominant disorder affecting the receptor-mediated pathway for LDL metabolism in the human body. Homozygous FH patients have very high levels of LDL due to the lack of synthesis of LDL receptors.

As a result, LDL is not cleared by the liver, resulting in increased LDL levels. The defect in LDL uptake also causes extra-hepatic tissues to switch on their endogenous cholesterol biosynthesis. These explain the extremely high levels of LDL in homozygous patients, who are at very high risk of coronary heart disease, with the majority dying in their early twenties. Heterozygous also have high cholesterol levels and have a 50% chance of having a myocardial infarction by the age of 50.

8. Lead inhibits three key enzymes involved in haem synthesis, resulting in an accumulation of intermediates:

   i.   ALA dehydrase, leading to the accumulation of ALA, which can be measured in urine.
   ii. Coproporphyrinogen III oxidase, leading to the accumulation of coproporphyrinogen III.
   iii. Ferrochelatase, leading to the accumulation of protoporphyrin IX in erythrocytes, causing fluorescence.

   The result is the inhibition of haem synthesis and thus of haemoglobin production. This leads to anaemia unless treated. Treatment is with lead chelators such as Ca-EDTA or d-penicillamine. They bind lead, forming a complex that can be excreted in the urine.

9. The easiest and quckest way to do this is to draw it (see Fig. 2). N.B. Also refer back to Fig. 2.34 for details.

10. Jaundice occurs when there is an increased concentration of bilirubin in the blood. Bilirubin can be present in two forms; either as free unconjugated bilirubin or conjugated bilirubin. A patient might be jaundiced because of:
    a. haemolytic anaemia, where erythrocytes undergo rapid lysis which overwhelms the conjugating system of the liver.
    b. impaired bilirubin uptake from the blood into the liver
    c. impaired conjugating activity in the liver
    d. obstruction of bile flow from the liver to the gallbladder and gut.

11. a. Fed state (0–4 h after a meal): Exogenous glucose (carbohydrate in the diet) provides the main fuel.
    b. Fasted state (4–12 h after a meal): The breakdown of liver glycogen stores provides glucose for oxidation, mainly by the brain. Stores are only sufficient to last between 12 and 24 h.
    c. Early starved (12 h to 16 days): Once most of the liver glycogen has been used up, glucose is formed from non-carbohydrate precursors via gluconeogenesis. Protein breakdown in muscle releases amino acids, mainly alanine and glutamine, and the hydrolysis of triacylglycerol in liver and adipose tissue releases glycerol. Along with lactate formed in muscle, they are all used to form glucose. The rate of gluconeogenesis is greatest after about 2–6 days of fasting and then starts to fall off.
    d. Late starved (longer than 16 days): In prolonged starvation, the breakdown of muscle protein, and

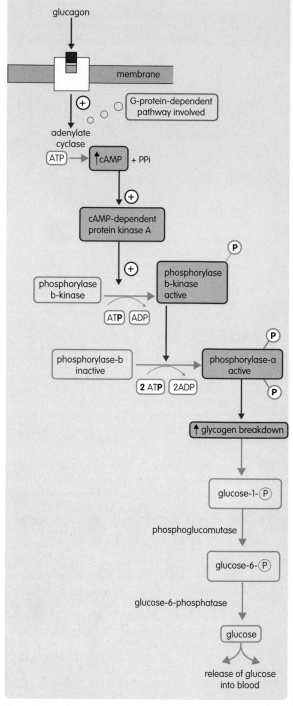

Fig. 2. Answer to Question 9.

thus gluconeogenesis, slow down. There is less need for glucose because the brain adapts to using more ketone bodies, namely acetoacetate and β-hydroxybutyrate.

12. In adults, vitamin K deficiency is rare because most of our vitamin K is synthesized by bacteria in the gut. However, newborn babies have sterile guts and therefore cannot initially make vitamin K, and human milk is a very poor source. Newborn babies may develop vitamin K deficiency, resulting in the condition known as haemorrhagic disease of the newborn. They have low levels of vitamin K-dependent clotting factors (II, VII, IX and X) and thus an increased bleeding tendency. Bleeding is usually minor, but in some cases can lead to major bleeds, causing intracranial haemorrhage and death. Therefore, every baby in the UK is given prophylactic intramuscular or oral vitamin K shortly after birth to prevent haemorrhagic disease.

13. Vitamin B_1 (thiamine), in the form of thiamine pyrophosphate (TPP), is a cofactor for four key enzymes:
   a. Pyruvate dehydrogenase, which converts pyruvate into acetyl CoA.
   b. α-Ketoglutarate dehydrogenase (TCA cycle).
   c. Branched-chain amino acid α-ketoacid dehydrogenase.
   d. Transketolase, an enzyme of the pentose phosphate pathway (PPP).
   In thiamine deficiency, the activity of all four enzymes is reduced. The decreased activities of pyruvate dehydrogenase and α-ketoglutarate dehydrogenase result in a decrease of acetyl CoA and ATP formation, and thus a fall in acetylcholine. Decreased activity of transketolase results in decreased activity of the PPP, leading to a decrease in the NADPH necessary for fatty acid synthesis. This results in decreased synthesis of myelin, causing a peripheral neuropathy.
   Neurological disorders caused by thiamine deficiency include:
   (i) Dry beriberi, characterized by gradual, symmetrical, ascending peripheral neuropathy.
   (ii) Wernicke's encephalopathy which, untreated, may progress to Korsakoff's psychosis, a severe, irreversible amnesic syndrome.

14. a. Niacin is part of the cofactors NAD and NADP. These cofactors play an important role in glycolysis, gluconeogenesis, pentose phosphate pathway and TCA cycle.
   b. Pyridoxal plays a very important role in amino acid catabolism as pyridoxal phosphate is involved in amino acid transamination and decarboxylation. Folate and vitamin B_{12} play a role in one-carbon metabolism.

15. a. Modifiable cardiovascular risk factors include smoking, hyperlipidaemia, (high LDL and low HDL concentration), hypertension and diabetes mellitus. Non-modifiable risk factors include age, sex and family history of premature atherosclerotic disease.

Fig. 3. Part of answer to Question 15.

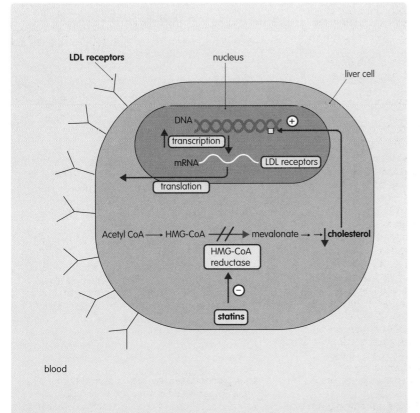

253

b. The first course of action is diet modification. The diet should be low in cholesterol and saturated fat. Drugs such as statins are also given.

c. It is important to elicit whether there is a history of familial hypercholesterolaemia or hyperlipidaemia. Such patients generally present in childhood, so it is likely that he has inherited a mild form.

d. Statins, for example, simvastatin or pravastatin, help to reduce plasma cholesterol. They reversibly inhibit HMG-CoA reductase, the rate-limiting enzyme of cholesterol synthesis. This decreases cholesterol synthesis in cells. The cells compensate for the low intracellular cholesterol by stimulating transcription of the LDL receptor gene. This increasing LDL receptor synthesis, resulting in increased cholesterol uptake, thus leads to decreased plasma cholesterol (see Fig. 3).

16. a. The most likely diagnosis is gout. It occurs predominantly in middle-aged men, and is an obvious inherited condition in some families. It is also more common in New Zealand. In gout, high levels of insoluble uric acid can precipitate out to form sodium urate crystals, which may become deposited in joints, causing damage.

b. Poor diet, alcohol, exercise and stress all increase lactic acid level, which increases the precipitation of uric acid (lactic acid competes with uric acid for excretion in the kidney). It might also be caused by an increase in purine turnover resulting from leukaemia, myeloproliferative disorders, or the use of cytotoxic drugs in the treatment of cancers. Drugs such as thiazide diuretics decrease the excretion of uric acid. Lead toxicity has a similar effect.

c. Treatment is aimed at reducing uric acid levels. The most common acute treatment is non-steroidal anti-inflammatory drugs such as indometacin, which provide relief within 24–48 hours.

d. Allopurinol is the main drug used in the prophylaxis of gout. It is an analogue of hypoxanthine and a competitive inhibitor of xanthine oxidase. It decreases the amount of insoluble uric acid formed and increases the amount of its soluble precursors hypoxanthine and xanthine, which are easily excreted in the urine. There are two other actions:
   i. Salvage enzyme (HGPRT) catalyses addition of ribose-5-phosphate to allopurinol, forming allopurinol ribonucleotide which can inhibit PRPP amidotransferase, the rate-limiting enzyme of purine synthesis.
   ii. Allopurinol can be metabolized by xanthine oxidase to oxypurinol, an even stronger inhibitor of xanthine oxidase.

17. a. Type 1 diabetes can present for the first time with diabetic ketoacidosis. This is the most likely diagnosis in this case. In Type 1 diabetes there is an absolute deficiency of insulin caused by the auto-immune destruction of the β cells of the islets of Langerhans in the pancreas. Insulin normally facilitates the uptake of glucose by peripheral tissues. In its absence, glucose remains in the blood, resulting in low tissue availability of glucose but a high plasma concentration of glucose. Ketoacidosis is caused by an increase in triacylglycerol hydrolysis in adipose tissue, releasing fatty acids, and an increase in ketone body synthesis in the liver.

b. Long-term treatment of diabetes consists of diet modification, insulin and patient education. Patients must ensure the correct content and timing of meals:
   i. The diet should be high in fibre and unrefined carbohydrate, low in saturated fat and refined carbohydrate.
   ii. Insulin is available in short, intermediate and long-acting preparations. Discussion will be needed with the patient to decide on the most appropriate and acceptable regimen for her lifestyle.
   iii. Patients must understand their condition and feel in control of management if suitable compliance with treatment is to be achieved.

18. a. Iron deficiency anaemia causes a microcytic, hypochromic anaemia.

b. The most common cause of deficiency is inadequate intake, particularly in a vegan diet. In addition you must enquire about blood loss. Heavy periods or loss from the gut due to ulcers, hernias or ulcerative colitis are possibilities. You must also ask about pregnancy.

c. Treatment for iron deficiency anaemia is normally oral iron supplements such as ferrous sulphate or gluconate. If malabsorption is suspected, such as in this case, intramuscular or intravenous iron should be used. Iron is given long enough to replenish stores as well as to correct the haemoglobin level. This normally takes 3–6 months after the haemoglobin level is back within the normal range.

19. a. The most likely diagnosis is rickets. This is common in developing countries and results from a dietary deficiency of calcium. The clinical features include failure to thrive, bowed legs, craniotabes (skull bones easily indented by finger pressure), rickety rosary (expansion and swelling at costochondral junctions), Harrison sulcus (indrawing of softened ribs along attachment of diaphragm), expansion of metaphyses and delayed dentition. Low calcium results in decreased neuromuscular transmission and therefore the patient may present with seizures.

b. There will be decreased serum calcium and phosphorus and an increased alkaline phosphatase. ALP is secreted by osteoblasts to compensate for the low calcium and to increase bone formation. X-rays will show defective mineralization of the pelvis, long bones and ribs.

c. Osteomalacia is particularly seen in the elderly, usually secondary to vitamin D deficiency. It causes spontaneous, incomplete fractures, often in long bones or pelvis, bone pain and weakness of proximal muscles, causing a proximal myopathy with a characteristic waddling gate.

20. a. You will need to take a full history and perform a complete examination. For every lump, you must define the site, size, shape, surface, colour, temperature, edge composition, reducibility and state of overlying and adjacent tissues. Ask the patient to swallow, as all thyroid lumps ascend on swallowing because they are attached to the trachea.

   b. Endemic goitre. This occurs in areas where the soil and water lack iodine, such that daily intake is less than 70 μg. Iodine is necessary to make thyroxine and triiodothyroxine. Low levels of iodine decrease thyroxine formation, so it cannot exert its normal negative feedback effect on thyroid releasing hormone and thyroid stimulating hormone. The resulting high levels of TSH overstimulate the thyroid gland, causing hyperplasia of the thyroid epithelium and generalized enlargement.

   c. Pregnant mothers who are deficient in iodine may give birth to babies who are hypothyroid. Growth and mental development is severely impaired. The Guthrie test is performed on all neonates born in the UK, to screen for raised TSH levels. Treatment is lifelong oral replacement of thyroxine.

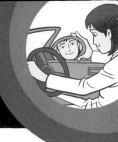
1. Clinical aspects of diabetes

1. **B** **Autoimmune disease with peak age of onset at 15–20 years.** Type 1 diabetes, also known as insulin-dependent diabetes or juvenile-onset diabetes, typically occurs in childhood or puberty.

2. **J** **Injection of insulin preparations.** In type 1 diabetes, there is a complete deficiency of insulin that can only be corrected by life-long insulin treatment.

3. **C** **Diet and weight reduction.** Type 2 diabetes is typically associated with obesity, and diet management is often the only treatment necessary when patients are first diagnosed. Weight loss can prevent or delay the development of type 2 diabetes.

4. **G** **Hypoglycaemia.** Hypoglycaemia causes unpleasant autonomic symptoms, such as sweating, nausea and palpitations, and more severe neuroglycopenic symptoms as a result of a decrease in glucose supply to the brain: drowsiness, unsteadiness, confusion and coma.

5. **K** **Measurement of glycated haemoglobin.** The concentration of glycated haemoglobin provides a measure of the average blood glucose concentration over the preceding 4–6 weeks, that is, the lifetime of an erythrocyte.

2. Metabolic transformation

1. **C** **Fatty acid synthesis.** The production of malonyl CoA from acetyl CoA is an irreversible, rate-limiting step of fatty acid synthesis.

2. **L** **Urea cycle.** The carbamoyl group is transferred to ornithine by ornithine transcarbamoylase to form citrulline.

3. **K** **Transamination.** Amino groups are transferred to α-ketoglutarate to form glutamate.

4. **G** **Glycolysis.** A sequence of 10 reactions that break down one molecule of glucose (six carbons) to two three-carbon molecules of pyruvate.

5. **B** **Cholesterol synthesis.** Following the formation of acetoacetyl CoA, HMG-CoA synthase catalyses the addition of a third molecule of acetyl CoA to form HMG-CoA.

3. Control of carbohydrate and lipid metabolism

1. **E** **Glucokinase.** The low affinity of glucokinase for glucose enables the liver to respond to high blood glucose levels that occur after a meal.

2. **D** **Fructose 1,6-bisphosphatase.** The hydrolysis of fructose 1,6-bisphosphate by fructose 1,6-bisphosphatase bypasses the phosphofructokinase reaction (a rate-limiting step of glycolysis) in gluconeogenesis.

3. **A** **Acetyl-CoA carboxylase.** Acetyl CoA carboxylase is controlled by hormone-dependent reversible phosphorylation. Glucagon activates a cAMP-dependent protein kinase which phosphorylates acetyl CoA carboxylase, inactivating it. Insulin promotes dephosphorylation and activation of the enzyme.

4. **F** **Glucose transporter 4 (GLUT-4).** Following insulin stimulation, GLUT-4 is recruited to the cell membrane to increase glucose uptake by peripheral tissues.

5. **C** **Fatty acid synthase.** Fatty acid synthase is a dimer of two identical subunits, each with seven different enzymatic activities which each catalyse a different reaction of fatty acid synthesis and each subunit contains the acyl carrier protein.

4. Inadequate or excessive micronutrient intake

1. **J** **Vitamin D.** The main role of vitamin D is in calcium homeostasis, where a severe deficiency causes rickets in children and osteomalacia in adults.

2. **G** **Thiamine.** Deficiency of thiamine causes two types of beri-beri: wet beri-beri which results in oedema and heart failure, and dry beri-beri which causes muscle wasting and peripheral neuropathy.

3. **H** **Vitamin A.** Deficiency of vitamin A results in an increase in epithelial keratinization of the cornea leading to xeropthalmia.

4. **C** **Folic acid.** A deficiency in folic acid results in decreased synthesis of purines and pyrimidines, leading to a decrease in nucleic acid synthesis and cell division. This shows up mostly in cells that rapidly divide such as

red blood cells, presenting as large, immature red blood cells.

5. A **Calcium.** There is a progressive reduction of total bone mass, due to the effects of oestrogen deficiency in post-menopausal women, and calcium deficiency increases the risk of osteoporosis.

5. Liver and alcohol abuse

1. D **Bilirubin.** Jaundice refers to the yellow pigmentation of skin or sclerae of the eyes due to a raised plasma bilirubin level.

2. H **Thiamine.** Alcohol inhibits the uptake of thiamine.

3. L **Vitamin K.** Vitamin K is a coenzyme required for the γ-carboxylation of clotting factors II, VII, IX and X, activating them and thus, the clotting cascade.

4. A **Albumin.** With reduced levels of serum albumin, fluid may escape into tissues to cause oedema or into body cavities to cause ascites or pleural effusions.

5. B **Alcohol.** Regular consumption of moderate amounts of alcohol, i.e. one glass of red wine a day has been found to have a protective effect against heart attacks and strokes.

6. Locations of metabolic processes in organs and tissues

1. A **Adipose tissue.** During prolonged periods of fasting, fatty acids stored in adipose tissue are mobilized to provide energy.

2. F **Intestine.** Chylomicrons are assembled in intestinal mucosal cells from dietary fat.

3. G **Liver.** The urea cycle occurs in liver hepatocytes, mainly in the periportal cells.

4. D **Erythrocytes.** Glycolysis is modified by the bisphosphoglycerate shunt in erythrocytes.

5. J **Mitochondria.** Ketone body synthesis occurs in liver mitochondria.

7. Causes of anaemia

1. I **Sickle-cell anaemia.** A vaso-occlusive crisis occurs when the microcirculation is obstructed by sickled erythrocytes, causing ischaemic injury to joints, resulting in pain. The spleen can undergo a sudden very painful enlargement due to pooling of large numbers of sickled cells. This phenomenon is known as splenic sequestration crisis.

2. L **Vitamin B_{12} deficiency.** B_{12} deficiency causes secondary folate deficiency, which leads to decreased production of DNA and defective cell division. As a result, the developing

erythrocytes are megaloblastic, where the nuclei mature more slowly than the cytoplasm.

3. D **Glucose-6-phosphate dehydrogenase deficiency.** Anti-malarial treatment is a precipitating factor here, resulting in oxidative stress and haemolysis of erythrocytes. Damage to the haemoglobin causes its oxidation to methaemoglobin, and the globin chains are precipitated as Heinz bodies.

4. K **Thalassaemia.** The patient has β-thalassaemia, resulting in a deficiency of β-globin chains. As a result, fetal haemoglobin (HbF) persists in the circulation.

5. H **Pernicious anaemia.** An auto-immune condition in which antibodies are made to intrinsic factor; preventing vitamin B_{12} absorption.

8. Nutritional deficiencies

1. G **Vitamin A.** Vitamin A is required for proper function of 11-*cis* retinal, which binds to opsin to form rhodopsin, the visual pigment of rod cells in the retina involved in night vision.

2. I **Vitamin C.** A deficiency in vitamin C results in scurvy which typically presents with swollen, sore, spongy gums with bleeding and loose teeth.

3. F **Thiamine.** A deficiency of thiamine results in Wernicke's encephalopathy which typically presents with ataxia, nystagmus and opthalmoplegia.

4. K **Vitamin K.** Vitamin K is a coenzyme required for the γ-carboxylation of clotting factors II, VII, IX and X, activating them and thus, the clotting cascade.

5. C **Nicotinic acid.** Isoniazid treatment for tuberculosis inhibits nicotinic acid, which results in pellagra which presents with dermatitis, diarrhoea and depression.

9. Clinical investigations

1. E **Glycated haemoglobin.** The concentration of glycated haemoglobin provides a measure of the average blood glucose concentration over the preceding 4–6 weeks, that is, the half-life of an erythrocyte.

2. J **Schilling test.** The Schilling test measures the absorption of vitamin B_{12} and is usually used to diagnose pernicious anaemia.

3. F **Guthrie test.** A sample of capillary blood is taken from a heel-prick at 5–10 days after

birth and screened for phenylketonuria and hypothyroidism.

4. G **Lipid profile.** Patients in 'at risk' groups have their cholesterol levels monitored routinely.

5. L **Uric acid.** The patient has clinical symptoms of gout, which is usually due to a high level of uric acid in the blood which has precipitated out to form crystals.

10. Disorders of metabolism

1. I **Phenylketonuria.** Phenylketonuria is an autosomal recessive disorder due to a deficiency of the enzyme phenylalanine hydroxylase, which results in accumulation of phenylalanine. Patients are advised to be on phenylalanine-restricted diet.

2. B **Alkaptonuria.** Alkaptonuria is caused by a deficiency of the enzyme homogentisic acid oxidase. This results in the accumulation of homogentisate which is excreted in the urine, resulting in the urine turning black due to formation of alkapton.

3. A **Albinism.** Albinism is a deficiency of the enzyme tyrosinase which converts tyrosine to melanin. People with pale skin which makes them more prone to sunburn and skin cancer, thus they are often advised to use high sun protection when going out.

4. G **Maple syrup urine disease.** Patients with this disease excrete branched-chain amino acids in the urine, which gives it a maple syrup smell.

5. F **Lesch–Nyhan.** A very rare X linked disorder caused by absence of the enzyme hypoxanthine guanine phosphoribosyl transferase. It results in hyperuricaemia causing kidney stones, arthritis and gout as well as severe neurological disturbances such as spasticity and self-mutilation.

Index

Note: Page numbers in *italics* refer to tables and figures.

A

AANAT (arylalkylamine N-acetyltransferase), 90
abdomen
  distension, *205*
  examination, 204–7, *205, 206, 207*
ACAT (acyl CoA:cholesterol acyl transferase), 75, *75*
acetaldehyde, 45, *46*
acetate, *46*
acetoacetate, 83
acetoacetic acid, 82
acetoacetyl CoA, 101, 102
acetoacetyl-ACP, 61–2
acetone, 82, 83
acetyl CoA, 28, 70, 102
  amino acid breakdown, 101
  central role of, 18, *19*
  formation of, 24
    HMG-CoA from, 72–3
    from pyruvate, 18–19, *20*
  gluconeogenesis, 100
  ketogenesis, 83–4
  lipid biosynthesis, 57–60, *58*
  oxidation of palmitic acid to, *25*
  pentose phosphate pathway, 50
  production of, 57–9, *59*
  pyruvate dehydrogenase, 19–20
  pyruvate-malate cycle, 50, *52*
  structure of, 17, *19*
  transport of, 59
  tricarboxylic acid (TCA) cycle, 23
acetyl CoA carboxylase, 59–60, *60*, 62, 70
acetyl transacylase, 61
acrodermatitis enteropathica, 179
ACTH (adrenocorticotrophic hormone), 70
activated partial thromboplastin time (APTT), *210*
acute intermittent porphyria, 126, *126*
acyl carrier protein, 60
acyl CoA, 17, 70
acyl CoA dehydrogenase, 69
acyl CoA oxidase, 70
acyl CoA:cholesterol acyl transferase (ACAT), 75, *75*
acyl transferase, 63
acylcarnitine, *68*
adenine phosphoribosyl transferase (APRT), 114
adenosine diphosphate (ADP), 26
adenosine monophosphate (AMP), 14, 26, 37, 67
adenosine triphosphate (ATP), 3

aerobic glycolysis, 11, *13*
anaerobic glycolysis, 11, *13*
balance in the urea cycle, 97
electron transport chain, 29–30
  uncoupling from phosphorylation, 30–1
fatty acid activation, 67
generation of, 25–31, 29–30
  respiratory control of, 31
  via a proton gradient, 30
glycolysis, 9, 11, *13*
inhibition of PFK-1, 14
pyruvate kinase deficiency, 17
structure of, *27*
synthesis of, 26–8, *28*
tricarboxylic acid (TCA) cycle, 23, 59
yield from oxidation of
  fatty acid palmitate, 69
  glucose, 23, *24*
  glycogen, 23, *24*
  ketone bodies, 83–4, *84*
adenosine triphosphate (ATP) synthase, 30
adenosine triphosphate (ATP)-citrate lyase, 24
adenyl cyclase, *38*
adenylsuccinate synthase, 115
adequate intake, 146
adipocytes, 140
adipokines, 151
adiponectin, 140
adipose tissue, triacylglycerols stores, 66
ADP (adenosine diphosphate), 26
adrenaline
  during exercise, 70
  glucose homeostasis, 135
  glycogen metabolism, 37, *38*
  synthesis of, 90, *90*
adrenocorticotrophic hormone (ACTH), 70
aerobic glycolysis, 9, 11
ALA *see* aminolevulinic acid (ALA)
alanine, 85
  amino acid metabolism, 106–7
  formation of, 88, *88*
  N-terminal, 94
  pyruvate formation, 101, *102*
  starvation, 98
  see also glucose-alanine cycle
alanine aminotransferase (ALT), 86
  normal (reference) value, *211*
albinism, *104*, 104–5, *105*
albumin, 151, 154, 179, 218
  normal (reference) value, *211*

W

wasting, 196, *196*
  see also weight loss
water babies, 154
water (H$_2$O)
  body, *148*
  tricarboxylic acid (TCA) cycle, 9
water-soluble vitamins, 155, 161–72
  symptoms of deficiencies, 189, *189*
  see also specific vitamin
weight loss, 185–6, *186*, 196, *196*, 216
Wernicke-Korsakoff syndrome, 162
Wernicke's encephalopathy, 161, 162, *163*
Wernicke's syndrome, 20
Wilson's disease, 180

X

xanthelasma, *201*
xanthine, 117, *117*, 118
xanthine oxidase, 118
xanthine oxidase inhibitors, 118

Y

yeast, anaerobic glycolysis, 12

Z

zinc, 172, 179, *179*
  deficiency, 179